Sandy Provance

Bottom Line's HEALTH BREAKTHROUGHS 2013

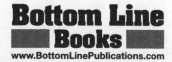

Bottom Line Books

www.BottomLinePublications.com

10 9 8 7 6 5 4 3 2 1

ISBN 0-88723-683-9

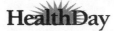

Articles in this book were written by reporters for HealthDay, an award-winning international
daily consumer health news service, headquartered in Norwalk, Connecticut.

Bottom Line Books® publishes the advice of expert authorities in many fields.
These opinions may at times conflict as there are often different approaches to solving problems.
The use of this material is no substitute for health, legal, accounting or other professional services.
Consult competent professionals for answers to your specific questions.

Telephone numbers, addresses, prices, offers and Web sites listed in this book are accurate
at the time of publication, but they are subject to frequent change.

Bottom Line Books® is a registered trademark of Boardroom® Inc.
281 Tresser Boulevard, Stamford, Connecticut 06901

www.bottomlinepublications.com

Bottom Line Books® is an imprint of Boardroom® Inc., publisher of print periodicals,
e-letters and books. We are dedicated to bringing you the best information from the most
knowledgeable sources in the world. Our goal is to help you gain greater wealth,
better health, more wisdom, extra time and increased happiness.

Printed in the United States of America

Contents

Contents

6 • DIABETES

7 • DIET, FITNESS & NUTRITION

8 • DRUGS

Contents

Contents

Preface

We are proud to bring you the all-new *Bottom Line's Health Breakthroughs 2013*. This collection represents a year's worth of the latest health news and scientific discoveries in a broad spectrum of fields.

When you choose a Bottom Line book, you are turning to a stellar group of experts in a wide range of specialties—medical doctors, alternative practitioners, renowned nutrition experts, research scientists and consumer-health advocates, to name a few.

We go to great lengths to interview the foremost health experts. Whether it's cancer prevention, breakthrough arthritis treatments or cutting-edge nutritional advice, our editors talk to the true innovators in health care.

How do we find all these top-notch professionals? Over the past 20 years, we have built a network of leading physicians in both alternative and conventional medicine. They are affiliated with the world's premier medical institutions. We follow the medical research, and

with the help of our partner HealthDay, an award-winning service that reports on evidence-based health news, we bring the latest information to our readers. We also regularly talk with our advisers in teaching hospitals, private practices and government health agencies.

Bottom Line's Health Breakthroughs 2013 is a result of our ongoing research and contact with these experts, and is a distillation of their latest findings and advice. We hope that you will enjoy the presentation and glean helpful information about the health topics that concern you and your family.

As a reader of a Bottom Line book, please be assured that you are receiving reliable and well-researched information from a trusted source. But, please use prudence in health matters. Always speak to your physician before taking vitamins, supplements or over-the-counter medication…changing your diet…or beginning an exercise program. If you experience side effects from any regimen, contact your doctor immediately.

The Editors, Bottom Line Books, Stamford, Connecticut.

Asthma, Allergies & Respiratory Disorders

Natural Relief for Asthma

So many Americans have asthma. Nearly one in 12 adults and one of every 10 school-age children has the condition, according to the Centers for Disease Control and Prevention. And incidence is on the rise. Natural therapies can be of tremendous help. *Here's what you need to know…*

To relieve symptoms of wheezing and gasping for breath, conventional medical doctors prescribe antihistamines, bronchodilators and inhaled corticosteroid medications, which are taken short- or long-term. These medications can cause serious side effects, such as digestive upset, increased heart rate, dizziness and tremor. Rather than simply suppressing the symptoms of asthma, the natural remedies I recommend lessen airway inflammation to such an extent that many of my patients are able to reduce or even eliminate their use of traditional asthma medications.

MY NATURAL ANTI-ASTHMA PROGRAM

My program can help children and adults. It also can help relieve symptoms in the case of a mild flare-up and may be used in combination with asthma medications. I recommend following this program for one to two months. It's best if you do this while supervised by a holistic doctor, although you also can start this program working with your primary doctor or asthma doctor. After about two months, you can see if you are able to reduce the amount or frequency of your asthma medications. Keep your rescue inhaler on hand just in case you need it.

ASTHMA-PREVENTIVE
LIFESTYLE

When I work with asthma patients, I make sure that they adopt an asthma-preventive lifestyle that includes diet changes and stress management, because diet and stress are two major

Mark A. Stengler, NMD, naturopathic medical doctor in private practice, Encinitas, California…adjunct associate clinical professor at the National College of Natural Medicine, Portland, Oregon…author of *The Natural Physicians Healing Therapies* and coauthor of *Prescription for Natural Cures* (both from Bottom Line Books).

triggers for asthma. I ask patients to avoid foods that can aggravate asthma symptoms, including artificial sweeteners and preservatives, and, oftentimes, dairy products and foods containing gluten, a group of proteins found in the grains wheat, rye and barley. I also recommend that patients find and practice a stress-reduction method that works for them, such as yoga or biofeedback.

NUTRIENTS FOR ASTHMA

I recommend several lung-protective nutritional supplements that reduce inflammation and provide antioxidants because oxidative stress has been shown to play a significant role in airway inflammation. *These supplements, which have no side effects except as noted, include…*

•**Pycnogenol (pine bark extract),** which has a powerful anti-inflammatory effect on the respiratory system. In a study by researchers at Loma Linda University in California, children ages six to 18 years old who took Pycnogenol supplements had significantly more improvement in lung function and asthma symptoms and were more likely to be able to reduce or discontinue rescue inhaler use than children in the placebo group.

Dose: Take a supplement equal to about 1 milligram (mg) per pound of body weight daily. Pycnogenol has a blood-thinning effect, so people who take blood-thinning medication should take this supplement only while being supervised by a physician.

•**Fish oil.** The anti-inflammatory omega-3 fatty acids EPA and DHA in fish oil have many health benefits, including curtailing the inflammation that causes asthma symptoms. Research shows that a daily fish oil supplement reduces airway narrowing and coughing and can reduce the need for medication in children with asthma. Adults can get similar benefits.

Dose: Supplements containing 2,000 milligrams (mg) to 3,000 mg of combined EPA and DHA daily for adults…1,000 mg to 1,500 mg for children. Fish oil has a blood-thinning effect, so if you take blood-thinning medication, speak to your doctor about taking fish oil.

For a more aggressive approach, add…

•**Choline.** A nutrient in the B-vitamin family, choline has been found to reduce the frequency and severity of asthma flare-ups and the need for bronchodilators. A study in *Immunobiology* found that choline reduced inflammation and oxidative stress in patients with asthma.

Dose: 1.5 grams (g) to 3 g daily. Start with the smallest dose, and increase to 3 g if symptoms don't improve in one month.

•**Glutathione.** This very potent antioxidant also revitalizes other antioxidants, boosts the immune system and breaks down environmental toxins in the body. Follow instructions on the label for dosages for adults and children.

Or take either one of the following supplements that boosts the body's glutathione levels…

•**N-acetylcysteine (NAC).**

Dose: 1,000 mg to 2,000 mg daily for adults…500 mg to 1,000 mg for children.

•**Alpha-lipoic acid (ALA).**

Dose: 100 mg to 300 mg daily for adults. It has not been studied in children. ALA can reduce glucose levels, so you should be monitored while taking this supplement if you have diabetes.

If you have exercise-induced asthma, add…

•**Lycopene.** This antioxidant, which is a powerful carotenoid, is known to improve lung function. A study published in *Allergy* found that more than half of people with exercise-induced asthma had significantly fewer symptoms after taking lycopene for one week, compared with those taking a placebo.

Dose: 30 mg daily for adults…15 mg for children.

If you get frequent respiratory infections that trigger asthma, add…

•**Astragalus.** This herb, which often is used in traditional Chinese medicine, helps to enhance the immune system's protective effects. Studies have shown that people with impaired immunity have fewer colds when they take astragalus, compared with people with impaired immunity who don't take the herb.

Dose: 500 mg to 1,000 mg twice daily for adults…250 mg to 500 mg twice daily for children.

My asthma patients are now breathing easier because of these supplements—and you will be, too.

■ ■ ■ ■

Asthma Pills Versus Inhalers

Investigators followed 650 chronic asthma patients (ages 12 to 80) for two years to compare oral medications, such as *montelukast* (Singulair) and *zafirlukast* (Accolate), with steroid inhalers.

Result: Asthma symptoms improved just as well for patients taking daily pills as for those who used steroid inhalers.

Reason: Taking pills was easier for about 60% of patients, since it meant not having to worry about proper inhaler technique.

David Price, MD, professor of primary care respiratory medicine, University of Aberdeen, Scotland.

Why Your Asthma Drugs May Not Work

John V. Fahy, MD, director, Airway Clinical Research Center, University of California, San Francisco.
Len Horovitz, MD, internist and pulmonary specialist, Lenox Hill Hospital, New York City.
American Journal of Respiratory and Critical Care Medicine, online

---

Almost half of patients with mild or moderate asthma may have a different type of disease than those with more severe symptoms, perhaps explaining why common treatments often don't work well, research suggests.

Asthma is a chronic disease involving inflamed airways. As the airways become more swollen, the muscles around them can tighten when something triggers symptoms such as coughing, wheezing and shortness of breath.

"We are beginning to understand that different 'flavors' of asthma probably have different molecular mechanisms," said John Fahy, MD, director of the Airway Clinical Research Center at the University of California, San Francisco. He is the senior author of the recent asthma study, published in the *American Journal of Respiratory and Critical Care Medicine*.

Current anti-inflammatory treatments target a condition called *eosinophilic airway inflammation*, which is common in asthma. *Eosinophils* are a type of white blood cell that help fight off infection and play a role in the immune response.

However, the recent research finds that nearly half of the 995 patients studied did not have this condition.

STUDY DETAILS

Dr. Fahy's team repeatedly measured these white blood cells in sputum samples of the volunteers with asthma who were enrolled in nine clinical trials. Nearly half, or 47%, had no airway eosinophilia on any test of their sputum. Some had the condition intermittently and some had it on each test.

The investigators found that only 36% of those not taking an inhaled corticosteroid, an anti-inflammatory, had the condition, while 17% of those who used the inhaled steroids did.

After two weeks of giving the participants anti-inflammatories and bronchodilator therapy, Dr. Fahy found those with the airway eosinophilia responded and had better airflow. But those who didn't have the condition did not respond. The responses to the bronchodilators—other medicines commonly used for asthma that work by helping to open the bronchial tubes—were similar in both groups, however.

Previous studies looked at a single sample to assess whether those with asthma had the white blood cell involvement, Dr. Fahy explained, while this study looked at many over time.

"This study reinforces the idea that asthma is not a one-type disease," he said.

STUDY AUTHORS EVALUATE RESULTS

Even within the nearly 50% without the white blood cell involvement, there are probably many different subtypes, Dr. Fahy noted.

The sputum test used in the study was complicated, Dr. Fahy pointed out, and it is not easily done in clinical practice.

Based on the study results, researchers might next work on a simpler test to determine if those with asthma have involvement of these white blood cells, he said. Eventually, the findings may help doctors better individualize asthma treatment.

The findings suggest that a sizeable group of people with mild to moderate asthma have a type of disease that is not typical, with poorly understood mechanisms, and that new treatments will be needed, Dr. Fahy concluded.

EXPERT COMMENTARY

"The finding that half of these had the absence of eosinophils in the sputum was a little surprising," said Len Horovitz, MD, pulmonary specialist at Lenox Hill Hospital in New York City. "It's higher than I thought." The "cascade" of inflammation in asthma—what happens to bring on the symptoms—has been well studied, he noted. However, "we can't guarantee that our current regimen of bronchodilators plus inhaled corticosteroids is going to work, even in mild asthma," Dr. Horovitz explained.

Doctors should ask their patients with asthma if they produce a lot of sputum, Dr. Horovitz suggested. If they do, they tend to respond to the corticosteroids.

info To learn more about asthma, visit the Web site of the American Academy of Allergy, Asthma and Immunology at *www. aaaai.org/conditions-and-treatments/asthma. aspx.*

Home Visits Reduce Asthma Problems

Children's Hospital Boston, news release

A home-visit program for children with asthma reduced hospitalizations and emergency department visits, improved patient outcomes and saved $1.46 for every dollar spent, according to a recent study.

Researchers examined the impact of the Community Asthma Initiative, a community-based asthma care program for low-income families, developed and implemented in 2005 by a team at Children's Hospital Boston.

WHAT THE STUDY REVEALED

The study included 283 families with children who had been hospitalized or who had made emergency department visits for asthma. Of those children, 43% had moderate or severe asthma. Over one year, the families received an average of 1.2 home visits.

After one year, the researchers saw a 68% decrease in asthma-related emergency department visits, an 85% drop in asthma-related hospitalizations, a 43% reduction in the percentage of children who had to limit physical activity on any day, a 41% decrease in reports of missed school days and a 50% fall in parents having to miss work to care for their child.

The percentage of children with an up-to-date asthma care plan rose from 53% to 82%.

These improvements were evident within six months and persisted for as long as two years, the study authors noted in a Children's Hospital Boston news release.

The study appears in the journal *Pediatrics*.

PROGRAM DETAILS AND SAVINGS

The program includes nurse case management and care coordination combined with home visits by a nurse or community health worker to educate families about asthma, assess the home for asthma triggers, and provide materials and services to reduce asthma attacks, such as HEPA vacuums (which have high-efficiency air filters), special bedding covers and pest control.

The program cost $2,529 per child but yielded savings of $3,827 per child, due to fewer hospitalizations and emergency department visits. That means that $1.46 in health care costs was saved for every dollar spent on the program.

"This is a remarkable savings to society and reflects better health outcomes for the children," said program team coleader Elizabeth Woods, MD, associate chief, division of adolescent/young adult medicine, Children's Hospital Boston.

info Visit the American Lung Association Web site (*www.lung.org/lung-disease/asthma/ taking-control-of-asthma/for-parents-of-children- with-asthma*) for more information about asthma and children.

....

Ancient Asthma Remedy

Indian frankincense may relieve asthma. Boswellia, a white resin from the frankincense tree, is a potent anti-inflammatory that may make breathing easier for people with asthma.

Recent finding: Breathing eased and frequency of attacks dropped in 70% of asthma patients who took boswellia daily for six weeks. Ask your doctor about taking 300 milligrams (mg) to 400 mg of a standardized extract with at least 60% boswellia acids three times a day.

Laurie Steelsmith, ND, a naturopathic doctor and acupuncturist in private practice, Honolulu. *www.drsteel smith.com*

....

Belly Fat Is Linked to Asthma

Norwegian University of Science and Technology researchers have found that people who had excess belly fat (but were not obese) were 1.4 times more likely to develop asthma than those who didn't have excess belly fat. Excess belly fat refers to waist circumference of at least 40 inches in men and 35 in women. Researchers are not sure why the link occurs, although fat cells are known to produce inflammatory compounds.

B. Brumpton, "A Prospective Study of Central Obesity, Overall Obesity and Incident Asthma in Adults," European Respiratory Society's Annual Congress, Amsterdam (2011).

Soft Drinks Bubble Up Respiratory Ills

Respirology, news release

Drinking a lot of soft drinks may increase the risk for asthma and/or chronic obstructive pulmonary disease (COPD), a recent study suggests.

STUDY DETAILS

Nearly 17,000 people aged 16 and older in South Australia were asked about their consumption of soft drinks such as Coke, flavored mineral water, lemonade, Powerade and Gatorade.

More than 10% of the participants said they drank more than half a liter of soft drinks a day, according to the study, which was published in the journal *Respirology.* That's a little more than two 8-ounce glasses of soft drinks.

The researchers found that 13.3% of the participants with asthma and 15.6% of those with COPD consumed more than half a liter of soft drinks a day.

People who consumed that amount were 1.2 times more likely to have asthma and 1.7 times more likely to have COPD than those who did not consume soft drinks, the researchers said.

WHAT FINDINGS MEAN

"Our study emphasizes the importance of healthy eating and drinking in the prevention of chronic diseases like asthma and COPD," said study leader Zumin Shi, MD, PhD, of the University of Adelaide.

The researchers said the risk was dose-related, meaning the more soft drinks consumed, the greater the odds of having COPD or asthma.

However, the study merely points out an association and does not establish a cause-and-effect relationship. It's possible, for example, that people who drink large amounts of soft drinks have poor diets, or other bad habits, that may cause the observed increase in lung disease.

Smoking increased the risk even further, especially for COPD. People who smoked and consumed more than half a liter of soft drinks a day had a 6.6 times greater risk of COPD than those who didn't smoke and didn't consume soft drinks.

info For more information on COPD, visit the American Lung Association Web site, *www. lung.org/lung-disease/copd.*

■ ■ ■ ■

COPD Inhaler Warning

COPD inhalers may cause urinary difficulty. According to a recent study, among more than 500,000 patients ages 66 and older with chronic obstructive pulmonary disease (COPD), men who had just started using anticholinergic inhalers were 42% more likely than those who did not use inhalers to develop acute urinary retention, or difficulty urinating. Risk was almost twice as high in men with enlarged prostate. There was no increased risk for women.

Theory: Inhaled anticholinergic medications can be absorbed into the bloodstream and affect other organs such as the bladder.

Anne Stephenson, MD, PhD, respirologist, St. Michael's Hospital, Toronto.

Herbal Paste Eases Winter Breathing

Yongjun Bian, MD, clinical researcher in the respiratory department of Guang'anmen Hospital in Beijing, China, and a research fellow for a study of 125 COPD patients.

For people with chronic obstructive pulmonary disease (COPD), an incurable condition characterized by chronic bronchitis and/or emphysema, winter often brings a worsening of symptoms such as coughing, wheezing, shortness of breath, fatigue and recurrent respiratory infections. Steroids help control symptoms but can have side effects… antibiotics fight infection but increase the risk for antibiotic resistance.

Good news: A recent study has provided scientific evidence of the effectiveness of a topical herbal remedy called Xiao Chuan paste (XCP), which has been used in China for more than 1,000 years to treat COPD and other breathing problems.

Researchers randomly assigned COPD patients to receive either XCP or a placebo paste. As is traditional, the paste was applied to three specific pairs of acupuncture points on the back…the treatment was given four times during an eight-week period in July and August. Then participants were monitored from November through February.

Results: Compared with patients who received the placebo, those who received XCP were significantly less likely to experience an exacerbation of symptoms requiring steroids, antibiotics and/or hospitalization…and they reported a significantly higher quality of life. The only side effect—a mild skin reaction that cleared up without treatment once XCP was discontinued—occurred in just 2% of users.

XCP is made from herbs native to China, including *Asarum heterotropoides*, *Ephedra vulgaris* and *Acorus gramineus Soland*. Researchers theorize that the herbs have properties that affect immune regulation.

You can learn more about XCP by consulting a practitioner of traditional Chinese medicine who is knowledgeable about herbal therapies.

info To find a practitioner of traditional Chinese medicine, contact the National Certification Commission for Acupuncture and Oriental Medicine (*www.nccaom.org*) or the American Association of Acupuncture & Oriental Medicine (*www.aaaomonline.org*).

Antibiotics May Not Be Best for Cystic Fibrosis Patients

University of Michigan, news release

Antibiotics can prolong the lives of individuals with cystic fibrosis, but the drugs also allow treatment-resistant bacteria to thrive in the lungs, a recent, small study suggests.

Cystic fibrosis is a chronic disease in which the body produces thick, sticky mucus that clogs the lungs. The accumulation of the mucus leaves people prone to serious, hard-to-treat and recurrent infections. Eventually, the repeated infections destroy the lungs.

The findings from the 10-year investigation suggest, but do not prove conclusively, that the current standard of aggressive antibiotic treatment for cystic fibrosis patients may not always be the best approach.

Aggressive use of antibiotics actually lowers the diversity of lung bacteria, resulting in infections that are increasingly difficult to treat. A more diverse community of lung bacteria may help keep the most dangerous strains in check, the researchers noted.

STUDY DETAILS

In the study, researchers examined bacteria from six patients collected over eight to nine years. Half of the patients had a relatively stable type of cystic fibrosis and the others had the more typical, faster-progressing form. The investigators conducted DNA analysis on bacteria in 126 sputum samples.

Over time, the researchers found that bacterial diversity declined, yet the overall level of bacteria remained fairly constant. The study authors explained that this means a small number of organisms multiply to take the place of those that have been killed off by antibiotics.

IMPLICATIONS

"The conventional wisdom has been that as patients with cystic fibrosis age and become sicker, their lung disease progresses and more bacteria move in," John LiPuma, MD, research professor of pediatrics and communicable diseases at the University of Michigan Medical School in Ann Arbor, said. "But our study—which was the first to examine the bacterial communities in cystic fibrosis patients' lungs over a long period of time—indicates that's not what happens.

"What we normally do is essentially carpet bombing with antibiotics," Dr. LiPuma explained. "However, what we found is that over time this ultimately assists treatment-resistant bacteria by getting rid of their competition."

He said the findings may be a first step toward developing new treatment methods, such as more focused use of antibiotics or even distribution of beneficial bacteria to cystic fibrosis patients.

The study was published in the *Proceedings of the National Academy of Sciences*.

info For more information on cystic fibrosis, visit the US National Heart, Lung, and Blood Institute's Web site at *http://www.nhlbi. nih.gov/health/health-topics/topics/cf/*.

Breakthrough Treatments For Sleep Apnea

David M. Rapoport, MD, associate professor of medicine and director of the sleep medicine program at New York University School of Medicine, New York City.

If you're one of the 18 million Americans who have been diagnosed with moderate-to-severe sleep apnea, chances are your doctor has suggested that you try a continuous positive airway pressure, or CPAP (pronounced "SEE-pap"), machine.

Problem: Many people complain that the CPAP face mask is too uncomfortable to wear and often causes problems such as mouth dryness.

Solution: There are now many ways to make CPAP treatment less uncomfortable—or, if necessary, you can use one of various alternative therapies that are effective when CPAP is not tolerated.

WHAT IS SLEEP APNEA?

Sleep apnea occurs when breathing temporarily stops multiple times during sleep. Symptoms may include snoring, gasping, choking and daytime drowsiness. At least 10% of adults over age 65 are believed to have the most common form, obstructive sleep apnea, though the majority of them don't know it. The condition affects men and women.

THE SLEEP APNEA CHALLENGE

Sleep apnea frequently goes undiagnosed. Even though snoring is a telltale symptom in some sufferers, not everyone who snores has sleep apnea—and not everyone with sleep apnea snores.

Red flag: If you have chronic snoring loud enough to wake your bed partner, you may have sleep apnea.

Don't ignore this condition: If you have moderate-to-severe sleep apnea (20 or more interruptions in breathing per night), be sure to seek medical treatment. Sleep apnea causes severe sleepiness and has been linked to impaired cognitive function (including memory loss), elevated blood pressure, increased stroke and heart attack risk and a higher mortality rate.

CPAP—IF YOU CAN TOLERATE IT

Use of a CPAP machine is widely considered the most effective treatment for moderate-to-severe sleep apnea. If you're overweight, weight loss also helps.

CPAP increases the pressure of the air being breathed, which helps keep the airway open. The CPAP machine—about the size of a dictionary—pumps air into a hose that is connected to a face mask (nasal or full-face covering the nose and mouth). *Modifications that make CPAP more user-friendly include…*

•**More comfortable mask designs** are available in a variety of designs from Respironics…ResMed…and Fisher & Paykel Healthcare, as well as from specialty manufacturers, such as Dreamweaver and CPAP Pro.

•**Humidifying feature to fight mouth dryness**—some CPAP machines are built with features to maximally humidify or to allow an external humidifier to be attached, while others come with an internal humidifier. Humidifying CPAP machines and attachments can be found at *www.directhomemedical.com*, 888-505-0212.

•**Bilevel positive airway pressure** (BiPAP and others) and C-Flex are modified versions of CPAP that reduce air pressure as the wearer exhales, which some patients find more comfortable. (CPAP provides constant and steady air pressure, whereas bilevel devices provide varying pressure.) Bilevel machines cost more than those used for CPAP, starting at about $1,700 versus about $800.

New: CPAP can be modified with a breathing sensor called SensAwake that detects when the user's breathing pattern becomes irregular (indicating partial wakefulness) and drops the pressure.* The CPAP resumes full pressure only when regular breathing indicates the patient is

*Dr. Rapoport has a financial interest in SensAwake.

asleep. CPAP with SensAwake is available from Fisher & Paykel Healthcare for $629.

CPAP ALTERNATIVES

If you still find CPAP too uncomfortable to use, consider…

•**Oral appliances.** These hinged mouthpieces, which are worn during sleep, pull the lower jaw (and base of the tongue) forward to keep the upper airway open. Oral appliances are typically custom-made by a dentist. The initial cost of an oral appliance (usually about $1,000) is similar to that of CPAP, but patients usually need a half dozen follow-up dentist visits to adjust the appliance.

•**Nasal devices.** Provent (Ventus Medical) is a disposable device that's attached to the nostrils at night, then thrown away in the morning. The opening of the device narrows during exhalation, which increases pressure in the airway. It is believed that this makes the airway less prone to collapse. Provent, which must be prescribed by a doctor, was recently approved by the FDA.

The good news: It costs just $2 a day ($730 a year) and can easily be tried for a week.

•**Sleep position products.** Sleep apnea worsens when the sufferer is lying on his/her back. That's because gravity makes it more likely that throat muscles will collapse and block the person's airway.

Products that help people stay off their backs during sleep include an "antisnore" T-shirt (with pockets sewn on the back to hold inflatable or Styrofoam "bumpers"). It is available from Rematee, 877-753-6844, *www.rematee.com*, for $56.79. Or sew a pocket on the back of a T-shirt and place a tennis ball inside.

Several pillows that are designed to promote side sleeping also are available.

Examples: Sona Pillow, 800-366-2324, *www.sonapillow.com*, for $59.99…and Splintek Sleep Right Side Sleeping Pillow, *www.amazon.com*, $78.95.

SURGERY: A LAST RESORT

If noninvasive approaches don't relieve sleep apnea symptoms, there are surgical options. These include a procedure that removes tissue from the throat and mouth (with a success rate of up to 40%) and another that remolds the lower and upper jaw to increase airway space (with a success rate of up to 90%).

Exciting new approach: An experimental implant, which is about the size of a matchbox and known as a hypoglossal nerve stimulator, is implanted under the collarbone to electrically stimulate the throat's nerves so that the tissues won't collapse and block the airway.

The implant has shown promising results in early trials but is not yet available.

One catch: The battery needs replacing every three to five years, requiring another small operation.

• • • •

Sleep Apnea Returns Quickly If CPAP Stops

Sleep apnea returns quickly if CPAP stops. Continuous Positive Airway Pressure (CPAP), in which a machine blows air continuously into a patient's airway through a tube and a mask, is effective at relieving obstructive sleep apnea. But once people are established users of CPAP, withdrawal of the treatment leads to rapid recurrence of apnea and sleepiness within days.

Malcolm Kohler, MD, senior consultant, Sleep Disorders Centre and Pulmonary Division, University Hospital, Zurich, Switzerland, and leader of a study published in *American Journal of Respiratory and Critical Care Medicine.*

Stop Summer (and Fall) Allergies…Without Medication

Richard Firshein, DO, director of the Firshein Center for Comprehensive Medicine, New York City, *www.drfirshein.com.* He is board-certified in family medicine and a licensed acupuncturist. Dr. Firshein is author of *Reversing Asthma* (Warner).

Springtime is considered the worst time of year for allergy sufferers due to the abundance of grass and tree pollen. But it doesn't stop there. In virtually all parts of the US, pollen from various grass and weed species is a problem throughout the summer and into the fall, keeping many people miserable as late as October in some parts of the US.

Often mistaken for a "summer cold," allergies that occur in the summer usually cause the same symptoms triggered by spring pollen—runny nose, itchy eyes, sneezing, wheezing and shortness of breath.

The antihistamines that most allergy sufferers reach for, such as *loratadine* (Claritin), *fexofenadine* (Allegra) and *cetirizine* (Zyrtec), work by blocking the effect of inflammatory compounds called *histamines,* which produce allergy symptoms. A newer, even more powerful class of medications, including *montelukast* (Singulair) and *zafirlukast* (Accolate), block the action of a different group of inflammatory compounds called *leukotrienes.*

Problem: These medications suppress symptoms but don't halt the underlying allergic event. Stop taking them at any point during allergy season, and symptoms come back worse than ever because the body overcompensates for a lack of response to the histamine production.

Solution: By combining preventive strategies with the right natural remedies, most people can establish a simple regimen that keeps even severe allergies under control without resorting to drugs.

Step 1: Reduce your exposure to certain foods. Many people with seasonal allergies have cross-sensitivities to foods containing proteins similar to the airborne allergens they're sensitive to. These foods may cause no problems the rest of the year, but during allergy season, they can make typical pollen allergy symptoms significantly worse and may also trigger symptoms of their own.

This phenomenon, known as oral allergy syndrome, causes symptoms such as tingling, itching or swelling of the mouth, tongue or throat, itching of the scalp or skin, wheezing and/or unusual fatigue.

Raw foods (especially their skins) are more likely to trigger allergic reactions.

Foods that can trigger cross-sensitivity reactions include…

•**Fruits,** especially apples, bananas, melons and peaches.

•**Certain vegetables,** including cucumbers, tomatoes and zucchini.

•**Foods that are made from grain** (particularly wheat).

•**Milk from grass-fed cows**—it may contain microscopic undigested grass particles.

My advice: Keep a food diary during allergy season, and note the foods that seem to worsen symptoms. If you suspect that a food is affecting you, avoid it for several days to see if symptoms improve.

Also, avoid red meat, sugar and junk foods, all of which have inflammatory effects that contribute to allergy symptoms.

Step 2: **Reduce your exposure to pollen.** *Best approaches…*

•**Don't exercise outdoors in the morning.** Exercising between 5 am and 10 am can increase your pollen exposure tenfold.

•**Keep windows shut during this same period** (or all day, if possible) to keep pollen out of your home.

•**Use a HEPA filter.** It's the most effective device for removing pollen from the air in your bedroom and other heavily used rooms.

Good brands: Austin Air and Honeywell.

•**Remove outer clothes when coming inside** after you have been outside for an hour or more.

•**Vacuum often** (every day if pollen levels are high) with a HEPA-filter vacuum.

Step 3: **Try allergy-fighting supplements.***
Supplements of the nutrient *quercetin* (300 mg to 600 mg daily) and, if needed, extract of the herb stinging nettle (500 mg to 1,000 mg daily) both reduce the body's histamine response. It may take up to a week to see improvement in allergy symptoms.

If this combination doesn't provide relief, try adding the herb butterbur. Evidence suggests that it relieves pollen symptoms by reducing both histamine and leukotriene production. Butterbur may be toxic to the liver and kidneys in some people, so consult your doctor first.

Typical dose: 50 mg/day.

*Speak to your doctor before starting any supplement regimen. For children's doses, consult a physician.

For additional symptom relief, consider trying the following supplements—add them one at a time if you need greater symptom relief…

•**Vitamin C.** This powerful antioxidant helps stabilize the body's mast cells, which facilitate histamine release.

Typical dose: 1,000 mg to 2,000 mg/day. If you have kidney disease, be sure to consult your doctor before taking this dose.

•**Pycnogenol (pine bark extract).** This herb was found in a recent study to reduce hay fever symptoms.

Typical dose: 100 mg/day.

•**Bromelain.** This enzyme has anti-inflammatory properties and enhances absorption of quercetin.

Typical dose: 1,000 mg/day.

•**Resveratrol.** This grape derivative has potent immune-stimulating effects, which help stabilize your body's reaction to allergens.

Typical dose: 100 mg/day.

•**Fish oil capsules.**

Typical dose: 2,000 mg daily for anti-inflammatory benefits. Each capsule should contain a minimum of 250 mg of DHA and 100 mg of EPA.

•**Nux vomica.** This homeopathic remedy can help relieve seasonal allergy symptoms in some people. Consider adding it to the above regimen if you need additional relief.

Typical dose: 30C up to four times daily. Do not exceed this dose. Nux vomica is a highly diluted remedy derived from seeds containing the poison strychnine. Extreme overdoses could result in anxiety, muscle spasms or even death.

Step 4: **Consider allergy drops.** Most people know about allergy shots, but allergy drops are another natural therapy that can be administered year-round or only during allergy season. Sublingual allergy drops contain the same purified substances used in allergy shots and are a good option for people who strongly dislike shots. Drops are simply placed under the tongue daily.

Allergy sufferers who receive allergy shots get weekly injections containing small doses of the offending allergen. Over time, the immune system learns to stop overreacting to the allergens.

Bee Pollen—Taking the Sting Out of Allergies

Mark A. Stengler, NMD, naturopathic medical doctor in private practice, Encinitas, California…adjunct associate clinical professor at the National College of Natural Medicine, Portland, Oregon…author of *The Natural Physician's Healing Therapies* and coauthor of *Prescription for Natural Cures* (both from Bottom Line Books).

There's nothing more "made by nature" than bee pollen, the substance that clings to bees as they gather nectar from flowering plants. It is rich in vitamins A, B-complex and C as well as nutrients such as calcium, magnesium and potassium. Bee pollen also contains flavonoids that have been found to reduce inflammation. Bee pollen supplements mainly are used to reduce hay fever symptoms, treat arthritis and fight fatigue. Are they worth taking?

My experience: One spring, I had a terrible bout of hay fever. None of the natural treatments that I had successfully used in the past were of any help. I was miserable. I tried bee pollen supplements. Bee pollen supplements have a homeopathic effect—they help to desensitize the immune system to the allergic reaction. They contain small amounts of the allergen, which help the body build up its defenses against the allergen and prevent future allergic reactions. These supplements helped me when all else failed. Now I recommend them to prevent or treat flare-ups in some of my patients with hay fever.

My advice: If you suffer from hay fever, start taking bee pollen about two months before hay fever season begins. If it is effective at keeping hay fever at bay, continue taking it throughout hay fever season.

Dosage: Two to four capsules (500 mg to 1,000 mg) daily. To relieve acute symptoms, four to eight capsules can be taken as long as needed if no side effects are experienced. Do not take bee pollen supplements if you are allergic to bee stings. Even if you have never had an allergic reaction to a bee sting, test a small amount of bee pollen supplement before taking a whole capsule. To do this, open a capsule and place a small amount of the powder on your tongue. If you experience wheezing, a rash or any other reaction, do not take bee pollen supplements. If you experience digestive upset from taking bee pollen, stop taking it.

To ensure that a bee pollen product does not contain contaminants, such as pesticides, buy from companies that manufacture quality bee pollen supplements, such as Nature's Way (800-962-8873, *www.naturesway.com*) or Natural Factors (800-322-8704, *www.naturalfactors.com*).

■■■■

Some Hotels Cater to Guests With Allergies

In addition to cleaning rooms with hypoallergenic products and washing linens with fragrance-free detergents, Hyatt, Marriott and Hilton hotels now offer rooms that have medical-grade air purifiers and chemical- and fragrance-free bath products. These rooms cost $20 to $30 more per night. To see a list of all hotel locations that offer these types of rooms, go to *www.pureroom.com*.

The New York Times

Solving Adult Mystery Allergies

Michael S. Blaiss, MD, clinical professor of pediatrics and medicine at University of Tennessee Health Science Center, Memphis, and past-president of the American College of Allergy, Asthma and Immunology.

You never used to have allergies, but now you do—at least you think you do. You've got the symptoms—the sneezing, stuffiness and runny nose. Adults who suddenly are sensitive to things that didn't bother them before, such as fragrances, smoke, detergents, lotions or even aspirin, might have nonallergic *rhinitis*, a condition that mimics allergies but isn't quite the same.

The difference is important because many of the medications that are used to treat allergies don't work for nonallergic rhinitis even when the symptoms virtually are identical.

NO IMMUNE RESPONSE

True allergies are characterized by a release of *histamine*. Histamine is an inflammatory substance that causes irritation and swelling of the nasal tissues.

Nonallergic rhinitis is different. It causes irritation, but the irritation isn't related to histamine and the underlying cause is unknown. Unlike allergies, which usually develop in childhood, nonallergic rhinitis mainly occurs in adults, affecting up to 10% of American adults.

WHAT TO LOOK FOR

The only way to prove that someone has nonallergic rhinitis rather than an allergy is with skin-prick or blood tests. If you test negative, your symptoms probably are due to nonallergic causes.

Main symptoms: Most patients with nonallergic rhinitis suffer from nasal congestion, a runny nose and/or postnasal drip. Many patients also have conjunctivitis (eye inflammation), along with coughing and sometimes a headache.

They're somewhat less likely than allergy patients to be bothered by sneezing or nasal itching, and they're rarely bothered by watery eyes.

It's tricky to distinguish the two because many patients have mixed rhinitis, a combination of allergic and nonallergic reactions.

Example: One of my patients, a 46-year-old man, is sensitive to (not allergic to) detergents but also sneezes a lot because of allergies.

Self-test: Take a nonsedating oral antihistamine, such as *loratadine* (Claritin) or *fexofenadine* (Allegra), for a week or two. Medication will help only if you have allergies. It won't make a difference for nonallergic rhinitis.

PREVENTION

The most effective way to prevent symptoms is with avoidance…

•**Avoid colognes and other scented personal-care products.** Look for household products with no scent.

•**Don't burn candles indoors,** even unscented ones. All candles emit soot, which can trigger reactions.

•**Wear a mask or respirator** when working with wood, paints, varnishes and the like.

•**Switch to *acetaminophen* if you need a painkiller for another condition such as arthritis.** Nonsteroidal anti-inflammatory drugs (NSAIDs), such as aspirin and *ibuprofen*, can trigger nonallergic rhinitis.

TREATMENTS

Talk to your doctor about your choices, including…

•**Oral decongestants that contain pseudoephedrine** (such as Actifed and Sudafed) or phenylephrine (Neo-Synephrine).

•**Prescription antihistamine nasal sprays,** such as *azelastine* (Astelin). Unlike oral antihistamines, the sprays help relieve symptoms.

Are You Allergic to Your Cell Phone?

Thomas Brunoski, MD, a practitioner of nutritional and preventive medicine, Westport, Connecticut.

Cell phones regularly come under fire for raising the risk of brain cancer—an assertion that has created some controversy. One thing we know for sure is that heavy users can develop nasty skin rashes. The condition even has a name. Doctors in Italy documented the first case in 2000 and appropriately categorized it as "mobile phone dermatitis." Thomas Brunoski, MD, a practioner of nutritional and preventive medicine in Westport, Connecticut, explained that this cell phone allergy is actually people reacting to nickel, which is commonly found in the exterior casings, menu buttons, headset logos and the fancy trim on mobile devices. But, he adds, while the itchy, bumpy rash may be annoying, it is usually not severe.

What you can do: You can be tested for a nickel allergy. Many more women than men have nickel allergy, probably because of exposure during ear piercings. Another place nickel is typically found is in the cheap buttons on jeans, which cause a steady stream of complaints. Some women report that putting clear nail polish on jeans buttons helps with that problem, and they suggest that a similar tactic on cell phones might be useful, although there is no data on this. Another alternative is one of the many cell-phone covers that are commercially available. Or opt for a hands-free device (e.g., a Bluetooth wireless headset or wired headset). This will protect you from both the allergy and the cell phone's radiation.

How to Clean the Air You Breathe

Allen P. Rathey, president of The Healthy House Institute, an independent educational resource for creating healthier homes based in Boise, Idaho. *www.healthy houseinstitute.com*

It might not be pleasant to think about, but the air we breathe is full of contaminants—dust, pollen and mold, to name just a few, as well as noxious gases, such as formaldehyde.

Surprising fact: Air is actually the number-one way that our bodies are exposed to contaminants in the home—in fact, we inhale about 35 pounds of air per day.

Unfortunately, dirty air can have significant effects on your health. For example, several studies have strongly linked air pollution to heart disease, asthma and depression.

While you can't eliminate all airborne pollutants, it's always wise to take basic steps to improve your indoor-air quality. These include frequent vacuuming and dusting…as well as efforts to ventilate your home, such as opening windows and using a kitchen range hood and bathroom exhaust fans.

Air purifiers can also help. What's more, these devices can be especially beneficial for people with allergies or chemical sensitivities. What's right for you?

CHOOSING THE RIGHT AIR PURIFIER

Air purifiers are available in portable devices designed for individual rooms or whole-house units that are built into your central air-conditioning or forced-air heating system. If you want air purification in your entire home, it may be cost-effective if the air ductwork is built in. However, most people get good results in the areas where they spend the most time with one or more portable units.

Important: Because there are so many options when buying a portable air purifier, it's easy to make mistakes that end up costing you money and/or prevent you from getting the pollution-fighting features you really need…

Mistake 1: **Getting the wrong type of air purifier.** There are two main types of air purifiers—units that remove particles (such as dust, pollen, mold and pet dander) and those that remove gases/odors (such as paint fumes and formaldehyde from glue in wood furniture). Some units remove both particles and gases/odors.

To determine which type of air purifier you need, ask yourself, *What am I trying to get rid of?*

Allergy and asthma sufferers often will want an air purifier that removes particles…someone who is chemically sensitive will want to eliminate gases and odors.

Air-cleaning devices designed to capture tiny particles from the air typically use high-efficiency particulate air (HEPA) technology. HEPA filters remove 99.97% of particles as small as 0.3 microns. For reference, a single hair is about 70 microns wide.

Air purifiers designed to remove gases and odors typically use activated charcoal or other material that binds to the pollutants. If you want to get rid of particles and gases, look for a purifier with both HEPA technology and a material such as activated carbon.

Important: If germs are your concern—for example, if you live with a person who is chronically ill or who has a compromised immune system—you might opt for an air purifier that uses ultraviolet (UV-C) light technology. This type of air purifier is frequently used in hospitals and destroys germs such as certain types of viruses and bacteria. The "C" stands for the frequency of UV light that kills germs.

Mistake 2: **Not checking a unit's efficiency and certification.** A critical factor when selecting an air purifier is the device's Clean Air Delivery Rate (CADR), established by the Association of Home Appliance Manufacturers (AHAM). This numerical rating measures how quickly a portable air purifier can remove pollen, dust and tobacco smoke from a certain square-foot dimension. Specifically, it measures how much air is moving through the filter and the volume of filtered air delivered by an air purifier.

The higher the number, the better. Maximum CADR values are 450 for pollen and smoke and 400 for dust. For a list of certified air purifiers with their CADR values, visit the AHAM Web site, *www.cadr.org.*

Your room size helps determine the most appropriate CADR. If there's, say, a smoker in the home, the AHAM recommends looking for a unit with a "tobacco smoke CADR" of at least two-thirds of your room's area. For example, a 10-foot by 12-foot room (120 square feet) would require a CADR of at least 80.

If you're older, have a compromised immune system or are particularly sensitive to chemicals, be sure to look for a bigger filter, more powerful fan and a high CADR, and ask to see the filter itself. If it looks thin and flimsy, it probably won't clean the air very efficiently.

Two of the best: The RabbitAir MinusA2 Ultra Quiet HEPA Air Purifier, *www.rabbitair.com* (*cost:* $459.95) can be custom-designed to filter chemical gases, airborne bacteria, pet dander or tobacco smoke. The Idylis280 for medium-to-large rooms, *www.idylishome.com* (*cost:* $249) also includes a UV-C light.

If you have allergies or asthma, you may also want to visit *www.asthmaandallergyfriendly.com* to see whether the air purifier you're considering has been certified by the Asthma and Allergy Foundation of America (AAFA).

Mistake 3: **Not placing the air purifier in the right location.** It sounds obvious, but the key to achieving the cleanest air possible is to ensure that the polluted air actually passes through the filter. Many contaminants will never reach a small device that is located, for example, in the corner of your bedroom.

For the best coverage, you may wish to purchase several air purifiers depending on how big an area they can clean—or at least shut the door to the room with the single air purifier to keep out nonfiltered air.

Mistake 4: **Not changing the filter often enough.** Manufacturers provide a schedule of recommended times to change the filter—carefully follow these recommendations to keep your unit running in peak condition. Dirty filters lose effectiveness over time, and this could result in higher electricity costs if the air purifier has to run for longer periods of time to clean the air.

If your air is especially dirty, you might need to replace the filter every few months (or more often)…if it's reasonably clean, once a year (or less often) may be sufficient. Many units come with filter-change sensors that alert you when they're clogged, often based on airflow reduction.

Chronic Sinusitis? Alternative Medicine To the Rescue

Jeffrey Suh, MD, assistant professor, rhinology and skull-based surgery, department of head and neck surgery, University of California, Los Angeles.

Jordan Josephson, MD, sinus and allergy specialist, Lenox Hill Hospital, New York City, and director, NY Nasal and Sinus Center.

Archives of Otolaryngology

When used in tandem with standard Western treatments, alternative therapies such as acupuncture, acupressure and dietary changes may spell significant relief for patients battling chronic sinusitis, a recent pilot study suggests.

The authors say that their study is the first to explore the potential of combining Western medicine with Eastern therapies among these patients, who experience swollen and inflamed sinuses, facial pain, headaches and impaired breathing.

"Our study was small, looking at a handful of patients who were not benefiting that well from standard treatment," acknowledged study author Jeffrey Suh, MD, an assistant professor of rhinology and skull-based surgery in the department of head and neck surgery at the University of California, Los Angeles.

"And my take on alternative treatments is that Western medicine is effective for the majority of patients," he added. "But for those who don't get complete relief, adding in a more holistic Eastern approach that includes exercise, improved sleep, a better diet, and acupuncture and self-administered acupressure seems to provide an alternative that can have great benefit."

BACKGROUND

The authors point out that chronic *rhinosinusitis* is a very prevalent condition in the United States, with nearly 30 million American adults diagnosed with the disease in 2010 alone, according to the US Centers for Disease Control and Prevention.

The acute version of the disease is typically due to infection, experts say. However, the chronic form (namely, cases enduring past 12 weeks) is thought to stem from a variety of environmental and anatomical causes (such as the presence of polyps or a deviated nasal septum), thereby complicating treatment efforts.

Such efforts usually include the use of nasal corticosteroid sprays and nasal irrigation, while in some instances surgical intervention is required. Despite such efforts, some patients remain debilitated.

STUDY DETAILS

Dr. Suh and his team focused on 11 such individuals (eight men and three women), between the ages of 32 and 70. Many had struggled with the condition for years. None had had any kind of surgery in the three months before the study started. Similarly, no one had undergone acupuncture or acupressure intervention in the two months beforehand.

During the study, all previous treatments were continued. However, patients were offered eight weekly 20-minute sessions of therapeutic acupuncture and acupressure massage, performed by licensed therapists. Counseling was also offered to teach patients how to self-administer acupressure at home.

A dietary analysis was conducted, and patients were given nutritional guidance that tracked traditional Chinese approaches toward food consumption. Stress management was also discussed, as were the benefits of regular exercise.

BENEFITS OF ALTERNATIVE THERAPIES

The result: The team found that when applied alongside modern medicine, the use of such so-called "staples of Eastern medicine" appeared to be both safe and effective.

After two months, all the patients showed a statistically significant gain in terms of quality of life, with a drop in feelings of frustration and restlessness and a boost in their ability to concentrate.

What's more, patients were found to have less of a problem with runny noses, reduced sneezing and a subsequent reduced need to blow their noses. Facial pain and pressure also appeared to drop off somewhat.

Dr. Suh and his colleagues reported their findings in the *Archives of Otolaryngology.*

IMPLICATIONS

"These were the worst of the worst patients," Dr. Suh stressed. "And during treatment they got better. Now were they completely better? No. Only some of their symptoms improved. And those who did not keep up the lifestyle modifications like self-administered acupressure returned to their previous state after the study. But those who kept it up continued to see a benefit. So this offers some hope, and leads us to consider the next question, which is what might be possible with Eastern therapy alone?"

EXPERT COMMENTARY

Jordan Josephson, MD, a sinus and allergy specialist with Lenox Hill Hospital in New York City, cautioned that chronic sinusitis is a "very complex problem" for which there is no simple solution.

"Augmenting traditional medicine with Eastern therapies is a very wise thing to do for sinus sufferers," he said. "In my practice, I certainly do this. Because it's not a question of antihistamines or acupuncture.

"And the reason for that is that we're not talking about a cure," Dr. Josephson continued. "This is not a cold or a sniffle. If you have chronic sinusitis, it's chronic, like diabetes. So, the best thing to do is to treat patients with a combination of diet, antibiotics, antifungals, nasal sprays, allergy treatment, acupuncture, lifestyle changes, irrigation with saline and irrigation with medicines. You need a comprehensive plan for each individual patient that will give them the best chance at control."

■ ■ ■ ■

Quick Cure for Sinusitis

To reduce inflammation of the sinuses caused by viral, bacterial or fungal infection, use grapefruit seed extract nasal spray. It boosts the immune system and has antifungal and anti-microbial properties. Tilt your head back, and spray once into each nostril. Use once daily to prevent sinusitis (when you feel it coming on) or to treat it. Use it four times daily for acute infections. Grapefruit seed extract does not help sinus problems related to allergies. Available at health-food stores, it is safe for everyone and can be used with antibiotics.

Mark A. Stengler, NMD, licensed naturopathic medical doctor in private practice, Encinitas, California…adjunct associate clinical professor at the National College of Natural Medicine, Portland, Oregon…author of The Natural Physician's Healing Therapies and coauthor of Prescription for Natural Cures (both from Bottom Line Books).

Occasional Pot Smoking May Not Harm Lungs

Stefan Kertesz, MD, associate professor, University of Alabama at Birmingham.
Robert Hancox, MD, associate professor, department of preventive and social medicine, University of Otago, New Zealand.
Calvina Fay, executive director, Drug Free America Foundation, St. Petersburg, Florida.
Paul Armentano, deputy director of the national pro-marijuana group NORML.
Journal of the American Medical Association

Unlike the cigarette habit, occasional pot smoking does not seem to trigger declines in lung function that could lead to breathing problems, a recent 20-year study suggests.

"Tobacco takes you down that road toward breathlessness, but low to moderate levels of marijuana don't," said study coauthor Stefan Kertesz, MD, associate professor, University of Alabama at Birmingham.

OKAY TO PARTY IN MODERATION?

But there were limits to the study. For example, the findings do not indicate whether occasional (two or three joints a month) pot smokers face a higher risk of lung diseases such as cancer.

And it is clear that marijuana smoke irritates the lungs, causing coughing and sputum production, and addiction to marijuana obviously causes problems, noted Dr. Kertesz. However, as with alcohol and other drugs, the question of harm becomes more ambiguous when it comes to more occasional users who aren't addicted, he said.

"What about the adults who use three joints of marijuana a month for many years?" he said. "Clarifying that is actually quite difficult."

Nevertheless, the research should fuel the ongoing debate over medical marijuana, which critics say is too hazardous to serve as a drug to treat conditions such as pain.

STUDY DETAILS

In the recent study, researchers examined the findings of another study, which began in 1985, of more than 5,100 people ages 18 to 30 from California, Chicago, Minneapolis and Alabama. Researchers regularly asked participants about past and current use of cigarettes and marijuana.

Every few years over two decades, the participants took lung tests that measured their lung function through their ability to blow hard into a tube.

The typical tobacco user smoked eight to nine cigarettes a day, while the marijuana users in the study smoked about two to three times over the past 30 days. "That's really different from ['pothead' film icons] Cheech and Chong," he said. "Americans who smoke marijuana typically don't smoke it every day."

Respiratory risks did seem to rise with the intensity of marijuana use, however. The study authors found increasing evidence of lung trouble among people who smoked marijuana more heavily (20 or more times a month).

The study findings appeared in the *Journal of the American Medical Association*.

Dr. Kertesz said that research has consistently shown that "with tobacco smokers, the more use of tobacco that's accumulated, the more airflow and lung volume is lost over time." But that wasn't the case with mild to moderate users of marijuana, he and his colleagues found.

EXPERTS WEIGH IN

Robert Hancox, MD, associate professor, department of preventive and social medicine, University of Otago, New Zealand, praised the research. But he also believes that pot smoking has negative respiratory effects.

"Smoking marijuana definitely harms the lungs," said Dr. Hancox. "Several studies have clearly shown that even light marijuana smokers can develop severe bronchitis with symptoms of cough and phlegm production. Studies have also demonstrated that smoking marijuana leads to abnormal lung function, but using different tests than those used by this study. What this study shows is that the pattern of lung damage seen with marijuana is not the same as caused by tobacco."

And one advocate against drug abuse noted that the study has a variety of limitations.

"A significant problem is that cannabis use is often difficult to quantify precisely due to smokers sharing joints, different inhalation techniques and different ways of smoking cannabis, including joints, pipes and bongs," said Calvina Fay, executive director of Drug Free America Foundation. "By comparison, the average amount of tobacco in a commercial cigarette of standard length is 1 gram."

Also, Fay said, "it is important to not forget the numerous other serious consequences of marijuana use," such as cognitive and learning problems, psychosis, addiction, criminal behavior and impaired driving, "none of which were considered in this study."

On the other side of the argument is Paul Armentano, deputy director of the national pro-marijuana group NORML. He said that people can now virtually eliminate the lung-irritating effects of marijuana by using vaporizer devices.

Armentano added that, in his opinion, science has determined alcohol, tobacco and prescription drugs "to be far more dangerous and costlier to society than cannabis," but they are regulated instead of banned.

info For more information on marijuana, visit the Web site of the US National Institutes of Health (US National Library of Medicine) at *http://www.nlm.nih.gov/medlineplus/marijuana. html.*

■ ■ ■ ■

Use Zinc to Stop a Cold

Some studies show that people who take zinc within a day of the first evidence of illness develop milder symptoms and/or feel better more quickly. Try a lozenge or syrup to get the zinc into direct contact with the cold virus in your throat. The upper limit for zinc is 40 milligrams a day for adults, but many studies have used slightly higher amounts, which probably are safe if taken for only a few days.

Side effects: Nausea and bad taste in the mouth.

Carol Haggans, RD, scientific and health communications consultant, Office of Dietary Supplements, National Institutes of Health, Bethesda, Maryland. *www. ods.od.nih.gov*

■ ■ ■ ■

Three Great Herbal Cold Remedies

If you're concerned about the sleepy side effects from over-the-counter cold medicine, try the following herbal formulas…

•**Rosemary clears congestion.** Place one-half cup of crushed leaves in the toe of hosiery, and soak it in a tub of warm water for 20 minutes. Breathe in the aroma.

•**Sage relieves a sore throat.** Make a tea by steeping two teaspoons of crushed leaves in eight ounces of hot water for 20 minutes. Strain, and add one teaspoon of sea salt. Gargle with the liquid for 30 seconds, then spit it out. Repeat as necessary.

•**Thyme unplugs sinuses.** Pour three cups of boiling water over two tablespoons of crushed thyme leaves in a bowl. Cover your head with a towel, and lean over the bowl. (Don't let the steam burn you.) Close your eyes, and breathe in deeply for eight to 10 minutes.

Stephanie Tourles, licensed holistic esthetician, Orland, Maine, and author of *Organic Body Care Recipes: 175 Homemade Herbal Formulas for Glowing Skin & a Vibrant Self* (Storey).

Breathe Easier with Rolfing

Greg Brynelson, RN, a registered nurse and certified Rolfing practitioner based in San Francisco. *www.city rolfer.com*

Rolfing structural integration, a type of hands-on bodywork, is designed to improve posture, alignment, flexibility and movement as well as to ease tension and pain. A side benefit of the therapy is that it becomes easier to breathe—and typically that occurs after the first session.

Rolfing releases areas of restriction in the *myofascial* tissue, the weblike connective tissue that wraps around muscles, organs and bones. (Think of the thin white film you see just beneath the skin of a chicken breast as you prepare it for cooking.) Using fingers, hands and elbows, a certified Rolfing practitioner applies firm, steady pressure—slower, deeper and sometimes more uncomfortable than, say, a Swedish massage—to this tissue to stretch and loosen it.

Typically there are 10 hour-long sessions in a Rolfing series. Ida Rolf, PhD, who developed the Rolfing technique more than five decades ago, believed that, to prepare the body for this type of intense therapy, it is important to open up the ribcage. So at the initial appointment, the practitioner applies pressure to the front of the chest and the spaces between the ribs. When that first session is over, clients often find that they can take fuller, deeper breaths because their lungs literally have more room to expand.

info To find a certified Rolfing practitioner in your area, contact the Rolf Institute of Structural Integration (800-530-8875, *www. rolf.org*).

■ ■ ■ ■

Fight the Flu with a Humidifier

Recent evidence indicates that raising the humidity in your home will cause the flu virus to die and decrease person-to-person transmission. The humidity increase seems to deactivate airborne flu molecules, possibly by changing their size or shape. When using a humidifier, be sure to empty, dry and refill it daily to prevent the buildup of mold and bacteria.

Jeffrey Shaman, PhD, assistant professor, College of Oceanic and Atmospheric Sciences, Oregon State University, Corvallis, and leader of a study of the effects of humidity on flu mortality, published in *PLoS Biology*.

■ ■ ■ ■

Hum for Better Breathing

Humming may reduce risk for sinus infections. More than 37 million Americans suffer the pain, headaches and congestion caused by sinus infections each year.

Recent finding: Humming increases airflow between the sinus and nasal cavities, keeping the sinuses healthy and reducing the likelihood of infection.

Jon O. Lundberg, MD, PhD, professor, department of physiology and pharmacology, Karolinska Institute, Sweden, and coauthor of a study published in *The European Respiratory Journal*.

Blood Pressure & Cholesterol

Salt Shake Up: It May Not Be So Bad

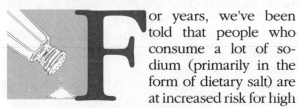

For years, we've been told that people who consume a lot of sodium (primarily in the form of dietary salt) are at increased risk for high blood pressure (hypertension).

Now: The Journal of the American Medical Association recently published a European study that suggests the issue may be more complex than previously believed—a finding that may mean that many of us can safely use more salt.

Recent finding: In an eight-year study, which followed more than 3,600 men and women ages 60 and younger (all of whom had normal blood pressure at the start of the research), researchers found that the one-third of study participants who had the highest sodium intake experienced only a slight rise in systolic (top number) blood pressure and no rise in diastolic (bottom number) blood pressure.

Those in the highest intake group consumed an average of 6,000 mg of salt daily, which is more than twice the daily recommendation for adults in general. Even more surprising, the research found that the one-third of study participants with the lowest salt intake (an average of 2,500 mg daily) were 56% more likely to suffer a heart attack or stroke than the group consuming the most salt.

Lower sodium levels reduce blood pressure but also increase resistance to insulin and sympathetic nervous system activity, including heart rate. If sodium levels fall too much, it can damage the cardiovascular system.

What does this new research mean for people who are concerned about controlling their blood pressure…and avoiding heart attack and stroke?

The results of the European study are controversial—some scientists point out that many of the people with low-sodium intake had

---

Michael Alderman, MD, distinguished emeritus professor of medicine and population health at Albert Einstein College of Medicine in New York City and editor of the *American Journal of Hypertension*.

pre-existing health problems that caused them to curtail their salt intake. The findings also call into question one of the most basic premises of good medicine—that a low-sodium diet helps prevent high blood pressure, which is itself a significant risk factor for heart attack and stroke.

In fact, the CDC urges adults in general to not exceed 2,300 mg of sodium per day (about one teaspoon of salt). If you have hypertension or are among those at increased risk for it—such as adults ages 51 and older and African-Americans of any age—the CDC recommends no more than 1,500 mg per day.

As a physician and researcher who has closely followed the scientific evidence on sodium consumption for the past 35 years, I believe this latest study simply confirms that the salt issue is not as straightforward as it might seem. In fact, there have been mixed results from about 15 major studies conducted over the past several years on the health effects of sodium consumption. Roughly one-third of those studies found no association between salt intake and mortality…one-third found that people who consumed more sodium (6,000 mg to 8,000 mg per day) were more likely to die…and one-third found, like the recent European study, that high salt intake does not increase one's risk for death.

Also recently, a review prepared by The Cochrane Collaboration of existing research involving 6,250 people found that cutting salt intake lowered blood pressure but had no effect on cardiovascular deaths. In fact, lower sodium increased risk for those with congestive heart failure.

It's important to remember that none of this research is definitive—all of the studies are observational, which means that researchers draw inferences about behaviors of people in the general population without creating a controlled environment. This type of research is limited in its ability to reveal a causal relationship between a biological factor—in this case, sodium intake—and a complex condition with many contributing factors, such as heart attack or stroke.

Bottom line: Since there is currently no definitive evidence showing that reducing sodium saves lives or prevents heart attack and stroke

among healthy adults—and a number of studies suggest that sodium restriction actually may be dangerous to at least some people's health—there still are many unanswered questions.

So, what should you do about salt? *Important points to consider…*

1. Sodium intake is not the only factor that contributes to high blood pressure and related ailments. Over the past two decades, the percentage of American adults with high blood pressure has risen from one in four to about one in three—a trend that sodium-reduction advocates blame on our increased sodium intake from processed and fast foods.

Problem with this theory: A recent analysis by Harvard nutritionist Walter Willett, MD, based on 24-hour urine samples (the best way to measure sodium consumption), found that US average sodium intake has remained quite steady over the past 50 years, at around 3,500 mg per day. This suggests that sodium is not the main reason for the higher incidence of hypertension and that other factors, such as rising rates of obesity and diabetes—both of which harm cardiovascular health in other ways—may be more to blame.

2. Sodium has many important functions in the body. Most people are well aware of the research suggesting that reducing sodium intake lowers blood pressure—mainly by decreasing fluid retention, which in turn decreases blood volume.

What is less well-known is that reducing sodium intake increases insulin resistance, triglycerides and sympathetic nervous system activity, all of which are harmful to the cardiovascular system. Reducing sodium also activates the renin angiotensin system, a network of hormones that controls blood pressure and fluid balance in the body. When this system is activated, it triggers the release of substances that cause the blood vessels to constrict and blood volume to increase—both of which promote increased blood pressure. This explains why blood pressure goes up in some people when they cut back on salt.

3. People react to sodium differently. A significant percentage of people (including many with high blood pressure) are "salt-sensitive"—

meaning that their blood pressure reacts more strongly than does the average person's to increases in sodium.

Others, however, are "salt-resistant" and need higher levels of sodium to maintain normal, healthy physiological functions.

At present, we have no good way of determining which individuals are salt-sensitive or salt-resistant, though genetics, age, race and body mass all appear to play a role. People who are salt-sensitive tend to have relatively low levels of potassium in their diets, are over age 55, are obese, have hypertension or a family history of hypertension and/or are African-American.

Research suggests that there is likely a range of healthy sodium intake that we instinctively aim for in our individual diets—and that if your sodium intake is either above or below this range, health problems, such as dehydration, high blood pressure and fluid retention, can occur. The health risks tend to occur when the kidneys are unable to excrete excess salt (for example, in people with kidney disease), so it accumulates in the blood, causing fluid build-up. This range will vary among individuals—it's most likely about 2,000 mg to 4,000 mg a day for individuals who are not salt-sensitive—making it impossible to come up with a "one-size-fits-all" recommendation on sodium intake.

Very important: There's enough evidence to show that a low-sodium diet should be tried as part of any treatment plan for the one-third of Americans with hypertension (blood pressure of 140/90 mmHG and above) and the one-quarter of Americans with prehypertension (systolic pressure of 120 mmHG to 139 mmHG and/or diastolic pressure of 80 mmHG to 89 mmHG).

But right now, there's no good scientific evidence to suggest that people with normal blood pressure who are not at risk for hypertension should reduce sodium intake to a certain predetermined number—this practice may do more harm than good. Ask your doctor what your target sodium levels should be based on your personal medical profile.

Why You Must Get a Blood Pressure Reading In Both Arms

Gregg Fonarow, MD, professor, cardiology, University of California, Los Angeles, and spokesperson, American Heart Association.

William O'Neill, MD, professor, cardiology, and executive dean, clinical affairs, University of Miami Miller School of Medicine.

Christopher Clark, MD, clinical academic fellow, Peninsula College of Medicine and Dentistry, University of Exeter, England.

The Lancet, online

People whose systolic blood pressure—the upper number in their reading—is different in their left and right arms may be suffering from a vascular disease that could increase their risk of death, British researchers report.

The arteries under the collarbone supply blood to the arms, legs and brain. Blockage can lead to stroke and other problems, the researchers noted, and measuring blood pressure in both arms should be routine.

"This is an important [finding] for the general public and for primary care doctors," said William O'Neill, MD, a professor of cardiology and executive dean of clinical affairs at the University of Miami Miller School of Medicine.

The arteries that run under the collarbone can get blocked, especially in smokers and people with diabetes, he noted. "If one artery is more blocked than the other, then there is a difference in blood pressure in the arms," Dr. O'Neill explained.

"Doctors should, for adults—especially adult smokers and patients with diabetes—at some point check the blood pressure in both arms," he said. "If there is a difference it should be looked into further."

The report appeared in an online edition of *The Lancet*.

THE STUDY

A team led by Christopher Clark, MD, from the Peninsula College of Medicine and Dentistry at the University of Exeter in England, reviewed 28 studies that looked at differences in systolic blood pressure between arms.

The analysis found that a difference of 15 millimeters of mercury (mmHg) or more between readings was linked with an increased risk of narrowing or hardening of the arteries supplying the lower limbs, called peripheral vascular disease.

The risk of reduced blood flow to the legs and feet was increased 2.5 times and the risk of decreased blood flow to the brain was increased 1.6 times, the researchers found.

The difference in blood pressure was also associated with a 70% increased risk of dying from cardiovascular disease and a 60% increased risk of death from any cause, the authors added.

The risk of having peripheral vascular disease was also increased with a 10 mmHg difference in blood pressure between arms, the researchers noted.

It makes no difference which arm has the higher or lower pressure, it's the difference between them that matters, the study authors said.

CONCLUSIONS

Finding peripheral vascular disease early and treating it by lowering blood pressure and cholesterol as well as giving up smoking can help reduce the risk of death, Dr. Clark's group said.

"Our findings suggest that a difference in [systolic blood pressure] of 10 mmHg or more between arms could identify patients at high risk of asymptomatic peripheral vascular disease and mortality who might benefit from further assessment," the researchers concluded.

"Findings from our study should be incorporated into future guidelines for hypertension [high blood pressure] and blood pressure measurement," they added.

Another expert agreed that when it comes to blood pressure monitoring, both arms matter.

"These findings further reinforce blood pressure measurement guidelines of the American Heart Association, World Health Organization, International Society of Hypertension and European Society of Hypertension, which recommend that blood pressure should be measured in both arms at initial assessment," said Gregg Fonarow, MD, a professor of cardiology at the University of California, Los Angeles, and spokesperson for the American Heart Association.

According to Dr. Fonarow, individuals found to have differences in systolic blood pressure in between arms of greater than 10 or 15 mmHg should see their doctor for further tests.

info For more information on high blood pressure, visit the American Heart Association's Web site, *www.heart.org*, and search "Every step counts."

Lower Your Blood Pressure While You Sleep

Mark Houston, MD, associate clinical professor of medicine at Vanderbilt University School of Medicine and director of the Hypertension Institute at Saint Thomas Hospital, both in Nashville.

The supplemental form of melatonin (the "sleep" hormone) may alleviate nocturnal hypertension (a form of high blood pressure that occurs during sleep). In most people, blood pressure drops by 10% to 20% during sleep. But about one-quarter of people with prehypertension or hypertension are "non-dippers"—their sleeping pressure is about as high as or higher than their waking pressure.

High blood pressure during sleep (which is diagnosed by a 24-hour blood pressure monitor) is particularly common among blacks and people with chronic kidney disease, and it worsens their risk for heart attack, stroke and kidney failure. Researchers at Boston's Brigham and Women's Hospital have found that 2.5 mg of melatonin, taken one hour before bedtime, may lower systolic (top number) pressure by an average of 6 mmHg and diastolic (bottom number) pressure by 4 mmHg during sleep.

My advice: If you know that you have nocturnal hypertension, or if you have hypertension plus insomnia or chronic kidney disease, ask your doctor about taking melatonin. At the very least, it may help you sleep better.

■ ■ ■ ■

Tea That Lowers Blood Pressure

Among 95 tea drinkers (average age 56.5), those who drank three cups of black tea daily for six months saw their systolic (top number) and diastolic (bottom number) blood pressure readings drop by three and two points, respectively. Even such small drops in blood pressure translate into a 7% to 10% drop in risk for cardiovascular disease.

Theory: Flavonoids in black tea may improve the functioning of endothelial cells that line the blood vessels.

Jonathan Hodgson, PhD, research professor, The University of Western Australia, Perth.

■ ■ ■ ■

Pop a Purple Potato to Lower Blood Pressure

In a recent study, 18 overweight people with high blood pressure ate about seven golf ball–sized purple potatoes twice daily for a month. The potatoes with skins were cooked in a microwave.

Result: The study participants' diastolic (bottom number) blood pressure readings dropped 4%, on average, and their systolic (top number) readings were 3.5% lower. None of the participants gained weight. Purple potatoes are available at specialty-food stores and some supermarkets.

Joe Vinson, PhD, professor of chemistry, The University of Scranton, Pennsylvania.

■ ■ ■ ■

A Delicious Way to Reduce Blood Pressure by 10%

In one of the first population-based studies to look at the effect of flavonoids on high blood pressure, researchers from the University of East Anglia in England found that blueberries' powerful antioxidant flavonoid anthocyanin can help keep pressure down. Eat one-half cup of blueberries (fresh or frozen) five times weekly.

A. Cassidy, et al., "Habitual Intake of Flavonoid Subclasses and Incident Hypertension in Adults," *American Journal of Clinical Nutrition* (2011).

Could Soy Help Lower Your Blood Pressure?

Suzanne Steinbaum, DO, director of Women and Heart Disease, Heart and Vascular Institute, Lenox Hill Hospital, New York City.
American College of Cardiology, news release

Isoflavones—a compound found in foods such as soy milk, green tea, tofu and peanuts—may help lower blood pressure in young adults, recent research suggests.

The researchers also found that isoflavones may be of particular benefit for black American adults, nearly 42% of whom are estimated to have high blood pressure, also known as hypertension.

Isoflavones "dilate the vessels by increasing the release of nitric oxide," explained Suzanne Steinbaum, DO, director of women and heart disease at Lenox Hill Hospital in New York City. She said the study "brings to light a compelling dietary recommendation that can help control hypertension in younger patients."

STUDY FINDINGS

In the recent study, investigators examined data from more than 5,000 participants in a major study funded by the US National Institutes of Health.

The analysis revealed that those who consumed the highest amounts of isoflavones per day (more than 2.5 milligrams [mg]) had an average 5.5 mmHg lower systolic pressure (the top number in a blood pressure reading) than those who consumed less than 0.33 mg of isoflavones per day.

To understand what that means to the everyday diet, an eight-ounce glass of soy milk has about 22 mg of isoflavones and 100 grams of roasted soybeans have as much as 130 mg of isoflavones, the researchers explained.

IMPLICATIONS

"What's unique about this study is that the results are very applicable to the general population. Our results strongly suggest a blood pressure benefit for moderate amounts of dietary isoflavone intake in young black and white adults," said lead investigator Safiya Richardson, a graduating medical student at Columbia University's College of Physicians and Surgeons in New York City.

"Our study is the first to show a benefit in African-Americans, who have a higher incidence of high blood pressure, with an earlier onset and more severe end-organ damage," she added.

The findings "could mean that consuming soy protein, for example, in combination with a DASH diet—one that is high in fruits and vegetables, low-fat dairy and whole grains—could lead to as much as a 10 mmHg drop in systolic blood pressure for pre-hypertensives [people on the threshold of high blood pressure], greatly improving their chances of not progressing to hypertension," Richardson said.

"Any dietary or lifestyle modification people can easily make that doesn't require a daily medication is exciting, especially considering recent figures estimating that only about one-third of American hypertensives have their blood pressure under control," she added.

info To learn more about preventing and treating high blood pressure, visit the American Heart Association Web site, *www.heart.org,* and search "prevention and treatment of high blood pressure."

■ ■ ■ ■

Diuretics May Boost Gout Risk

Researchers analyzed data on 5,789 patients (average age 55) who had high blood pressure, but not gout, at the beginning of a nine-year study.

Finding: Patients who took diuretics to control their blood pressure were twice as likely to develop gout during the study.

Theory: Diuretics increase uric acid levels, which can trigger gout.

Self-defense: If your doctor suggests a thiazide or loop diuretic, such as Lozol, Hydro-DIURIL or Demadex, ask about gout risk. Other blood pressure drugs may be more appropriate.

Mara McAdams DeMarco, PhD, instructor, Johns Hopkins University, Baltimore.

More Than 80% of Blood Pressure Readings Are Wrong

Steven Burgess, MD, chief resident in family medicine at Texas Tech University Health Sciences Center, School of Medicine, Amarillo.

Here's a disturbing bit of news. A recent study reports that 81% of blood pressure measurements taken by doctors and nurses are done improperly, resulting in numerous misdiagnoses. This means that many people are taking medications that they really don't need!

The American Heart Association has published guidelines recommending a particular methodology to follow when taking blood pressure measurements in a clinical setting, such as a doctor's office. In an earlier study, researchers evaluated pressure-taking techniques of 172 doctors and nurses and reported that none were following guidelines set by the American Heart Association—this inspired Steven Burgess, MD, chief resident in family medicine at Texas Tech University Health Sciences Center, School of Medicine in Amarillo, to undertake a study to evaluate how these potentially erroneous measurements impact patient care.

What he learned is disconcerting. He said that the mistakes made when taking blood pressure readings were significant enough to change treatment recommendations for more than half the patients in the study! "My study showed that if someone initially has elevated blood pressure and we redo the reading in accordance with the guidelines, over 50% of the time the new 'correct' pressure puts the patient into a different category, which would cause treatment to be different," he said, noting that the pressure is virtually always lower when taken "correctly."

MISTAKES ARE MADE

The most common blood pressure measurement mistake being made by health-care practitioners is to take a blood pressure reading immediately after a patient sits down. The guidelines say that patients should rest quietly for five minutes first. Why? Because physical activity raises blood pressure, often by 10 mmHg or more.

In his 18-month study of 56 patients, Dr. Burgess found that when blood pressure is measured properly, the average patient's systolic (top number) reading is 15.7 mmHg lower than when the guidelines aren't being followed. For more than half (56.4%) of the patients, using the correct technique—compared with doing it the wrong way—meant that patients were fine without medication or changes to their current therapy.

MEASURE BY MEASURE

Here are the American Heart Association's guidelines regarding the proper technique for measuring blood pressure…

•**Patients should not exercise, drink caffeine or smoke for 30 minutes** prior to measurement and should sit quietly for five minutes immediately before.

•**While the measurement is being taken, the patient should be comfortably seated with his/her back supported** (not perched on a stool or a table) and with feet flat on the floor. The patient's bare arm (the sleeve can be rolled up or, if it is too constricting, the shirt can be removed) should be supported at the level of his heart. In other words, the patient should lean his arm on an armrest or table or the doctor or nurse taking the reading should hold the patient's arm, not let it hang at the patient's side.

•**The cuff must fit properly according to specific guidelines.** For most people, a standard cuff will satisfy these guidelines, but large or obese patients or those who are unusually small require special-sized equipment.

For professional equipment (what's used by a health-care professional), the cuff should be placed one inch above the elbow. For digital monitors designed to be used at home, the cuff should be centered over the inside of the elbow.

•**No talking—by either the patient or the practitioner.** Speaking not only raises blood pressure, it also interferes with the practitioner's ability to focus on your pulse while taking a reading.

•**At an initial visit, two readings should be taken and the results should be averaged.** If the readings differ by more than 5 mmHg, a third reading should be taken and averaged with the other two. (*Note*: At subsequent visits, a single reading may be sufficient.)

HOMEWORK

Lots of people now monitor their blood pressure at home—so it's important that everyone recognizes that these readings must be done in the proper way. Be sure you are using the right type of equipment and following instructions. Also check to see whether your equipment gives you readings that match those taken in your doctor's office.

Better Blood Pressure Readings—Ask Your Doctor About This Device Now

George Bakris, MD, director of the Hypertension Center, The University of Chicago Medical Center.

You may have heard of the phenomenon "white-coat hypertension," which describes people who only experience high blood pressure in the doctor's office. The issue has drawn so much attention that Britain's National Institute for Health and Clinical Excellence started recommending that all patients suspected of having hypertension in the doctor's office (a reading of 140/90 mmHg or higher) should wear a device called an ambulatory blood pressure monitor (ABPM) for 24 hours to see if the high blood pressure diagnosis is the real thing.

The question is why aren't doctors in the US already routinely using this device?

READINGS AROUND THE CLOCK

Hypertension specialist and ABPM expert George Bakris, MD, director of the Hypertension Center at The University of Chicago Medical Center, said that the monitor provides doctors with invaluable health information. "Blood pressure is variable throughout the day in all of us," he said, "and it is the extent of the variability that causes hypertension and helps predict risk for stroke and other cardiovascular problems. We can't know what that variability is without information from a 24-hour monitor." *The ABPM also can reveal the following...*

•**Masked hypertension.** Doctors have identified this problem, which is essentially the opposite of white-coat hypertension, in just the last decade. Let's say that there's a person who doesn't have a stressful life, but he happens to have a stressful job, which causes his blood pressure to soar to dangerous levels in the middle of the day. Readings at a doctor's office may not reveal this, so this condition is called "masked hypertension," and it's potentially fatal. So doctors may soon require certain patients with normal readings in the doctor's office to use the ABPM.

•**Hyper-dipping.** At night, blood pressure normally settles into lower numbers, but some people are "hyper-dippers." That means that their blood pressure sinks far below normal and puts them at risk for stroke and other cardiac events—possibly because their blood flow isn't strong enough to get through the vessels that feed the heart if they are blocked, Dr. Bakris said.

•**Non-dipping.** Then again, some people are "non-dippers," meaning that their blood pressure fails to fall at night. This also increases the risk for stroke or other cardiac events. A non-dipper might be able to avoid this danger with judicious use of medication taken at bedtime.

HOW IT WORKS

The ABPM is made up of two elements—a waist device with tubes leading up to an upper-arm cuff that can be programmed to automatically inflate every 15 to 30 minutes during the day and once an hour at night. This pattern of inflation may be annoying for light sleepers, but doctors need at least six nocturnal readings to get an accurate picture and, as Dr. Bakris noted,

one night's discomfort is a small price to pay for (potentially) a lifetime of better health.

WHAT DOES THE FUTURE HOLD?

Right now in the US, these ABPM devices are used only by hypertension specialists—doctors who are specially trained to interpret the readings accurately. Some private US insurers and Medicare are beginning to recognize the value of the ABPM and cover at least some of the cost of the monitoring. But until these devices become cheaper to use and until more general practitioners are trained to use them, it's unlikely that you'll be able to request an ABPM at a doctor's appointment anytime soon.

But, in the long run, the monitor would likely save the health-care system money by curtailing unnecessary and risky treatment for people who don't need it and preventing stroke and other cardiac events in people whose blood pressure is silently but surely putting them at risk.

■ ■ ■ ■

Keep Still

For an accurate blood pressure reading, empty your bladder because a full bladder can affect the reading. Avoid smoking, drinking anything caffeinated and exercising 30 minutes before the test. Keep your feet flat on the floor for five minutes prior to checking your blood pressure. During the reading, keep still and rest your arm on a table so that it is at heart level.

Consumer Reports on Health, www.consumerreports. org/health

Midlife Blood Pressure Control Can Lower Lifetime Heart Risk

Robert Graham, MD, internist, Lenox Hill Hospital, New York City.

Norrina Allen, PhD, assistant professor in the department of preventive medicine at the Northwestern University Feinberg School of Medicine, Chicago.

Circulation, news release

Blood pressure changes in middle age can affect your lifetime risk for heart disease and stroke, a recent study suggests.

"This study adds to our existing knowledge that hypertension is the most important modifiable risk factor for cardiovascular disease, including coronary heart disease and stroke," said Robert Graham, MD, an internist at Lenox Hill Hospital in New York City.

"Unfortunately, many patients do not take this 'silent disease' seriously because they usually don't see or feel the effects of their hypertension until some catastrophic outcome has occurred," he added.

STUDY DETAILS

US researchers analyzed data from almost 62,000 people whose blood pressure readings were tracked for an average of 14 years.

People who kept or lowered their blood pressure to normal levels by age 55 had the lowest lifetime risk (22% to 41%) for heart disease. The risk for people who had high blood pressure at age 55, however, was 42% to 69%.

When all blood pressure levels were factored in, the overall lifetime heart disease risk for people over the age of 55 was about 53% for men and about 40% for women.

Among the other findings...

•**Women generally had higher increases in middle age than men,** and women who have high blood pressure by early middle age (average age 41) have a higher lifetime risk for heart disease (49%) than those who have maintained normal blood pressure up to age 55.

•**At an average age of 55, 26% of men had normal blood pressure,** as did 41% of women, while about 49% of men and 48% of women had prehypertension.

•**Nearly 70% of men who develop high blood pressure in middle age** will experience a cardiovascular event such as a stroke or heart attack by age 85, the team found.

The study appeared in the journal *Circulation*.

MIDDLE-AGE BLOOD PRESSURE DETERMINES RISK AND CARE

"Taking blood pressure changes into account can provide more accurate estimates for lifetime risk of cardiovascular disease, and it can help us predict individualized risk, and thus, individualized prevention strategies," explained study author Norrina Allen, PhD, assistant professor in the department of preventive medicine at the Northwestern University Feinberg School of Medicine, in Chicago.

"Both avoiding hypertension during middle age or delaying the onset of the development of hypertension appear to have a significant impact on an individual's remaining lifetime risk for CVD," Dr. Allen noted.

Dr. Graham agreed. He said that hypertension in middle age "can affect one's lifetime risk for heart disease and stroke. Fortunately, with medications and lifestyle changes, patients who control their blood pressure during middle age had the lowest lifetime risk of cardiovascular disease, while those with an increase in blood pressure had the highest risk."

info The US National Heart, Lung, and Blood Institute offers a guide to lowering high blood pressure at its Web site *http://www.nhl bi.nih.gov/hbp/*.

Why Low Cholesterol May Not Be Good for You

Mark A. Stengler, NMD, naturopathic medical doctor in private practice, Encinitas, California...adjunct associate clinical professor at the National College of Natural Medicine, Portland, Oregon...author of *The Natural Physicians Healing Therapies* and coauthor of *Prescription for Natural Cures* (both from Bottom Line Books).

When it comes to cholesterol, the message that most of us have been hearing for years is—"lower your cholesterol, lower your cholesterol." But what happens when cholesterol gets very low? You would think that would be good news—and good for your health. In fact, the opposite is true.

What most people don't know: Reducing cholesterol levels too much carries its own health risk. *Here's why...*

WHAT TOO LOW CAN DO

It is important to remember that some cholesterol is needed by the body—and that cholesterol, including LDL (so-called "bad") cholesterol—plays an important role in our health.

Reducing cholesterol too much can impair the body's immune system response and increase susceptibility to infection and even cancer. This is especially worrisome because target cholesterol levels have been progressively lowered in recent years.

Today, many doctors are encouraging their patients to drive their levels of both total cholesterol and LDL cholesterol lower than ever. People at very high risk for heart disease, including those with diabetes, are being told to lower their total cholesterol to 160 mg/dL or less and their LDL to 70 mg/dL or less. People at lower risk are being told to reduce their LDL to less than 100 mg/dL.

I think it's unwise to bring cholesterol levels down that far. Based on the research I've seen and my own clinical experience, I believe that reducing LDL cholesterol to below 100 mg/dL or total cholesterol to below 160 mg/dL poses a risk to many people. This is especially true for seniors who generally are more susceptible to infection.

WHY YOU NEED
SOME CHOLESTEROL

Cholesterol in general (including both LDL and HDL) actually is one of the most important substances in the body. It's found in every cell membrane and is used by the body to manufacture brain cells and to metabolize vitamin D, sex hormones (including testosterone and estrogen), stress hormones and bile acids used for digestion. It's involved in conducting nerve impulses and in the healing process, including the repair of damage to the lining of blood vessels.

Even LDL cholesterol plays an important role. It fights infection, binding to and neutralizing various bacteria such as *Staphylococcus aureus.* It also transports essential fatty acids and fat-soluble vitamins, including A, D, E, K and co-enzyme Q10, throughout the body to fuel the cells of the immune system.

In one study published in *Annals of Clinical and Laboratory Science,* researchers examined the medical histories of more than 200 patients and found that those with LDL cholesterol levels of 70 mg/dL or lower had significantly increased risk for fever, sepsis (severe infection) and hematologic (blood) cancer. Studies have shown

that people whose LDL cholesterol is lower than 70 mg/dL are at increased risk for severe pneumonia and influenza and urinary tract, viral and skin infections. They also are at higher risk for death from respiratory and gastrointestinal infections. There is substantial data linking significantly reduced total cholesterol levels and LDL levels to increased risk for cancer and higher rates of depression, anxiety, suicide and poor memory—possibly because LDL cholesterol specifically enhances activity of serotonin, the brain neurotransmitter found to play a central role in preventing depression.

GET IN THE RANGE

If you have no known heart disease and are taking statins or other cholesterol-lowering drugs simply to bring down your cholesterol values preventively, there's a real concern that you may be putting your health in danger. Other people who may be in danger are those who eat a very low-fat vegan diet.

In my view, an LDL level in the range of 105 mg/dL to 130 mg/dL and total cholesterol between 160 mg/dL and 200 mg/dL are best for most people.

And research now shows that it's the size of your cholesterol particles that is the key to your cardiovascular health, not how much total cholesterol you have.

If your total cholesterol and/or LDL are too low, you should talk to your doctor about stopping your statin drug (if you take one). You also can eat healthful foods with saturated fat, such as grass-fed meat, eggs, coconut oil and butter. Be sure to have your cholesterol levels monitored while you do this to ensure that you reach optimal levels without going too high.

If your total cholesterol is above 200 mg/dL, you may want to consider having your LDL particle size tested and, if necessary, working to reduce the size of your LDL particles with natural therapies. I recommend that all my patients have their LDL particle size tested, regardless of their total cholesterol values.

THE REAL CULPRIT: INFLAMMATION

If high cholesterol is not to blame for heart disease, then what is? Studies have shown that fully half of all heart attacks occur in people whose cholesterol is within "normal" range, which further calls into question the role cholesterol plays in heart disease. Why is this? As much research now shows, other factors play a role—most notably, inflammation-related damage to the artery walls, which can have a number of underlying causes that have nothing to do with cholesterol. The danger from inflammation is why C-reactive protein (CRP), a sign that inflammation is present, is now (or should be) routinely measured as part of your annual physical exam.

New Treatment Lowers Tough-to-Treat Cholesterol As Much as 72%

Gregg C. Fonarow, MD, director, Ahmanson-UCLA Cardiomyopathy Center, codirector, UCLA Preventative Cardiology Program.
James McKenney, PharmD, chief executive officer, National Clinical Research Inc.
Brian A. Ference, MD, director, cardiovascular genomic research center, Wayne State University School of Medicine, Detroit.
Journal of the American College of Cardiology, online

Researchers report that injections of a novel "monoclonal antibody" lowered LDL cholesterol levels in patients with high cholesterol by as much as 72%.

This treatment could help lower levels of "bad" cholesterol for the one in five people who don't respond to the commonly prescribed cholesterol-lowering drugs known as statins. It may also be helpful for patients who can't get their cholesterol low enough with statins alone, the researchers added.

"If this pans out, it will be a whole new approach to lowering cholesterol," said James McKenney, PharmD, chief executive officer of National Clinical Research Inc. A report on the findings was published in the *Journal of the American College of Cardiology.*

The experimental compound appeared to lower LDL cholesterol by making it easier for the liver to remove LDL cholesterol from the bloodstream, McKenney said. Monoclonal antibodies are antibodies cloned from a single cell,

which are all identical because they are cloned, the researchers explained.

The study was funded by the drug's manufacturers Sanofi US and Regeneron Pharmaceuticals. The research company that McKenney works for has also received funding from both drugmakers.

STUDY DETAILS

For this phase 2 study, McKenney's team randomly assigned 183 patients with high cholesterol who had been treated with *atorvastatin* (Lipitor) for more than six weeks, to one of six groups.

Three groups were given injections of the new drug in high, medium or low doses every two weeks. Two other groups were given very high doses of the drug every four weeks. The sixth group received a placebo.

After 12 weeks, the researchers found those who received the low dose of the monoclonal antibody saw their LDL levels drop by 40%. For those given the medium dose, LDL levels decreased 64% while those given the high dose saw their cholesterol levels drop by 72%.

For those in the two groups taking very high doses every four weeks, the drops in LDL cholesterol were 43% and 48%, the researchers said.

IMPLICATIONS

McKenney noted that more research is needed before this drug is ready for public use. Since it would need to be taken regularly, he sees it as akin to insulin, where the patient injects the drug in measured doses.

In terms of cost, it's far too early to say what a patient would have to spend for this therapy, the researchers said.

Longer trials have been planned. The study authors said they feel confident that the drug is safe and effective, but they need to confirm the results over the long-term.

EXPERT RESPONSE

Gregg Fonarow, MD, director of the Ahmanson-UCLA Cardiomyopathy Center and codirector of the UCLA Preventative Cardiology Program, said that "statin therapy has been remarkably effective in reducing fatal and nonfatal cardiovascular events."

Yet, many patients cannot achieve optimal reduction in LDL cholesterol levels with statins and some patients do not tolerate statins well, he noted.

"This novel therapy is exceptionally promising," Dr. Fonarow said. "Achieving LDL cholesterol reductions of up to 72% on top of statin therapy is very impressive."

"If further studies demonstrate the long-term safety, efficacy and effectiveness of this therapy, this will represent a tremendous advance in preventing and treating cardiovascular disease, which has remained the leading cause of premature death and disability in men and women," Dr. Fonarow added.

Results of another study also due out soon suggest that starting a type of statin therapy early in life might significantly reduce the risk for heart disease. Rather than actually treating patients with statins, the researchers looked at changes in DNA that, in this case, were linked to lower levels of cholesterol.

Since one has these mutations at birth, it's like being blessed with naturally low cholesterol. These mutations stand in for statin therapy, according to lead researcher Brian Ference, MD, director of the cardiovascular genomic research center at Wayne State University School of Medicine in Indiana.

"This research is a way of finding out the effects of lowering cholesterol early without having a lengthy clinical trial," Dr. Ference said.

The researchers looked at genes from participants of several studies, one including more than 350,000 patients, and found nine specific mutations.

For each single measure of reduced lifetime exposure to LDL cholesterol associated with having the mutations, the researchers found a 50% to 60% reduction in heart disease risk.

info For more about cholesterol, visit the US National Library of Medicine Web site at *www.nlm.nih.gov/medlineplus/cholesterol.html.*

■ ■ ■ ■

Drink OJ to Lower Bad Cholesterol

Drinking orange juice made from concentrate lowers cholesterol levels. A recent study of people with both high and normal cholesterol found that those who drank three cups of orange juice from concentrate daily had a significant improvement in HDL "good" cholesterol levels. Those with high cholesterol also had a drop in their LDL "bad" cholesterol levels. Other types of orange juice besides concentrate were not studied.

Thaïs B. César, PhD, associate professor, food and nutrition department, São Paulo State University, Brazil, and leader of the study published in *Nutrition Research.*

■ ■ ■ ■

Eat Dark Meat for a Healthier Heart

Dark meat may lower coronary heart disease (CHD) risk.

Background: Taurine is a nutrient found in the dark meat of chicken and turkey as well as in some fish and shellfish.

Recent study: Researchers took blood samples to measure levels of taurine in 223 women (average age 59) with CHD.

Finding: Women with high cholesterol and high levels of taurine were 60% less likely to develop CHD over a 20-year period than similar women with low taurine levels.

Yu Chen, PhD, MPH, associate professor of epidemiology, New York University School of Medicine, New York City.

Breast Cancer

Are Women Getting Breast Cancer Younger?

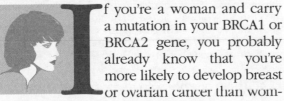

If you're a woman and carry a mutation in your BRCA1 or BRCA2 gene, you probably already know that you're more likely to develop breast or ovarian cancer than women who don't carry such a genetic mutation. But what you probably didn't know is that if you have either one of those mutations and your mom or aunt had breast or ovarian cancer, then there's a good chance that you could be diagnosed with cancer nearly eight years earlier than your mom or aunt was, according to a recent study from the University of Texas MD Anderson Cancer Center in Houston. This research adds to the small but growing body of reports about this trend.

Lead study author Banu K. Arun, MD, associate professor of breast medical oncology and clinical cancer prevention and codirector of the Clinical Cancer Genetics program at the university, and her colleagues analyzed 132 women with breast cancer who tested positive for either a BRCA1 or BRCA2 mutation between 2003 and 2009—these women served as the "younger" generation in the study. Of these women with both breast cancer and a BRCA mutation, 106 had aunts or mothers who had had either breast or ovarian cancer, so their aunts and mothers made up the "older" generation in the study. By analyzing the ages of cancer diagnosis among the families in both generations, Dr. Arun and her team found that the median age of the cancer diagnosis was 7.9 years earlier for women in the younger generation.

WHY THE SHIFT?

Several relatively recent trends may have helped lead to earlier BRCA-related cancer diagnoses in younger women, said Dr. Arun, including…

•**An increase in BRCA mutation awareness,** plus an increase in the availability of

---

Banu K. Arun, MD, professor of breast medical oncology and clinical cancer prevention and codirector of clinical cancer genetics, The University of Texas MD Anderson Cancer Center, Houston.

genetic tests (both of which may have led to an increase in genetic testing).

• **Improvements in imaging techniques** (which has likely led to getting more accurate diagnoses).

• **More environmental influences,** such as taking estrogen replacement hormone therapy or exposure to estrogen-like substances in the environment (which some studies have associated with an increased risk for breast cancer).

Another reason that BRCA-related cancer diagnoses are happening earlier in some women's lives, she said, may have something to do with what epidemiologists call *anticipation*. It's an unfortunate phenomenon in some inherited diseases in which DNA instability causes an illness to strike at a younger age and/or with increased severity in subsequent generations. (This happens with Huntington's disease, for example.)

In other words, these findings are not necessarily dire. They could mean that women are developing the disease at younger ages or that they're simply discovering it sooner—or both. Since all of those reasons listed above probably play a role, said Dr. Arun, the study's findings are likely due to a mixture of factors.

One limitation of the study is that the researchers assumed that the older generation's breast or ovarian cancer was caused by a BRCA1 or BRCA2 mutation—but there was no way to know for sure (because in some cases, the aunts and moms had already passed away and, in other cases, they never took genetic tests). So the younger generation's cancer may have been hereditary or those women may have been the first generation in their families with the mutation.

KNOW YOUR RISK

For women who have a BRCA mutation and are therefore at high risk for both breast and ovarian cancer, the question is: How soon and how frequently should you get screened?

• **How soon to start.** The American Cancer Society (ACS) recommends that high-risk women begin getting screened for both types of cancer at age 30, but they caution that it's a good idea to discuss the best age with your doctor—because if your mom or aunt got either disease at a young age, you may want to start getting screened earlier.

• **How often to go.** The ACS recommends that high-risk women get yearly breast screenings that should include a magnetic resonance imaging (MRI) scan, a mammogram and a clinical breast exam (where a doctor examines your breasts). A pelvic exam done by your doctor during your annual gynecological exam is usually the best way to get screened for ovarian cancer—your doctor might also want to give you a CA-125 blood test, which checks for the level of a certain protein found on the surface of ovarian cancer cells.

In spite of the questions this study raises, it is clear on one point—those at high risk for breast cancer must be aggressive in their screening and do all that they can to reduce environmental and lifestyle risk factors for the disease.

Get Through the Mammogram Maze

Mark A. Stengler, NMD, naturopathic medical doctor in private practice, Encinitas, California...adjunct associate clinical professor at the National College of Natural Medicine, Portland, Oregon...author of *The Natural Physicians Healing Therapies* and coauthor of *Prescription for Natural Cures* (both from Bottom Line Books).

There has been so much controversy lately about mammography for detecting breast cancer—whether to have a mammogram at all and if so, what type to have and when. It is difficult to make sense of recent studies.

RISK VS. BENEFIT

For a long time, the medical establishment believed that regular breast screening with mammography reduced the death rate from breast cancer by almost one-third in women over age 50 and caused them little harm. Then, in 2009, the US government came out with its controversial recommendation that women ages 40 to 49 with no family history of breast cancer and at average risk for the disease should not get routine annual mammogram screenings. Women ages

50 to 74 were advised to get screenings every two to three years…and women over age 74 were told that they do not need routine screening. In late 2011, the Canadian government basically echoed these recommendations.

Reasoning: Research seemed to point to the idea that the risks of testing outweighed the benefits.

One of the risks: Greater lifetime exposure to radiation. Another study, this one from England, published in *British Medical Journal* in 2011, identified a number of other harms associated with mammography, most notably negative effects on quality of life due to false-positive results and unnecessary surgeries, such as biopsies. These researchers determined that having regular mammograms over a 10-year period actually might result in more harm than good. The American Cancer Society (ACS) is one group that does not agree with the government's recommendations. The ACS maintains that all women should have annual mammograms after age 40. And certain studies support the idea of yearly mammograms.

TIMING IS EVERYTHING

While the benefits and frequency of mammography remain under debate, other researchers are taking a closer look at when mammography is performed during a woman's monthly cycle. A study by researchers at Group Health Research Institute in Seattle, reported in *Radiology*, found that in premenopausal women, mammograms appear to be more sensitive at detecting breast cancer when the screening is performed during the first week of the menstrual cycle (when you have your period). Premenopausal women often have dense breast tissue, which can make detection with mammogram difficult, resulting in a high number of false-positive results. With most women, breast tissue is less dense during the first week of the menstrual cycle, so premenopausal women should schedule a mammogram for that time. Since postmenopausal women don't have many hormonal changes, the timing of their mammograms is not as important.

WHICH SCREENING IS BEST

Researchers from the University of North Carolina School of Medicine looked at the diagnostic accuracy of film and digital mammography, which are both a form of X-ray. Film mammography has long been the standard, but it is not as good at detecting cancer in women with dense breasts as digital mammography (an electronic image of the breast stored on a computer), which provides doctors with greater detail. Researchers found that digital mammography was more accurate than film in pre- and perimenopausal women younger than age 50 with dense breasts. There was no difference between the two methods for women ages 50 to 65. For women over age 65 with fatty breasts, film was slightly more accurate because it gave a better view of problem areas.

In a study by Spanish researchers, published in *Radiology*, false-positive results were slightly higher for film mammography (7.6%) compared with digital mammography (5.7%). The researchers found no difference in cancer detection between the two types of mammography. Film mammography exposes women to slightly more radiation than digital mammography

OTHER TESTS

Other types of tests are sometimes recommended instead of, or to complement, mammography. Not all techniques are covered by insurance. *Basic techniques include…*

•**Digital breast tomosynthesis (DBT).** In 2011, the FDA approved a device that performs DBT, a form of 3-D imaging (mammography is 2-D). Studies show that DBT provides 7% better detection than other methods because it enables radiologists to pinpoint the location, size and shape of tumors more accurately than mammography can. The procedure does use more radiation than mammography—up to twice the amount. Currently available in a handful of hospitals around the country, DBT is recommended by some doctors for young women with especially dense breasts.

•**Thermography.** This technique uses infrared technology to assess variations in body heat. Areas of abnormal heat are considered to be areas that may be cancerous. Like many holistic doctors, I recommend that all women use thermography annually to detect any changes in breast tissue. There is no radiation exposure at all.

- **Ultrasound.** This technique, which is commonly used in conjunction with mammography, uses sound waves to make a picture of breast tissue. It emits no radiation.
- **Magnetic resonance imaging (MRI).** This technique provides details of the breast's internal structure. It can help physicians identify abnormalities not picked up by other techniques. There is no radiation exposure at all.

MY ADVICE

In addition to thermography for women with dense breasts, I often recommend ultrasound as a screening test. You can speak to your doctor about the screening test that will provide the clearest view of your breast tissue.

Women of any age who have a family or personal history of breast cancer or other cancer should talk with their doctors about the annual use of thermography, because it can detect early, slight changes in breast tissue. Then, based on your circumstances, you and your doctor can determine if you need a mammogram every one to three years. You and your doctor will also need to discuss the timing and type of mammogram that is best for you.

Experimental Drug Shows Promise for Certain Breast Cancers

Kimberly Blackwell, MD, professor of medicine and an assistant professor of radiation oncology at Duke Cancer Institute in Durham, North Carolina.

Daniel F. Hayes, MD, clinical director, Breast Oncology Program, University of Michigan Comprehensive Cancer Center, Ann Arbor.

American Society of Clinical Oncology, news release

An experimental drug designed to treat patients with a specific kind of breast cancer known as HER2-positive appeared to boost survival compared with a standard treatment, a recent study shows.

The drug, known as *trastuzumab emtansine* (T-DM1), is in the final stage of research necessary before the US Food and Drug Adminis-

tration can approve its sale (as of September 2012).

Patients with HER2-positive breast cancer have a protein called *human epidermal growth factor receptor 2* that promotes cancer cell growth.

The drug T-DM1 is a dual drug made up of the antibody *trastuzumab* (Herceptin) and the cytotoxic drug *emtansine* (DM1).

STUDY DETAILS

In the study, nearly 1,000 patients received either T-DM1 or a regimen of *capecitabine* (Xeloda) and *lapatinib* (Tykerb), a combination referred to as XL. They took the assigned treatment until the disease got worse or side effects became unmanageable.

After two years, 65.4% of those who took T-DM1 were alive, compared with 47.5% of those who took the other treatment.

The median progression-free survival time was 9.6 months for those who got T-DM1, compared with 6.4 months for the others.

The T-DM1 regimen was generally well tolerated by study participants, the researchers said. Those who got the standard treatment were more likely to experience diarrhea, stomach upset and redness, swelling and pain in their palms and the soles of their feet.

MORE EFFECTIVE, LESS TOXIC

Daniel Hayes, MD, clinical director of the breast oncology program at the University of Michigan Comprehensive Cancer Center in Ann Arbor, said the study suggests that T-DM1 will provide us with yet another effective and meaningful agent to use in women with HER2-positive breast cancer.

"The drug worked. It was significantly better than a very effective approved therapy for HER2-overexpressing metastatic breast cancer," said study author Kimberly Blackwell, MD, a professor of medicine and an assistant professor of radiation oncology at Duke Cancer Institute in Durham, North Carolina.

"Also, as a clinician who takes care of a lot of breast cancer patients, I'm pleased that this drug has very little dose-limiting toxicity," she added. "Patients don't lose their hair from this drug. For patients facing metastatic breast cancer, this is a breakthrough."

■ ■ ■ ■

Blood Test That Detects Cancer

Breast cancer may be detected by a blood test that detects prostate cancer in men.

Recent finding: Levels of prostate-specific antigen (PSA) are more than three times higher in women who have breast cancer than in women who do not have the disease.

Chien Chou, PhD, professor, Graduate Institute of Electro-Optical Engineering, Chang Gung University, Taiwan, and leader of a study published in *Analytical Chemistry*.

Reduce Your Breast Cancer Risk by 23%

Lila Nachtigall, MD, professor, obstetrics and gynecology, NYU Langone Medical Center, New York City.

Garnet Anderson, PhD, principal investigator, Women's Health Initiative Clinical Coordinating Center, Fred Hutchinson Cancer Research Center, Seattle.

Stephanie Bernik, MD, chief, surgical oncology, Lenox Hill Hospital, New York City.

The Lancet Oncology, online

Some women who take estrogen-only hormone replacement therapy to stave off hot flashes, night sweats and other symptoms of menopause may be at lower risk for developing breast cancer down the road, a recent study says.

BACKGROUND

Hormone replacement therapy (HRT) fell from grace rather dramatically after a large government-run trial, the US Women's Health Initiative, was stopped early in 2002 because HRT was shown to increase the risk of strokes and breast and ovarian cancer. Since that time, however, some subtleties have emerged as researchers parsed the evidence further. For example, short-term use of HRT is now deemed fairly safe for some women who have severe menopausal symptoms.

RECENT FINDINGS

The study shows that longer-term use of estrogen-only therapy may actually lower a woman's odds of developing breast cancer. Estrogen-only therapy is reserved for women who have had a hysterectomy; women with an intact uterus who use HRT must take the hormone progestin with estrogen to prevent uterine cancer.

"Women who have had a hysterectomy may be reassured that taking estrogen by itself, short term, to relieve menopausal symptoms will not increase their risk of breast cancer," said study author Garnet Anderson, PhD, of the Women's Health Initiative Clinical Coordinating Center at the Fred Hutchinson Cancer Research Center in Seattle. Women should not take estrogen to prevent breast cancer, she stressed.

The findings were published in an online edition of *The Lancet Oncology*.

The North American Menopause Society recently released a position statement that backs up these findings. The group said starting combination hormone therapy (both estrogen and progestin) around the time of menopause to treat symptoms and stave off the brittle-bone disease osteoporosis is safe for some women for three to five years. Estrogen alone can be used for longer than the combination HRT, according to the society.

STUDY DETAILS

The study, which was partially funded by drug manufacturer Wyeth (which is now a part of Pfizer Inc.), included more than 7,500 women from the Women's Health Initiative who took estrogen for about six years. Roughly five years after stopping treatment, the women were 23% less likely to develop breast cancer when compared with their counterparts who never used HRT.

Women in the estrogen group who did develop breast cancer were 63% less likely to die from the disease, compared with women who never took it. The lower risk of breast cancer was seen only among women without risk factors for breast cancer, such as a history of benign breast disease or a strong family history of breast cancer, the study showed.

IMPLICATIONS

"The story is pretty clear about estrogen plus progestin—no matter the age of the women, estrogen plus progestin increases [the risk of] breast cancer, heart disease, stroke and blood clots," Dr. Anderson said. "These risks outweigh the benefits for all age groups."

Why estrogen alone may lower breast cancer risk while adding progestin seems to increase the risk is the million-dollar question.

"There are hypotheses about the role of estrogen in breasts after a woman has gone through menopause," Dr. Anderson said. For example, "her breast tissue, including any precancerous cells, may go through changes as a result of menopause that make them susceptible to estrogen in a way that discourages cell growth."

Estrogen-only therapy is not without risks, however. For estrogen alone, the Women's Health Initiative data showed no overall effect of estrogen on heart disease, but an increased risk of strokes and blood clots.

RECOMMENDATIONS

Women are understandably confused about whether they should take hormones to treat their menopausal symptoms, and for how long they can safely use the therapy.

"The best use of estrogen-alone is in women with a hysterectomy who need relief of hot flashes and night sweats and related menopausal symptoms," Dr. Anderson said. These benefits need to be weighed against a woman's risk of stroke or developing blood clots.

Lila Nachtigall, MD, a professor of obstetrics and gynecology at NYU Langone Medical Center in New York City, agreed that, when used on its own, estrogen can still be safe and effective in treating the symptoms of menopause in women who do not have a uterus.

"It looks very definite that the bad guy is progestin, not estrogen," Dr. Nachtigall said. Her advice is to use the lowest effective dose for the shortest amount of time. If more women took estrogen, she said, there would be a dent made in the epidemic of osteoporosis. "Millions of women who never went on estrogen, even for a few years, are really losing bone," she said.

IMPORTANT

That said, estrogen does increase the risk for blood clots. "Women with blood-clotting disorders should not take it," Dr. Nachtigall said.

Commenting on the study, Stephanie Bernik, MD, chief of surgical oncology at Lenox Hill Hospital in New York City, said, "If you are looking to reduce menopausal symptoms and don't have an intact uterus, [estrogen] is an option." But estrogen-only therapy should not be prescribed indiscriminately, she added.

"This applies only to women who have severe menopausal symptoms. We are not saying that we should give women estrogen to reduce the risk of breast cancer," Dr. Bernik added.

info Learn more about the benefits and risks of hormone therapy at the North American Menopause Society's Web site, *www.menopause.org/HTbenefits_risks.aspx.*

Finally! Help for Hot Flashes After Breast Cancer

Myra Hunter, PhD, professor, clinical health psychology, King's College London, Institute of Psychiatry, London.
Holly G. Prigerson, PhD, director, Center for Psycho-Oncology and Palliative Care Research, Dana-Farber Cancer Institute, Boston.
The Lancet Oncology, online

After breast cancer treatment, many women suffer from hot flashes and night sweats, but a type of "talk therapy" might relieve these symptoms for some women, British researchers suggest.

In a recent study, women who received this form of psychotherapy, known as cognitive behavioral therapy, had reduced their symptoms by half within six months. Cognitive behavioral therapy helps a person become aware of inaccurate or negative thinking, and to change behavior effectively.

ABOUT HOT FLASHES AND NIGHT SWEATS

"Hot flashes and night sweats are distressing symptoms, which cause social embarrassment and sleep problems, and they are challenging to treat, especially for women who have had breast cancer" because hormone replacement therapy is generally not recommended for these women, explained lead researcher Myra Hunter,

PhD, professor of clinical health psychology, King's College London.

According to background information in the study, which is published in *The Lancet Oncology,* 65% to 85% of women have hot flashes after breast cancer treatment.

Group cognitive behavioral therapy is a safe and effective treatment for women who have hot flashes and night sweats following breast cancer treatment, Dr. Hunter said, with additional benefits to mood, sleep and quality of life.

"The women in this trial reported frequent and problematic symptoms and relatively low quality of life," said Dr. Hunter.

STUDY DETAILS

Dr. Hunter's team randomly assigned 96 women who had been treated for breast cancer and suffered from night sweats and hot flashes to either "talk therapy" or usual care.

The 47 women who received the therapy attended weekly 90-minute sessions for six weeks. For the others, usual care consisted of access to nurses and oncologists, telephone support and cancer support services, the researchers noted.

The therapy sessions included psycho-education, paced breathing and behavioral strategies to manage hot flashes and night sweats, as well as interactive PowerPoint presentations, group discussion, handouts and weekly homework, Dr. Hunter said.

In addition, participants learned how to handle the stress associated with hot flashes and night sweats, and found new ways to decrease anxiety, she explained.

The women were also taught to manage hot flashes in social situations and to understand night sweats and improve sleep habits using mental and behavioral strategies.

STUDY RESULTS

The investigators found that the women who had received the cognitive behavioral therapy significantly reduced the number of hot flashes and night sweats they experienced in the nine weeks after the start of the study.

This reduction in symptoms lasted for 26 weeks. At nine weeks there was a 46% reduction in symptoms and a 52% reduction at 26 weeks, Dr. Hunter's team found.

Among women receiving usual care, hot flashes and night sweats decreased by only 19% after nine weeks and 25% after 26 weeks.

"These reductions were sustained and associated with significant improvements in mood, sleep and quality of life," Dr. Hunter said. "This is a safe, acceptable and effective treatment option, which can be incorporated into breast cancer survivorship programs and delivered by trained breast cancer nurses."

EXPERT COMMENTARY

Holly G. Prigerson, PhD, director of the Center for Psycho-Oncology and Palliative Care Research at the Dana-Farber Cancer Institute in Boston, said "Hot flashes and night sweats are very common, distressing and persistent—women reported being troubled by them for an average of two years after breast cancer treatment."

Dr. Prigerson, who wrote an accompanying journal editorial, noted that the study provides sound evidence upon which to recommend cognitive behavioral therapy for breast cancer patients suffering from these symptoms.

Adaptations to an online, self-management version of the treatment the cognitive behavioral group received would allow for more flexible scheduling and greater access at a potentially lower cost, Dr. Prigerson said. Combining this treatment with medications that effectively treat hot flashes and night sweats might produce the most dramatic effects with reductions in symptoms as well as the distress caused by them.

Dr. Prigerson said this type of therapy might also be used to treat postmenopausal women suffering from these symptoms.

"Of course, scientifically, we can't generalize beyond the sample of women who experience menopausal symptoms as a result of treatment for breast cancer," she said. "But given that they found that [this type of therapy] worked on the distress associated with hot flashes and night sweats, then it would seem likely to generalize to menopausal symptoms experienced outside of this context."

 For more about cognitive behavioral therapy, visit the US National Institute of Mental

Health Web site, *www.nimh.nih.gov/health/topics/psychotherapies.*

Amazing Cancer Vaccine Shows Promise

James L. Gulley, MD, PhD, director, clinical trials group and deputy laboratory chief, Laboratory of Tumor Immunology and Biology, US National Cancer Institute, Bethesda, Maryland.

Elizabeth Poynor, MD, gynecologic oncologist and pelvic surgeon, Lenox Hill Hospital, New York City.

David Fishman, MD, professor of obstetrics, gynecology and reproductive science, Mount Sinai Medical Center, New York City.

Clinical Cancer Research

A vaccine that coaxes the body to attack tumor cells has shown promise in a small study of advanced breast and ovarian cancer patients, improving overall survival times and stopping the disease for a handful of breast cancer patients.

The PANVAC vaccine, administered to 26 women through monthly shots, helped the body's immune system recognize proteins produced specifically by cancer cells, said study author James L. Gulley, MD, PhD, director of the clinical trials group and deputy laboratory chief at the Laboratory of Tumor Immunology and Biology at the US National Cancer Institute.

STUDY DETAILS

All of the women had breast or ovarian cancer that had spread to other organs and were considered "heavily pre-treated" with other therapies, with 21 having received at least three chemotherapy regimens. In addition to the four breast cancer patients whose disease stopped progressing, one woman with breast cancer experienced a "complete response," meaning her cancer disappeared.

Among the 12 study participants with breast cancer, the median time before the disease continued to progress was 2.5 months and the median overall survival was 13.7 months. For the 14 patients with ovarian cancer, the median time to progression was two months and the median overall survival was 15 months.

Side effects from the vaccine were exceedingly mild, with minor injection-site reactions the most common problem reported.

The study was published in the journal *Clinical Cancer Research.*

PREVIOUS COLORECTAL CANCER STUDY FINDINGS

The PANVAC vaccine, containing certain genes that encourage the immune system to recognize and destroy tumor cells, was previously studied in 70 patients with advanced colorectal cancer, Dr. Gulley said. While the time before disease progression was similar between patients who did and did not receive the vaccine, the overall survival time in the vaccine group was "strikingly better," he noted.

IMPLICATIONS

"Anytime we have one type of biologic treatment demonstrate some success, it's exciting," said Elizabeth Poynor, MD, a gynecologic oncologist and pelvic surgeon at Lenox Hill Hospital in New York City, who was not involved in the study. "No matter how small the study is—and early studies will be small—when we have positive results on a particular technique, it's a very hopeful thing. These are our most difficult patients to treat; they have failed multiple therapies."

Indeed, most participants—whose average age was 57—had exhausted other forms of treatment, Dr. Gulley said, which likely hampered their immune systems from responding as fully to the vaccine as they otherwise might have. As therapeutic vaccines become more established, Dr. Gulley said they might prove even more effective in patients whose disease is less advanced.

"That's exactly what I'd like to eventually see—the vaccine used earlier in the disease process before other [toxic drugs] that can damage the immune system," he said. "I think it makes more sense, when the immune system is more likely to overcome a lower tumor burden. Until recently we haven't seen a lot of substantial clinical impact of vaccines."

"This is an exciting step forward," said David Fishman, MD, a professor of obstetrics, gynecology and reproductive science at Mount Sinai Medical Center in New York City. "The ultimate goal would be to identify unique proteins in an individual patient's cancer and use vaccines unique to that patient."

Info To learn more about cancer vaccines, visit the Web site of the US National Cancer Institute, *www.cancer.gov/cancertopics* and search "cancer vaccines."

What You Must Know Before Having a Partial Mastectomy

Laurence McCahill, MD, medical director of surgical oncology, The Lacks Cancer Center and professor of surgery, Michigan State University College of Human Medicine, Grand Rapids.
Monica Morrow, MD, chief, breast service, Memorial Sloan-Kettering Cancer Center, New York City.
Journal of the American Medical Association

Nearly one-fourth of women who opt for breast-conserving surgery instead of mastectomy as an initial treatment for breast cancer need a second surgery to ensure all of the cancer cells are removed, a recent study says.

New research has found that nearly 23% of women undergo a second procedure (medically known as re-excision), even though surgeons try to remove a clear "margin"—a thin rim of normal tissue—around the tumor to catch any stray cancer cells.

ABOUT BREAST-CONSERVING SURGERY

Breast-conserving surgery, also called partial mastectomy, is a very common choice for initial breast cancer treatment. Surgeons attempt to leave as much normal breast tissue as possible to preserve the cosmetic appearance of the breast.

The challenge is that it's very difficult for surgeons to see what's normal tissue and what's not once a tumor is removed. After surgery, a pathologist tests cells from the margin. If any are cancerous, this is known as a positive margin. If they're not cancerous, it's a negative margin.

Monica Morrow, MD, chief of the breast service at Memorial Sloan-Kettering Cancer Center in New York City, said, "You can't see where the negative margin begins when you're in surgery.

"What you take out is based on what you feel is abnormal with a margin of normal tissue around it. But, the more tissue you take out, the worse the breast looks," added Dr. Morrow, co-author of an accompanying journal editorial.

STUDY DETAILS

Laurence McCahill, MD, medical director of surgical oncology at The Lacks Cancer Center in Michigan, and his colleagues included data in the study from more than 2,200 women with newly diagnosed invasive breast cancers from four areas across the country. Information about the women, whose average age was 62, came from medical records (both in-hospital and outpatient), and surgical, pathology and radiology reports.

Overall, 22.9% of the women (509) had to have at least one additional surgery on the affected breast.

Re-excision can cause additional psychological, physical and economic stress, according to the study. It can also delay the use of other therapies, such as radiation or chemotherapy.

Most of the women only needed one re-excision, but about 10% needed two or more, the researchers found. For 8.5% of the women, a total mastectomy was eventually needed.

Re-excision rates were 85.9% for initial positive margins; 47.9% for a margin of less than 1.0 millimeter (mm); 20.2% for margins of between 1 mm and 1.9 mm; and 6.3% for 2-to-2.9 mm margins, reported the study.

The researchers noted a wide variation in the re-excision rate based on surgeon and institution, but not based on the number of surgeries a particular surgeon had performed.

Results of the study were published in the *Journal of the American Medical Association*.

IMPLICATIONS

"We shouldn't have the degree of variations that we demonstrated. We need to come up with a more acceptable range," Dr. McCahill said. "I think this should be more standardized. But, the debate about whether or not just getting a negative margin is good enough has been going on for more than two decades."

Dr. Morrow said it would be very difficult to set a standard for what a particular margin in every woman should be, because there are so many variables at play.

And, she said, she doesn't think re-excision rates are a good measure of the quality of surgery you're getting. "Re-excision rates would be way down on my list of the things women need to be concerned about," said Dr. Morrow.

While the authors found wide variations in re-excision rates around the United States, whether too many or too few re-excisions are performed is still unknown.

"We don't yet have the answer as to what serves women best," said Dr. McCahill, the study's lead author. "We do know from other research that positive margins left behind have a high recurrence rate," Dr. McCahill said. "But, we don't necessarily know if re-excision makes a significant difference in outcomes."

info To learn more about breast cancer surgery options, visit the Web site of the American Cancer Society, *www.cancer.org,* and search "surgery for breast cancer."

▪ ▪ ▪ ▪

Better Breast Cancer Treatment

An analysis of 17 randomized trials involving 10,801 women found that those who had breast-conserving surgery plus radiation had a 10-year recurrence rate of 19.3%, compared with 35% in the group that received surgery but no radiation. Risk for death after 15 years was 21.4% in the radiation group and 25.2% in the nonradiation group. This means that one death is prevented for every four recurrences.

Sarah C. Darby, PhD, professor of medical statistics, University of Oxford, UK.

Cadmium in Diet May Increase Breast Cancer Risk

Marisa Weiss, MD, director, breast radiation oncology and breast health outreach, Lankenau Medical Center, Wynnewood, Pennsylvania, and president/founder, Breastcancer.org.
Agneta Akesson, PhD, associate professor, Karolinska Institute, Stockholm, Sweden.
Johanna Lampe, PhD, public health sciences division, Fred Hutchinson Cancer Research Center, Seattle.
Stephanie Bernik, MD, chief, surgical oncology, Lenox Hill Hospital, New York City.
American Association for Cancer Research, news release.
Cancer Research

Consuming the toxic metal cadmium in the foods you eat may raise your risk for breast cancer, a recent Swedish study suggests.

ABOUT CADMIUM

Cadmium, which is found in many farm fertilizers, can make its way into soil and water, the researchers explained. Some of the main sources of cadmium in the diet are bread and other cereals, potatoes, root crops and vegetables. Once it enters the body, cadmium may mimic the effects of the female hormone estrogen, which can fuel the growth of certain breast cancers.

"Modern life has become increasingly dangerous for our breast health," said Marisa Weiss, MD, director of breast radiation oncology and breast health outreach at Lankenau Medical Center in Wynnewood, Pennsylvania. "Now, there's cadmium hanging onto our carrots and whole grains, the very vegetables that are supposed to be good for us," she noted.

"To help our patients reduce their exposure to environmental chemicals (like cadmium), which might increase their risk for breast cancer, we have to partner with our farmers to make sure our foods are grown in healthy soil without chemically loaded fertilizers," said Dr. Weiss, who is also president and founder of Breastcancer.org.

"Sticking to real, whole (unprocessed) foods remains a healthy strategy until we can be more sure of what's inside the package."

THE STUDY

In the Swedish study, the researchers followed nearly 56,000 women for more than 12 years. Women filled out food frequency questionnaires, which the researchers used to estimate how much cadmium they consumed in their diets. There were 2,112 breast cancer diagnoses during the follow-up period, including 1,626 estrogen receptor-positive and 290 estrogen receptor-negative cancers.

Women who had the highest amount of cadmium in their diets were 21% more likely to develop breast cancer than women who had the least amount of cadmium in their diets. This risk increased to 27% among women who were lean or normal-weight, the study showed. The risk was similar, 23%, for both estrogen receptor-positive and -negative tumors.

Those women who consumed higher amounts of whole grain and vegetables had a lower risk of breast cancer compared with women exposed to dietary cadmium through other foods.

"It's possible that this healthy diet to some extent can counteract the negative effect of cadmium, but our findings need to be confirmed with further studies," said study author Agneta Akesson, PhD, an associate professor at Karolinska Institute in Sweden. "It is, however, important that the exposure to cadmium from all food is low."

The findings were published in *Cancer Research*.

EXPERT COMMENTARY

Johanna Lampe, PhD, a member of the public health sciences division at Fred Hutchinson Cancer Research Center in Seattle, said the recent study adds to a growing body of research linking cadmium exposure to breast cancer risk. "It adds another grain of sand to the pile," she said. "We would benefit from more research in this area to understand these risks better."

The ideal study would use a more objective measure of cadmium exposure, such as cadmium levels in urine. "We could look at women years before they develop breast cancer and measure cadmium exposure at certain points in time," she explained.

In terms of lowering exposure to cadmium, Dr. Lampe said that smoking is the most important single source of cadmium exposure.

"Not smoking is a good place to start," she noted.

Stephanie Bernik, MD, chief of surgical oncology at Lenox Hill Hospital in New York City, said that it is too early to recommend making any dietary changes based on these findings. "We can't say we should limit intake of fiber and other things that contain cadmium yet," and some of the foods that contain cadmium are part of a healthy diet, Dr. Bernik stressed.

In the study, thinner women had a higher risk for breast cancer based on their exposure to cadmium. "Obesity overrides any effect that cadmium may have on breast cancer," Dr. Bernik said, adding that obesity is a greater risk factor for breast cancer than cadmium exposure, because "when people are overweight, they have more estrogen circulating in the body."

info To learn more about lowering your breast cancer risk, visit Breastcancer.org and *www. breastcancer.org/risk.*

Pregnancy Safe for Women With Estrogen-Sensitive Breast Cancer

European Breast Cancer Conference, news release

Pregnancy is safe for women with estrogen receptor-positive breast cancer, according to a recent study.

These types of breast tumors are especially sensitive to levels of estrogen in the body, and the findings address concerns that pregnancy could increase circulating estrogen and thereby cause the cancer to return.

This study's results suggest that becoming pregnant at any time after being diagnosed with breast cancer does not increase the risk of recurrence, even if the pregnancy occurs within two years after cancer diagnosis, according to the researchers.

In addition, breast cancer patients who become pregnant appear to survive longer than those who do not, according to Hatem Azim, Jr., MD, a medical oncologist at the Jules Bordet Institute in Brussels, Belgium, and colleagues.

STUDY DETAILS

Their study included 333 breast cancer patients who later became pregnant and 874 breast cancer patients who did not. Over an average of nearly five years of follow-up, breast cancer recurred in 30% of all the women.

Fifty-seven percent of the women in the study had estrogen receptor-positive breast cancer. Becoming pregnant made no difference in the length of time that patients with either estrogen receptor-positive or estrogen receptor-negative breast cancer survived without their cancer recurring. The study was presented at the European Breast Cancer Conference, in Vienna, Austria.

CONCLUSIONS

"We found that patients who became pregnant within two years of breast cancer diagnosis appeared to have a better disease-free survival compared with those who did not become pregnant," said Dr. Azim.

Because of the short length of the study, this finding should be interpreted with caution, Dr. Azim noted. Pregnancy within two years of diagnosis should be regarded as safe, and not as protective, he said.

info The American Cancer Society has more information about pregnancy and breast cancer at *www.cancer.org/cancer/breastcancer/moreinformation/pregnancy-and-breast-cancer*.

▪ ▪ ▪ ▪

Not All Surgical Breast Biopsies Are Needed

Researchers analyzed data on 172,342 breast biopsies of women with and without breast cancer.

Finding: Thirty percent of the biopsies were surgical as opposed to the less invasive needle biopsy, in which a tissue sample is obtained via a needle and syringe. Current guidelines recommend that only 10% of biopsies should involve surgery.

Theory: Doctors who overrely on surgery, which has a greater risk for infection than needle biopsy, might not have the resources to perform needle biopsies.

If you need a breast biopsy: Seek a doctor who is knowledgeable about surgical and needle biopsy.

Stephen Grobmyer, MD, associate professor of surgical oncology, University of Florida, Gainesville.

▪ ▪ ▪ ▪

Surgery Reduces Cancer Risk

For women with the BRCA-1 or BRCA-2 mutations, which increase risk for breast and ovarian cancer, surgery is more effective than rigorous screening.

Recent study: Four years after preventive double mastectomy, none of the high-risk women developed breast cancer...but 7% who had intensive screening without surgery did. Only 1% of women at high risk for ovarian cancer who had at least one ovary and fallopian tube removed developed the disease, versus 6% of women who did not have the surgery.

Claudine Isaacs, MD, medical director of cancer assessment and risk evaluation program, Georgetown Lombardi Comprehensive Cancer Center, Washington, DC, and coauthor of a study of 2,482 women at 22 cancer centers in the US and Europe, published in The Journal of the American Medical Association.

What to Expect with a Breast MRI

Rachel F. Brem, MD, professor of radiology and director of the Breast Imaging and Intervention Center at The George Washington University Medical Center in Washington, DC. She was named by Castle Connolly as one of America's Top Doctors for Cancer.

A breast MRI (magnetic resonance imaging) is a noninvasive test that uses a magnetic field, radio waves and a computer to produce detailed images that can reveal lesions not detectable with mammography or ultrasound.

For the test, a nonradioactive contrast agent (dye) must be injected into the bloodstream. Since cancerous areas have more blood vessels, more dye goes to those areas, making the resulting MRI images clearer.

A breast MRI may be prescribed if you…

•**Are at high risk because of a family history of breast cancer** or because genetic testing revealed that you carry a breast cancer gene.

•**Have a mammogram with inconclusive results that merit clarification.**

•**Are undergoing chemotherapy for breast cancer,** since MRI can reveal whether the disease is responding to treatment.

•**Were recently diagnosed with breast cancer**—because MRI may be useful for presurgical planning. In one recent study from the University of Rome involving 164 breast cancer patients, MRI detected 51 additional suspicious lesions not seen on other tests…and changed the proposed treatment for 20% of patients. In a second study from the same researchers, presurgical MRI was associated with a reduced risk for cancer recurrence. According to radiologist Rachel F. Brem, MD, director of the Breast Imaging and Intervention Center at The George Washington University (GWU) Medical Center, all GWU patients with newly diagnosed breast cancer have an MRI or other imaging test, though this is not the standard at all breast centers.

Risks: The MRI scan itself poses no danger. Possible side effects of the contrast agent include headache, nausea, chest pain, skin rash and irregular heartbeat. Your doctor can help you weigh the test's benefits against these risks.

MRI may not be safe or appropriate if you…

•**Have an implanted device** (pacemaker, cerebral aneurysm clip, cochlear implant, plate, screw or rod) made of any metal other than titanium anywhere in your body. Because MRI uses a powerful magnet, a nontitanium metal device could shift position during the test.

•**Are pregnant or breast-feeding** (the contrast agent could be toxic to the baby).

•**Have kidney problems.** Since patients with kidney disease eliminate the contrast agent from their bodies more slowly, they are at increased risk for side effects, including a serious condition that involves thickening of the skin and organ damage.

Note: Before undergoing a breast MRI, women age 50-plus routinely have a blood test to check for kidney problems.

•**Weigh 300 pounds or more**—you might have trouble fitting comfortably inside the MRI apparatus.

WHERE AND WHEN TO SCHEDULE YOUR MRI

Ask your doctor to refer you to an imaging facility that handles a large volume of breast MRIs, so the staff will have extensive experience with the test. GWU, for instance, does four to six breast MRIs daily, Dr. Brem said.

If you are having an MRI for screening purposes only and you are postmenopausal, simply schedule your MRI at your convenience. If you are premenopausal, the ideal time to have your MRI is between day seven and day 14 of your menstrual cycle (with day one being the first day of your period). Because this is when breasts are least affected by your natural hormones, the MRI results will be easiest to interpret. If you have an irregular cycle, just wait until you get your period and then schedule your MRI for day seven to 14.

Exception: If you have breast cancer or an inconclusive mammogram, do not wait for that day-seven-to-14 window—schedule your MRI immediately, Dr. Brem advised.

WHAT HAPPENS ON THE DAY OF THE TEST

You remove any metal you are wearing (jewelry, hairpins, eyeglasses), and an intravenous (IV) line is placed in your arm to deliver the contrast agent. You lie face-down on a padded table, face nestled into a donut-shaped pillow and breasts hanging freely into cushioned openings containing a signal receiver. Make sure you're really comfortable because you must remain motionless once the test begins. Then you are slid into the MRI tube, which encircles your entire body.

Do you get claustrophobic? Tell your physician ahead of time so he or she can prescribe a calming medication if necessary. To relax inside the tube, focus on your breathing (but don't take deep belly breaths, since staying still is paramount) or imagine yourself in a pleasant place (a mountaintop, a beach). Many imaging centers provide headphones so patients can listen to music, which camouflages the MRI machine's knocking and buzzing noises. The technician can see you and speak to you, and if you need to get out, you can signal the technician by squeezing a handheld device. (Test the signaling device before entering the MRI to make sure it works.)

After some initial images are taken, the dye is injected into your bloodstream via the IV. You may feel a spreading sensation of warmth and/or notice a metallic taste in your mouth. Expect to be in the tube for about 30 minutes as the MRI produces more than 3,000 images, each showing a thin slice of your breasts.

With so many images to interpret, it may take a few days to get your results. At that point, you and your doctor can discuss the appropriate next steps to take to safeguard your health.

■ ■ ■ ■

Hot Flashes? Night Sweats? It Could Be Good!

According to a recent study, women who experience intense hot flashes that wake them up at night and other severe symptoms of menopause, such as night sweats, vaginal dryness, bladder problems and depression, have up to 50% lower risk for breast cancer than women who don't have such symptoms. The protective effect increases with the number and severity of menopausal symptoms.

Possible reason: The symptoms occur as hormone levels fluctuate and drop. Women who have the intense symptoms may have lower levels of estrogen. High levels of estrogen are linked to breast cancer.

Christopher I. Li, MD, PhD, breast cancer epidemiologist, Fred Hutchinson Cancer Research Center, Seattle, and leader of a study published in *Cancer Epidemiology, Biomarkers & Prevention.*

■ ■ ■ ■

Better Breast Cancer Drug

Postmenopausal women with breast cancer do better with the drug *letrozole* (Femara) than *tamoxifen.*

Recent study: Women who had early-stage breast cancer who took letrozole were 21% less likely to die than women who took tamoxifen during the eight-year follow-up period, which included five years of treatment.

Meredith M. Regan, ScD, biostatistician at Dana-Farber Cancer Institute and associate professor of medicine at Harvard Medical School, both in Boston. She is lead author of a study of 8,010 postmenopausal women, published in *The Lancet Oncology.*

Vitamin D Eases Breast Cancer Drug Pain

Antonella Luisa Rastelli, MD, assistant professor of medicine in the section of medical oncology at Washington University School of Medicine in St. Louis, and leader of a study of 60 breast cancer patients.

Drugs called *aromatase inhibitors,* which are used to treat breast cancer, can make muscles and joints so painful and stiff that some women taking the medications say that they feel like they're 100 years old…many users experience bone loss, too. Yet because the medication is effective at halting breast cancer cell growth, shrinking tumors and reducing recurrence risk when taken for several years or more, discontinuing its use prematurely often is inadvisable.

Recent study: Recognizing that many breast cancer patients have low blood levels of vitamin D, Antonella Luisa Rastelli, MD, an assistant professor of medicine in the section of medical oncology at Washington University School of Medicine in St. Louis and her team of researchers tested a simple potential solution to the problem of drug side effects—vitamin D supplements.

STUDY DETAILS

Participants included 60 early-stage breast cancer patients with low vitamin D levels who had painful side effects from the aromatase inhibitor *anastrozole* (Arimidex). All received a standard daily dose of 400 international units (IU) of vitamin D-3 (the type typically found in supplements) and 1,000 mg of calcium. Half of the participants also received 50,000 IU of vitamin D-2 (a form that leaves the body more quickly than D-3) weekly for eight or 16 weeks, then monthly to the end of the six-month study period. The other half, serving as the control group, got a placebo weekly or monthly.

Results: After two months of weekly supplementation, the high-dose vitamin D groups reported significantly less musculoskeletal pain than the control group (though pain relief did not continue when participants switched to the monthly regimen).

Also: After six months, the high-dose vitamin D users showed no reduction in bone density, whereas the control group did have some bone loss.

Excessive vitamin D can have side effects of its own, including high levels of calcium in the urine that may increase the risk for kidney stones. Risks are thought to be lower with vitamin D-2 than with D-3—but even so, Dr. Rastelli cautioned that all patients taking high-dose vitamin D supplements must be monitored closely, as the study participants were.

■ ■ ■ ■

Dense Breasts and Tumors

Denser breasts may increase risk for agressive tumors, according to a recent study. Using mammogram data, researchers measured the breast density of 1,042 breast cancer patients (average age 60), comparing them with 1,794 healthy women.

Result: Women whose breast density exceeded 50% had more than three times higher risk for breast cancer than those with less than 10% density.

Also: Greater breast density was associated with more aggressive tumors. The link between breast density and cancer is not yet fully understood.

Rulla May Tamimi, ScD, assistant professor of medicine, Harvard Medical School, Boston.

Breast Cancer Treatment Side Effects May Last For Years

University of Pennsylvania, news release

Treatment-related complications are common in breast cancer patients long after their therapy has been completed, a recent study says.

There are 2.6 million breast cancer survivors in the United States, the authors noted in the news release.

"We can no longer pretend that the side effects of breast cancer treatment end after patients finish active treatment. The scope of these complications is shocking and upsetting, but a ready solution for many of them already exists in rehabilitative exercise," said study leader Kathryn Schmitz, PhD, MPH, associate professor of biostatistics and epidemiology at the University of Pennsylvania.

STUDY DETAILS

Researchers looked at 287 Australian breast cancer patients and found that more than 60% of them had at least one treatment-related complication up to six years after their diagnosis, and 30% had at least two complications.

Complications included skin reactions to radiation therapy, weight gain, fatigue, surgery-related issues, upper body symptoms and physical limitations, and lymphedema—a painful limb-swelling condition.

The study was published online in a special issue of the journal *Cancer* that focuses on the physical late effects of breast cancer treatment and ways to prevent, monitor and treat these conditions.

A CALL FOR PROPER MONITORING

Many factors can prevent proper monitoring of breast cancer survivors for the types of complications identified in the study, Dr. Schmitz and her colleagues said.

Patients may have fragmented care and receive different types of treatment at different hospitals, both patients and doctors may believe that certain complications are "expected" and "normal" and don't warrant treatment, and many breast cancer patients aren't aware of or referred to physical therapy professionals.

"Our work provides the first accounting of the true magnitude of the post-treatment problems suffered by breast cancer patients, and serves as a call to action for proper monitoring and rehabilitation services to care for them," said Dr. Schmitz, who is a member of the university's Abramson Cancer Center and serves as a senior scientist on a committee overseeing creation of a surveillance model for breast cancer survivors.

info The US National Cancer Institute has more about breast cancer at its Web site *www.cancer.gov/cancertopics/types/breast.*

Is There Breast Cancer In Your Family? Ask Dad!

J. Leonard Lichtenfeld, MD, deputy chief medical officer of the American Cancer Society in Atlanta. *www. cancer.org*

When it comes to physical traits, such as eye color or body type, many women are well aware that these can be inherited from either parent—but not so many realize that a genetic risk for breast or ovarian cancer is as likely to be passed down from your dad's side of the family as from your mom's.

Most inherited genetic predispositions to breast and ovarian cancers are caused by mutations in the BRCA1 and BRCA2 genes, and men are just as likely as women to pass on these mutations to their children. Yet, when researchers at Princess Margaret Hospital in Toronto examined records from their cancer clinic, they found that women were five times more likely to be referred for genetic counseling due to having a maternal history of cancer than they were if the disease occurred in their paternal line.

FATHERS HELPING DAUGHTERS

This has important implications—not only for women worried about their own health but also for fathers who want to be sure that their daughters are doing all that they can to protect themselves. J. Leonard Lichtenfeld, MD, deputy chief medical officer at the national office of the American Cancer Society in Atlanta, stressed the importance of learning as much as possible about both parents' family history. "Many fathers don't realize that they can be carrying genes for breast and ovarian cancer," he said, adding the surprising news that many healthcare providers don't know this either!

Of the 700,000 women worldwide diagnosed with breast cancer each year, 5% to 10% have a genetic predisposition, usually a mutation in one of the BRCA genes. Women with these mutations have a 55% to 87% risk for breast cancer and a 20% to 44% risk for ovarian cancer. In a commentary on the study published online in *The Lancet Oncology,* the researchers pointed out that if doctors don't ask about the medical history on the paternal side, women may not realize that they could be at high risk for breast or ovarian cancer—and that could prevent them from seeking genetic testing.

WHAT YOU CAN DO

Dr. Lichtenfeld urged women to invest some time in learning their family medical history—from both sides of the family tree. Ask questions of your relatives, and follow through to get as much information as you can. Be alert to other cancers connected to breast cancer on your father's side, such as colon and ovarian cancers.

"As you get older and relatives pass away, you'll find that the memory of the diseases they had and the causes of death disappear with them," Dr. Lichtenfeld pointed out. "If you discover a history of breast or ovarian cancer, especially premenopausal, on either side of your family, it's very important to get a consultation with an experienced genetic counselor who will discuss whether a test for the BRCA1 or BRCA2 mutation is appropriate and the implications of the results."

info To learn more about how to explore your family health history, go to the Web site for the Surgeon General's Family Health History Initiative at *www.hhs.gov/familyhistory*. You will be able to create, store and share an electronic record (and keep it confidential) for free. It may be the best thing you've ever done for yourself— and your family.

Mighty Mushrooms Combat Breast Cancer

Cynthia Bye, ND, naturopathic physician specializing in complementary cancer care at Journey to Wellness, her private practice in Vancouver, Washington. *www. cynthiabye.com*

A growing body of research suggests that certain mushrooms are powerful weapons in the fight against breast cancer and other cancers. *For instance, various mushrooms…*

•**Contain chemicals (including conjugated linoleic acid) that act as aromatase inhibitors.** Aromatase is an enzyme in fat tissue that converts testosterone to estrogen. Since estrogen fuels many breast tumors, certain mushrooms combat breast cancer by suppressing aromatase activity.

•**Increase apoptosis,** the natural programmed death of old, worn-out cells. This acts as a check against the cells becoming cancerous (since cancer cells proliferate instead of undergoing apoptosis).

•**Stimulate the immune response through the action of beta glucans,** substances that support the production and/or function of various disease-fighting cells, including white blood cells, T-cells and natural killer cells.

Simply eating more mushrooms may be good for you—but for maximum therapeutic effects, consider mushroom extracts.

Reason: The beta glucans are in the mushrooms' cell walls, which you cannot digest. To get the beta glucans, according to Cynthia Bye, ND, a naturopathic doctor based in Vancouver, Washington, you need mushroom supplements prepared through a process called hot water extraction.

Dr. Bye recommended using mushroom extracts only under the guidance of a naturopathic doctor who is trained in their use, to assure that you receive a formulation specifically tailored to your needs. Mushrooms come in many different varieties—coriolus, crimini, maitake, portobello, reishi, shiitake, white button, etc.—and each has its own distinct health benefits. The extracts best suited to helping a healthy person stay healthy are not the same as those that might be prescribed for a person with compromised immunity…or for a woman at high risk for cancer…or for a woman with a history of breast cancer who wants to reduce the risk for recurrence.

info To find a naturopathic doctor familiar with mushroom extracts, contact the American Association of Naturopathic Physicians (866-538-2267, *www.naturopathic.org*).

Cancer Breakthroughs

The New Anticancer Formula

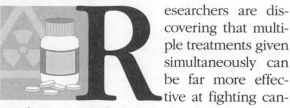 **R**esearchers are discovering that multiple treatments given simultaneously can be far more effective at fighting cancer than any single treatment. That's because a typical cancer involves an average of 63 genetic mutations, each of which works in different ways. A single treatment is unlikely to affect more than a few of these processes.

Better approach: Cancer "cocktails" that simultaneously attack abnormal cells in a multitude of ways.

Examples: A deadly form of blood cancer, multiple myeloma, now is routinely treated with drug combinations that have doubled survival rates. A French study, published in the *New England Journal of Medicine*, found that patients with pancreatic cancer who were given a combination of four drugs lived about 60% longer than those given standard chemotherapy.

For the most part, the conventional treatment strategy for cancer involves using one or two traditional treatments—surgery, radiation, chemotherapy or hormone therapy—one after the other. Only on occasion are different treatments used in combination simultaneously such as when radiation and chemotherapy are administered following a patient's surgery.

Many oncologists now believe that it's better to hit cancers all at once with a barrage of treatments—including, in some cases, unconventional treatments, such as vitamins, herbs, supplements and medications typically prescribed for other health problems.

Example: I might advise a cancer patient getting conventional treatments to include the arthritis drug *celecoxib* (Celebrex), which makes

Raymond Chang, MD, a faculty member at Weill Cornell Medical College, New York City, and a pioneer in the use of complementary and alternative treatments in oncology. He is author of *Beyond the Magic Bullet—The Anti-Cancer Cocktail: A New Approach to Beating Cancer* (Square One).

cancer cells more sensitive to radiation...the hormone melatonin (which decreases the growth of some cancers)...and vitamin D-3 (which may reduce cancer recurrence).

GETTING STARTED

Here's how to make this approach work for you...

•**Keep an open mind.** Ask your doctor if there are safe and effective treatments that he/she recommends that may be unconventional, including "off-label" drugs—medications that haven't been approved by the FDA specifically for your type of cancer. Doctors often know about new treatments that seem to work for a given cancer.

Important: Don't try any treatment without first checking with your doctor to make sure that it is safe for you. If it is, he/she can recommend the right dose and tell you when you should take it.

•**Start with conventional care.** I never advise patients to forgo appropriate standard cancer treatments such as chemotherapy and/or radiation. These approaches have been proven to improve survival. You can then supplement these approaches with off-label medications, herbs and/or supplements to help increase effectiveness.

•**Define your goals.** A cure isn't the only reason to use a medley of treatments. The right cocktail also can reduce treatment side effects and improve your quality of life.

Example: Patients with breast cancer may be given hormonal treatments that reduce tumor growth, but in premenopausal women, these treatments also induce early menopause—and the accompanying hot flashes, night sweats and "brain fog." To be more comfortable during the post-treatment period, you can take vitamin E to reduce hot flashes...ginkgo to improve memory...and herbs such as black cohosh to reduce vaginal dryness and night sweats.

INGREDIENTS TO CONSIDER

Ask your doctor what you can add to your current treatments to increase their effectiveness. Some of the most common medications in the US have been shown to help cancer pa-

tients, as have supplements. *Here, some unconventional treatments that can help...*

•**Vitamin D.** Studies have shown that vitamin D induces *apoptosis*, the death of cancer cells. This is important because one of the characteristics of cancer cells is the ability to avoid cell death. Using vitamin D along with chemotherapy, surgery and/or radiation could improve your outcome.

•**The ulcer medication *cimetidine*** (Tagamet) strengthens the immune system so that it can fight cancer cells. Studies have shown that patients who start taking cimetidine a few days before colon cancer surgery may be less likely to have a recurrence of the cancer.

•**Aspirin.** An analysis of data from the Harvard Nurses' Health Study found that breast cancer patients who took aspirin reduced the risk of the cancer spreading (metastasis) by nearly 50%.

•**Curcumin,** the active compound in the spice turmeric. Like aspirin, it's an anti-inflammatory that can reduce the invasion and spread of cancer cells. It also can inhibit *angiogenesis*, the development of blood vessels that nourish tumors.

•**Green tea.** This is one cancer-cocktail ingredient that everyone can "take." One cup of green tea has approximately 45 milligrams (mg) of *epigallocatechin 3-gallate* (EGCG), a compound that appears to reduce the growth of cancer cells. Dozens of studies have shown that green tea may be effective.

Example: A Mayo Clinic study found that the majority of leukemia patients who took EGCG showed clear improvement. Other studies have shown that it can reduce prostate-specific antigen (PSA), a substance that is elevated in patients with prostate cancer.

I recommend eight cups of green tea a day to fight cancer.

•**Red yeast rice.** This type of yeast, taken in supplement form, contains monacolin K, the same active compound that is used in lovastatin, one of the cholesterol-lowering statins. Red yeast rice is an anti-inflammatory that also affects immune response and cell signaling—actions that can help prevent and possibly treat some cancers.

Laboratory studies indicate that red yeast rice (as well as statins) might increase the effectiveness of radiation and chemotherapy.

As for statins, in studies involving nearly a half-million patients, the drugs have been shown to significantly reduce the incidence and recurrence of colon, breast, lung and prostate cancers.

GO SLOW

Mix the cocktail slowly. It's not good to start many treatments at the same time. You need to know if a particular ingredient is causing side effects.

Example: I might advise a patient to use Chinese herbs for a week. If he/she is doing well, I might add a second ingredient and then a third.

Good News for Lymphoma Sufferers

Craig Reeder, MD, assistant professor of medicine at the Mayo Clinic in Scottsdale, Arizona. Dr. Reeder is a hematologic oncologist who specializes in the treatment of lymphoma. He has published more than 100 articles in journals such as *The New England Journal of Medicine, Blood* and *Journal of Clinical Oncology.*

In 2011, about 75,000 Americans were diagnosed with lymphoma (cancer of the lymph nodes). The majority of these cases are non-Hodgkin's lymphoma (NHL).

WHAT IS LYMPHOMA?

Lymphoma is a cancer that affects *lymphocytes,* the white blood cells of the lymphatic system. Symptoms include a painless lump in the neck, armpit, groin or abdomen, unexplained weight loss, fever and night sweats. Hodgkin's lymphoma, which tends to strike adolescents and young adults, is highly treatable. Non-Hodgkin's lymphoma, on the other hand, can occur at any age and can be more difficult to treat depending on the specific type and how far it has progressed.

What you may not know: High-grade (aggressive) NHL is actually more curable than low-grade (slow-growing) lymphoma—with a 70% cure rate. That's because low-grade lymphoma, which may cause few symptoms, is usually quite advanced when it's diagnosed. While there's no cure for low-grade NHL, patients with these cancers can go into lengthy remissions.

Good news: Increasingly, doctors are finding that the old-standby treatments (radiation, chemo, immunotherapy and stem cell transplantation) can be enhanced with new medications to the point of curing (sending the cancer into permanent remission) a growing percentage of people with aggressive lymphoma, while low-grade lymphoma patients are living considerably longer than they used to.

The most promising newer medications...

NEW DRUG TREATMENTS

•**Monoclonal antibodies.** One of the key advances in lymphoma treatment involves immunotherapy drugs called monoclonal antibodies—injectable medications that attach themselves to a designated protein on the malignant cell's surface, making it easier for the immune system to attack the cell.

•*Rituximab* (Rituxan), one of the first monoclonal antibody drugs, attaches to the CD20 protein found only on B lymphocytes, a type of white blood cell. It is very effective at targeting tumor cells while sparing normal cells. Approved by the FDA in 1997, rituximab is considered the standard of care for B-cell lymphomas. It may be used alone for low-grade lymphomas or in combination with chemotherapy for high-grade forms.

What's new: The use of rituximab is continuing to expand as it is tried with different drug combinations.

Also: A recent study found that using rituximab to treat asymptomatic non-bulky follicular lymphoma, a slow-growing lymphoma that forms in B cells, instead of the traditional "watch and wait" protocol, extended the time before chemotherapy was needed from a median of 2.5 years to a median of four years.

•*Brentuximab vedotin* (Adcetris), another exciting new drug, consists of an antibody linked to an intracellular toxin. The drug, which targets CD30 receptor proteins on the tumor cell, has produced very good results in Phase I and Phase II trials.

What's new: The medication was approved August 2011 for relapsed Hodgkin's lymphoma (lymphoma that went into remission but then recurred), providing an important new therapy for these patients. It is now considered a first-line therapy for Hodgkin's and anaplastic large-cell lymphoma, a rare, aggressive form of lymphoma that affects T-cells.

•**Radioactive monoclonal antibodies.** Radioactively tagged CD20 antibodies are also being used to deliver doses of radiation to tumor cells.

What's new: The FDA has approved two such agents, *tositumomab* conjoined with radioactive iodine (Bexxar) and *rituximab* conjoined with Yttrium-90 (Zevalin), for relapsed low-grade lymphoma and transformed lymphoma (lymphoma that turns from low-grade into high-grade).

These treatments have somewhat better results than rituximab alone but also have more side effects (including low red or white blood cell or platelet counts) than rituximab alone and must be administered by a radiation oncologist.

•**Chemotherapy.** The four-drug chemotherapy known as CHOP (*cyclophosphamide,* Hydroxydoxorubicin, Oncovin and *prednisone*) has long been standard treatment for many types of NHL, including diffuse large B-cell lymphoma. In recent years, this protocol has been expanded to include rituximab (a combination called R-CHOP).

What's new: Phase III trials are under way comparing R-CHOP with a protocol that combines rituximab with a more aggressive chemotherapy treatment called EPOCH—CHOP plus a medication called *etoposide* (Etopophos). This study will tell us if it is more effective than the standard R-CHOP.

Also: *Pralatrexate* (Folotyn) recently received fast-track approval for peripheral T-cell lymphoma, an uncommon NHL that's more difficult to treat than the more common B-cell lymphoma.

DRUGS CURRENTLY BEING TESTED

In addition to the above drugs, all of which have been approved or are near approval, a number of very exciting lymphoma drugs are currently in Phase I and Phase II trials. *For example…*

•***Lenalidomide*** (Revlimid). This oral medication, already approved for multiple myeloma and *myelodysplastic syndrome,* a condition in which bone marrow produces misshapen blood cells, has also shown remarkable effectiveness as a single agent for some forms of relapsed lymphoma—including diffuse large B-cell lymphoma (28% improvement rate)…mantle cell lymphoma, a rare type of B-cell lymphoma (42% improvement rate)…and transformed lymphoma (45% improved response rate).

•***Everolimus*** (Afinitor). This oral medication, part of a class called mTOR inhibitors, which are a novel class of anticancer drugs, shows good effectiveness as a single agent when used to treat relapsed lymphoma.

Clinical trial information: Talk to your doctor to see if one is appropriate for you. Also visit *www.clinicaltrials.gov* and *www.mayo clinic.org* to find trials for a specific condition, eligibility requirements, locations and contact information.

Refined Sugar Raises Cancer Risks

Patrick Quillin, PhD, RD, CNS, clinical nutritionist and CEO of American Eagle Nutrition in Carlsbad, California. He is author of numerous books, including *Beating Cancer with Nutrition* (Nutrition Times).

With all the negative publicity that high-fructose corn syrup (HFCS) has been getting, an increasing number of food and beverage manufacturers are beginning to replace the processed sweetener with old-fashioned white sugar in products ranging from tomato sauce and soft drinks to salad dressing and bread.

But is sugar really more healthful than HFCS? The truth is, it can be harmful as well.

That's because every time a person eats a gooey donut packed with sugar or downs some other refined carbohydrate, such as a fluffy roll packed with bleached white flour, it can wreak havoc with his/her blood sugar (glucose) levels. We all know that elevated glucose levels can result in diabetes, but that's not the only risk.

Latest development: There is growing scientific evidence that consistently high levels of blood sugar may be linked to an increased risk for, and faster progression of, some cancers.

What you need to know: Reducing one's intake of any type of processed sugar and refined carbohydrates could reduce cancer risk and enhance cancer treatments in those battling the disease, according to many experts. Interestingly, the nutrients in fresh and frozen fruit, which are high in natural sugar, have been linked to reduced cancer risk.

KEY RESEARCH FINDINGS

Important studies have linked high blood glucose levels with…

•**Liver, gallbladder and other cancers.** In a study that appeared in the journal *PLoS Medicine*, Swedish investigators tracked blood glucose and rates of cancer and cancer deaths among more than 500,000 men and women for 10 years.

The researchers found that men with the highest blood glucose levels had a significantly higher risk of developing and dying of such cancers as those of the liver, gallbladder and respiratory tract than those with the lowest glucose levels. Women with the highest glucose levels had an increased risk of developing cancers of the pancreas and bladder and dying of cancers of the pancreas, uterus, cervix and stomach. In general, cancer risk increased right along with blood glucose readings for both men and women.

These risks were independent of body weight—an important point, since doctors have traditionally attributed any potential link between cancer and high intakes of dietary sugar and other refined carbohydrates to obesity, a known risk factor for various cancers.

•**Pancreatic cancer.** In a study published in *Cancer Epidemiology, Biomarkers & Prevention* in 2010, researchers followed more than 60,000 men and women in Singapore for 14 years and found that those who consumed two or more sugared sodas per week had almost twice the risk of developing pancreatic cancer as those who didn't.

The mechanisms linking high sugar intake to increased cancer risk are still being studied. But the likeliest reason is that it leads to higher circulating levels of insulin, as well as a related hormone, known as insulin-like growth factor, both of which scientists think may promote the growth of some cancers, including malignancies of the pancreas and colon.

Elevated blood glucose also suppresses the immune system. Perhaps even more important, cancer cells are believed to feed directly on blood glucose, which means that elevated blood glucose ensures a ready supply of "fuel" for cancer growth.

CANCER-FIGHTING ACTION PLAN

Even though the scientific evidence linking cancer to sugar consumption is not yet definitive, I believe that it's prudent for everyone to take steps to regulate blood glucose levels to reduce cancer risk. It's also wise for cancer patients to follow these steps, as an adjunct to their cancer treatment, to help the disease from progressing. *My advice…*

•**Adopt a low-glycemic-index diet.** Glycemic index (GI) indicates how quickly your digestive tract converts a given food into blood glucose. High-GI foods cause blood glucose (and the insulin production that results) to spike sharply, while lower-GI foods produce a more gradual rise. *What to do…*

•Reduce your intake of refined simple carbohydrates, most of which have a high GI. Simple carbohydrates include sugared soda, candy and any other foods containing sugars, such as sucrose, fructose, corn syrup, dextrose and maltose…foods containing refined flour, which includes any type of flour not listed as "whole grain," such as white rice and white bread…processed snack foods… and high-GI vegetables, such as white and red potatoes, corn and turnips.

Important: Do not limit the amount of colorful fruits and vegetables you eat—the fiber in these foods will improve the GI, and their phytochemicals help prevent cancer.

•Eat more low-GI foods, which are typically high in protein and complex carbohydrates that produce a mild, gradual rise in blood glucose levels.

Good choices include: Legumes…nuts and seeds…low-fat proteins, such as fish, chicken and lean beef (some fatty fish, such as salmon, have fatty acids that may help guard against cancer)…cheese…nonsweetened yogurt…eggs…low-GI vegetables, such as artichokes, asparagus, bell peppers, broccoli, Brussels sprouts, cabbage, cauliflower and onions…and low-GI fruits, such as cherries, grapefruit, plums, apricots and oranges. To check the GI of various foods, consult the Glycemic Index and GI Database Web site at *www.GlycemicIndex.com.*

My advice: If you have cancer and receive intravenous nutrition at any point during your treatment, ask your doctor about receiving a low-glucose solution (40% glucose) to help control your glucose levels and replacing the calories with protein (amino acids) and fats (lipids). The typical IV solution is 75% glucose.

•**Take nutritional supplements.** If you have cancer or are concerned about your cancer risk, ask your doctor about taking magnesium and chromium supplements to help stabilize your blood glucose levels. Also discuss the dosages he considers most beneficial for you.

Important: If you have a chronic medical condition or take any prescription medication, be sure to consult your doctor before taking these or any supplements.

•**Get serious about exercise.** Regular exercise lowers blood glucose (because your muscles burn more glucose during activity) and makes your body more responsive to the blood sugar–regulating properties of insulin. Exercising (ideally, strength training plus a cardio routine, such as brisk walking) for 30 minutes three times a week will have maximum benefit, but any amount of exercise is better than none.

ON THE HORIZON

There's also growing interest among scientists as to whether drugs that affect blood glucose mechanisms can be used to treat cancer. *For example…*

Important finding I: A small study in Japan, which was published in *Cancer Prevention Research*, found that when people with precancerous colorectal cells received a low dose of the diabetes drug *metformin* (Glucophage)—which works, in part, by reducing circulating insulin levels—for one month, these cells were significantly reduced, compared with those in a control group.

More extensive trials of metformin's effects on lung, prostate and breast cancers are now being coordinated by the National Cancer Institute.

Important finding II: In a study published in *The Journal of Biological Chemistry* in 2010, researchers reported that by tweaking the structure of the experimental diabetes drug *ciglitazone*, they produced a compound that killed prostate and breast cancer cells in the lab by preventing glucose from entering the cancer cells and by suppressing their ability to metabolize glucose. More research on the drug is under way.

Remember: If you're getting too much sugar in your diet, diabetes may not be the only potential threat to your health.

Targeted Treatments Key To War on Cancer

Michael Link, MD, president, American Society of Clinical Oncology.

Neal Meropol, MD, chief, hematology and oncology, University Hospitals Case Medical Center & Case Western Reserve University, Cleveland.

John Mendelsohn, MD, codirector, Institute for Personalized Cancer Therapy, MD Anderson Cancer Center, Houston.

Report, "Accelerating Progress Against Cancer: ASCO's Blueprint for Transforming Clinical and Translational Cancer Research."

More targeted treatments and efficient clinical trials are needed to speed the progress in finding better cancer treatments, a recent report says.

In a report released 40 years after the start of President Nixon's "War on Cancer," the American Society of Clinical Oncology (ASCO) pinpoints specific areas that need improvement to advance the cause of "personalized" cancer care.

"If we begin to make the needed changes, we believe that cancer research and patient care can become more targeted, more efficient and more effective," said Neal Meropol, MD, one of the three executive editors of the report. "We have a clear opportunity to accelerate the path of progress."

ASSESSMENT OF PROGRESS

Tremendous progress has been made against cancer since President Nixon signed the *National Cancer Act* in December 1971, said ASCO President Michael Link, MD. That includes a record number of cancer survivors, a childhood cancer cure rate of 80% and a drop in death rates for many types of cancer.

Still, said Dr. Link, a pediatric oncologist at Stanford University, "We have a long way to go."

Researchers have learned that certain cancer drugs work very well in one person, but not in another because of differences in the genetic makeup of the tumor, among other factors.

One hopeful scenario outlined in the report: An oncologist tells a patient he has kidney cancer. Instead of determining treatment based on where the tumor is located, the oncologist runs a genetic test on the patient and the molecular characteristics of the tumor to determine how likely the cancer is to spread, and which of the available medications will work best in this specific situation.

THE WAY TO IMPROVEMENT

Though researchers are working to make those sorts of advances possible, progress is being hindered by a difficult-to-navigate regulatory maze and "years of under-funding" research, according to the report. Drug companies also lack incentives to share data and collaborate on research.

The blueprint recommends improvements in several key areas.

First, there's a need for developing new therapies based on a better understanding of cancer biology. That includes defining cancer based not just on where it's located in the body, but by the characteristics of the tumor itself and the "environment" the cancer is growing in, or the tissue around the tumor.

"We need to identify and prioritize molecular targets that have the greatest promise for improving survival," said Dr. Meropol, chief of hematology and oncology at University Hospitals Case Medical Center & Case Western Reserve University, Cleveland.

BETTER CLINICAL TRIALS

Second, more participants for clinical trials need to be recruited and more collaboration needs to occur between the research and industry communities to develop new combinations of drugs that could target multiple pathways at once.

The medical community needs to focus on "smarter, faster clinical trials so that we can move quickly to find out if new treatments are effective," Dr. Meropol said.

Patients for clinical trials should be selected primarily based on the molecular characteristics of their tumors, said John Mendelsohn, MD, codirector of the Institute for Personalized Cancer Therapy at MD Anderson Cancer Center in Houston.

Finally, the system needs to take advantage of innovations in health information technology such as electronic medical records as well as "rapid learning systems," that, among other things, could alert physicians and patients to relevant trials, Dr. Meropol said.

info To see a timeline of the progress that has already been made against cancer, visit the Web site of the American Society of Clinical Oncology, *www.cancerprogress.net/*.

How Chemo Causes Some Cancers to Return

Washington University School of Medicine in St. Louis, news release.

Louis J. DeGennaro, PhD, executive vice president and chief mission officer, Leukemia & Lymphoma Society, White Plains, New York.

The chemotherapy used to treat a form of adult leukemia sets a trap that can result in the return of the disease within years, a recent study suggests.

The finding confirms the suspicions of specialists who thought chemotherapy drugs could disrupt DNA through mutations and ultimately allow tumor cells to avoid the effects of the medications.

THE PRICE OF CHEMO DRUGS

"Chemotherapy drugs are absolutely necessary to get leukemia patients into remission, but we also pay a price in terms of DNA damage," study coauthor Timothy Ley, MD, a professor of oncology at Washington University School of Medicine in St. Louis, said in a university news release.

These drugs "may contribute to disease progression and relapse in many different cancers, which is why our long-term goal is to find targeted therapies based on the mutations specific to a patient's cancer, rather than use drugs that further damage DNA," Dr. Ley added.

BACKGROUND

The type of leukemia in question is known as acute myeloid leukemia. While chemotherapy treatment can send the cancer into remission, 80% of patients die within five years. In the United States, about 13,000 cases of acute myeloid leukemia are diagnosed annually, most often in people age 60 and older.

The researchers came to their conclusions after studying the genomes—the entire DNA, both healthy and cancerous cells—from eight patients with acute myeloid leukemia. They watched to see what happened after the patients received chemotherapy.

The investigators found that tumors essentially reappeared, according to the report published in the journal *Nature*.

MUTATIONS

"It's the same tumor coming back but with a twist," coauthor Richard Wilson, PhD, director of the university's Genome Institute, explained in the news release. It "comes back with new mutations that give the cells new strategies for surviving attack by whatever drugs are thrown at them. This makes a lot of sense but it's been hard to prove without whole-genome sequencing."

FOR THE FUTURE: TARGETED THERAPIES

Commenting on the report, Louis DeGennaro, PhD, executive vice president and chief mission officer of the Leukemia & Lymphoma Society, said the study "demonstrates the critical need to identify disease-causing mutations in acute myeloid leukemia so that therapies targeted specifically at these mutations can be developed."

Ultimately, he added, "that would allow us to avoid the use of chemotherapy, which may contribute to cancer relapse."

For now, Dr. DeGennaro said, "while current chemotherapy regimens have liabilities, they represent the best treatment currently available and may result in complete remission, which would allow eligible patients to receive a stem cell transplant, the only treatment capable of curing acute myeloid leukemia."

info For more about acute myeloid leukemia, visit the Mayo Clinic Web site at *www.mayoclinic.com/health/acute-myelogenous-leukemia/DS00548*.

Seven Common Myths That Can Increase Your Risk of Melanoma

Steven Q. Wang, MD, director of dermatologic surgery and dermatology at Memorial Sloan-Kettering Cancer Center in Basking Ridge, New Jersey. He is author of *Beating Melanoma: A Five-Step Survival Guide* (Johns Hopkins).

When the temperatures drop outside, most people assume that they're at much lower risk for sun-related conditions such as melanoma. But that's a myth.

What you may not realize: Temperature does not affect the intensity of ultraviolet (UV) radiation, so the sun exposure you get in the winter can be just as damaging as what you get in the summer.

Fortunately, there are plenty of steps you can take to minimize your risk for melanoma—the deadliest skin cancer—but you must be able to separate the myths from reality. *Seven common myths...*

Myth 1: Melanoma is a rare disease. Most Americans get regular cancer screenings, including mammograms and colonoscopies. Yet many of the same people have never been screened for melanoma. They assume that they don't need to be screened, especially if they're careful to avoid too much sun.

Fact: More than 70,000 Americans are diagnosed with melanoma annually. This exceeds the annual incidence of other cancers such as malignancies of the thyroid or pancreas and non-Hodgkin's lymphoma.

In addition to performing regular self-exams of their skin, most adults over age 50 should receive a head-to-toe annual skin exam by a doctor who can see places you can't. People with a family history (especially in a parent, sibling or child) of any type of skin cancer and those with fair skin, blond or red hair and/or light eyes should speak to their doctors for advice on screening frequency. Among Caucasians, the lifetime risk of getting melanoma is about one in 50. The risk is lower in Latinos and African-Americans.

Myth 2: You can't get melanoma if you avoid the sun. Reducing sun exposure—with sunscreen and protective clothing, for example—substantially lowers one's risk for melanoma but does not eliminate it.

Fact: Melanoma can occur on any part of the body, including places that sunlight doesn't hit, such as near the anus, between the toes and even on the genitals.

Research has shown that *intermittent* and *intense* sun exposure on areas that are usually covered, such as the trunk, arms or legs, is a major cause of melanoma.

Myth 3: Sunscreen prevents melanoma. It helps but is not a guarantee.

Fact: Most people who use sunscreen and then spend the day outside are probably exposed to enough UV radiation to increase their risk for melanoma or other skin cancers.

Reason: Every sunscreen has a sun-protection factor (SPF) number. In the laboratory, a high SPF translates into more sun protection, but most people don't understand how to achieve this in real life.

When manufacturers test sunscreens, they apply 2 mg of sunscreen per square centimeter of skin. Then a number is assigned to the product, depending on how quickly the skin shows UV-related changes. For the average adult to achieve the same level of protection, he/she would have to apply 1.4 ounces (the amount held in one shot glass) of sunscreen over his/her body.

Virtually no one uses that much. An average-sized tube would be gone after just three or four applications. A product with an SPF of 30 in the laboratory might rate only 10 in real-world applications.

Sunscreen does help but not as much as such protections as wearing tightly woven clothing (which doesn't have to be reapplied and isn't greasy) and staying in the shade (away from the reflection from snow, sand, etc.).

My advice: Opt for a sunscreen product with an SPF of at least 30…apply the amount recommended above…reapply it every two hours…and make sure that it provides protection against both UVB (sunburn-causing) radiation, which mostly damages the skin's superficial layers, and UVA (cancer-causing) radiation, which penetrates more deeply than UVB rays. For additional information on sunscreen, consult *www.SunscreenGuide.com*.

Recommended products: Coppertone UltraGuard…Neutrogena Ultra Sheer Dry-Touch Sunblock…and Banana Boat SunWear. These have been shown to provide good UVB/UVA protection.

Also be sure to use sunscreen throughout the winter months—and don't forget your lips, backs of your hands and tops of your ears. And wear sunglasses with total UV protection—excessive sun exposure may increase risk for melanoma in the eye and does increase risk for eye conditions such as cataracts. Even if you're trying to get your vitamin D from sun exposure, don't stay in the sun more than 10 minutes without protection.

Myth 4: Tanning booths are safer than they used to be. The tanning industry tells customers that getting an artificial tan will help prevent sunburns and cancer. They also claim that tanning is necessary to produce vitamin D.

Fact: The lights that are used in tanning booths primarily emit dangerous UVA radiation...vitamin D is mainly synthesized from exposure to UVB. Getting a tan never reduces the risk for melanoma—every tan is dangerous.

Important finding: In a study published in the *Journal of the National Cancer Institute*, people who used tanning salons at least once a month were 55% more likely to develop melanoma than those who don't get artificial tans.

Myth 5: **You're safe in the car.** Many people assume that they're protected from the sun when traveling in a car. However, during long car trips on sunny days, it's common for exposed skin to redden if it's near the car window.

Fact: Car window glass blocks UVB exposure but only 30% of UVA. But factory-coated windshields block most UVB and UVA radiation.

Important research: A study in the *Journal of the American Academy of Dermatology* that looked at melanomas that occurred on one side of the body found 52% on the left side. In Australia, where the driver's seat is on the right side of the car, more melanoma is found on that side.

Helpful: Tinting the side windows even further can help.

More important: Wear a long-sleeved shirt on long car trips...keep the window closed... and use sunscreen.

Myth 6: **Melanoma appears as an ugly black mole.** Some melanomas are ugly and some are black. Just as often, they're neither. People who don't know this can miss the chance for an early diagnosis.

Fact: Many melanomas are *amelanotic*—that is, they don't produce melanin, which means they can resemble normal skin. Or they might be pink, purple or red.

Important: Look for a mole or other type of skin change that looks different from other moles and skin in the same area.

When you examine your own skin once a month, also be alert for moles that could be described by A, B, C, D or E: Asymmetric, in which the two halves of a mole are different... an irregular Border...variations in Color...a Diameter greater than 6 mm (about one-quarter inch)...and Evolution, a change in the appearance over time.

Myth 7: **Melanoma is usually fatal.** Melanoma is often described as a lethal skin cancer.

Fact: It's a dangerous cancer because it's more likely to spread than many other cancers. Between 8,000 and 9,000 Americans die from melanoma every year.

Good news: More than 95% of melanoma patients survive if the cancer is detected and removed at an early stage, when patients need only minor surgery to remove the cancer and no chemotherapy or radiation. Once the cancer is removed, it's unlikely to return.

More advanced cancers don't respond as readily to treatment—but with new developments, the survival rate is increasing. For example, a study of 675 patients with particularly dangerous melanoma tumors found that the drug *vemurafenib* (Zelboraf) reduced the risk for death during a recent six-month study by 63%. The drug was approved by the FDA for late-stage melanoma in 2011.

■ ■ ■ ■

Guard the Left Side

Skin cancers are more common on the left side of the face.

Possible reason: When people drive, the left side of the face is exposed to more sunlight than the right.

Self-defense: Even when you are in the car, wear sunscreens that block both UVA and UVB rays.

Susan Butler, MD, dermatologic surgeon, California Skin Institute, San Francisco, California, and coauthor of a study of 1,047 Americans, published in *Journal of the American Academy of Dermatology*.

■ ■ ■ ■

Exfoliate to Stop Skin Cancer

Exfoliating helps prevent skin cancer. Exfoliants that contain glycolic acid have been shown to reduce the number of *actinic keratoses*—skin lesions that can develop into squamous cell cancer.

Best: Creams and gels with up to 20% glycolic acid, available online and at some cosmetics stores.

Neal Schultz, MD, cosmetic dermatologist in private practice in New York City and associate clinical professor of dermatology at Mount Sinai School of Medicine, New York City. He is coauthor of *It's Not Just About Wrinkles* (Stewart, Tabori and Chang). *www.dermtv.com*

■ ■ ■ ■

Device Helps Doctors Find Curable Melanomas

MelaFind—a device that creates digital images of suspicious skin growths and compares them with a database of thousands of scans to analyze for signs of melanoma skin cancer—has been approved by the US Food and Drug Administration.

The non-invasive diagnostic can help doctors decide whether to biopsy skin growths in their early stages, when skin cancer is nearly 100% curable, said Irvington, New York, device maker Mela Sciences in a news release.

Melanoma, if not caught in its earliest stages, is the deadliest form of skin cancer. It accounts for about 75% of skin cancer deaths, the company said.

While the new technology can recommend to doctors whether to perform a biopsy, it is *not* intended to confirm a clinical diagnosis of melanoma, according to a Mela Sciences spokeperson.

info Read more about melanoma at the US National Cancer Institute Web site, *http://www.cancer.gov/cancertopics/types/melanoma*.

Calcium + Vitamin D= Decreased Melanoma Risk

Jean Y. Tang, MD, PhD, assistant professor of dermatology, Stanford University School of Medicine, Redwood City, California.

If you've had a basal or squamous cell skin cancer removed, as so many people have, you know all about the anxiety that experience leaves you with. Will it come back? Will you get more of them? Or, worst of all, does this mean you are likely to get the far more serious and worrisome melanoma?

HERE'S THE TRUTH

Sadly, yes, people who have had basal or squamous cell skin cancers are statistically more likely to later develop the deadly skin cancer melanoma than those who haven't had any skin cancers. In fact, a history of any kind of cancer ups your statistical risk for having another—but research suggests that this is especially so with skin cancer.

Now comes the good news. A group of researchers at Stanford University's School of Medicine has found evidence that taking calcium and vitamin D supplements significantly cuts the risk of developing melanoma in a group of women who had previously had nonmelanoma skin cancers.

RESEARCH RESULTS

The researchers learned this by analyzing a large pool of data from the 15-year Women's Health Initiative—36,000 women, ages 50 to 79, were followed for an average of seven years. While the study was initiated to investigate the effects of calcium and vitamin D on hip fractures and colorectal cancers, researchers also looked at whether these supplements affect risk for melanoma—and the researchers were pleasantly surprised.

Half the women in the study took a daily supplement containing 1,000 mg of calcium and 400 IU of vitamin D, while the other half took a placebo pill.

Findings: Those who took calcium and vitamin D were half as likely to develop melanoma subsequent to their other skin cancers. Surprisingly, the researchers also learned that this protective effect helped only those who had had previous skin cancers. Calcium and vitamin D had no apparent effect on melanoma risk in those who had been skin-cancer free.

On the downside, there was a higher incidence of kidney stones among the calcium/vitamin D takers…and emerging research now suggests that very high levels of supplemental vitamin D may encourage certain skin cancers, so none of us should start gulping vitamin D without speaking to a doctor first. The results were published online in the *Journal of Clinical Oncology.*

QUESTIONS AND ADVICE

As noted by lead researcher Jean Y. Tang, MD, PhD, assistant professor of dermatology at the Stanford University School of Medicine, lots of questions remain. For one thing, men weren't included in the Women's Health Initiative, so it's unclear whether they would derive the same benefit from taking the calcium and vitamin D combo. It's also not known whether natural sources of vitamin D (such as sunshine) and calcium (such as from leafy greens and dairy) would have the same effect as the supplements.

Dr. Tang's advice: If you have had basal cell or squamous cell skin cancer…and spend your time indoors for the most part…and/or are a postmenopausal woman (since many are considering calcium supplementation anyway to protect against bone loss), you might discuss a low-dose calcium and vitamin D supplement with your health-care provider. She mentioned also that her team continues to study this issue—focusing particularly on the potential relationship between vitamin D and cancer prevention—with a study that will compare blood levels of vitamin D with the incidence of melanomas.

■ ■ ■ ■

Test Predicts Lung Cancer Survival

Two recent studies involving a total of 1,439 early-stage lung cancer patients found that a new test, known as a *molecular assay*, correctly predicts whether a patient's odds of death within five years of lung cancer surgery are low, intermediate or high by measuring the activity of 14 genes in cancerous tissue.

Benefit: Knowing a patient's prognosis helps doctors determine whether standard postoperative treatments, such as chemotherapy, should be considered.

David Jablons, MD, professor of thoracic oncology, University of California, San Francisco.

Breakthrough Test May End Colonoscopies

David A. Ahlquist, MD, gastroenterologist and professor of medicine, Mayo Clinic Medical School, Rochester, Minnesota

Colonoscopy has been the gold standard in colorectal cancer detection and prevention for a very long time—but it's by no means perfect, and some people will do just about anything to avoid keeping that appointment. Now along comes a new, noninvasive way to screen for colon cancer—stool DNA testing—a procedure that remarkably enough promises accurate detection without the discomfort. The question that naturally follows: Is it really effective?

MORE ACCURATE DETECTION

David A. Ahlquist, MD, gastroenterologist at the Mayo Clinic, explained that colorectal cancer is the second-leading cause of cancer deaths in the US, and colonoscopy—the examination of your colon through insertion of a long, flexible tube—so far represents our best weapon to catch and treat it early. But, he said, colonoscopy may miss some cancers and precancerous lesions, particularly those on the right side of the colon, which has more nooks and crannies, making the search for polyps a challenge. The right side also has a greater likelihood of hard-to-detect flat polyps.

In addition, colonoscopy is expensive. And, like any invasive procedure, it is associated with a risk for complications—bleeding, perforation or sedation-related heart problems occur in a small percentage of patients.

Dr. Ahlquist and his research team found that the new stool DNA test identifies cells that are continuously shed from the surface of growths. It detects target lesions—pre-cancers and cancers, no matter if they are on the left or right side of the colon and no matter what stage, which has been a problem for colonoscopy. Because stool DNA testing effectively detects precancerous polyps, this test has the potential to prevent cancer, much like Pap smears have done for cervical cancer. Add to that the fact that it can be done at home and mailed in for analysis… and it requires no medication or diet restrictions.

IS DNA STOOL TESTING RIGHT FOR YOU?

The Mayo Clinic has collaborated with Exact Sciences to develop the test, and that firm is already meeting with Medicare and major third-party payers to pave the way for coverage. Current guidelines call for colorectal cancer screening if you are 50 or older—earlier if you are at high risk. For example, if you have inflammatory bowel disease (IBD), you face a greater risk for colorectal cancer, and Mayo researchers have confirmed that stool DNA testing can detect cancer and precancer in people with IBD.

Could stool DNA testing ever come to replace rather than complement colonoscopy? Dr. Ahlquist believes the procedure must always be linked to colonoscopy, because those with positive test results will need to undergo colonoscopies both to locate the cancer or polyps that are present, and to remove them as well. But for initial screening, if it works as advertised, the stool test may well become the preferred choice for patients.

Editor's note: Mayo Clinic and Dr. Ahlquist have a financial interest in the technology referenced in this article. In compliance with the Bayh-Dole Act, this technology has been licensed to Exact Sciences, and both Mayo Clinic and Dr. Ahlquist have received royalties. Mayo Clinic holds an equity position in Exact Sciences.

■ ■ ■ ■

Better Colonoscopy Prep

Researchers administered either a full-liquid diet (including ice cream and creamed soup) or a clear-liquid diet (including clear broth and gelatin) to 34 volunteers (average age 53) before they had colonoscopies.

Result: The adequacy of bowel cleansing and the number of patients with detected polyps did not differ between the two groups.

Theory: The liquids in both diets were low residue and adequately washed away with laxatives.

If you are planning a colonoscopy: Talk to your doctor about the possibility of a full-liquid diet that includes milk-based foods, which are more filling than clear liquids.

Ellen Gutkin, DO, researcher, division of gastroenterology, New York Hospital Queens, Flushing, New York.

33% of Americans Skip Life-Saving Test

American Society for Gastrointestinal Endoscopy, news release

Approximately one in three US adults between the ages of 50 and 75 who should be screened for colorectal cancer have not been, according to the American Society for Gastrointestinal Endoscopy.

The society continues to remind older adults about the benefits of a colonoscopy exam to screen for colorectal cancer, which is largely preventable, while offering tips on getting screened.

"Colorectal cancer is one of the most preventable cancers because the majority of colorectal cancers arise from precancerous growths in the colon called polyps, which can be found during a colonoscopy screening exam and removed before they turn into cancer," said Gregory

Ginsberg, MD, president of the American Society for Gastrointestinal Endoscopy (ASGE).

HOW OFTEN
SHOULD YOU BE TESTED

ASGE experts say everyone should be screened starting at age 50, and repeat the screening once a decade thereafter if the initial test results come back normal.

Those with a family history of colorectal cancer should get screened starting at age 40. Other high-risk groups, such as African Americans and those with inflammatory bowel disease, should discuss getting screened sooner with their doctors.

Before the screening, it is important to follow pre-colonoscopy instructions carefully to ensure the colon is thoroughly cleaned so no polyps or cancers are missed during the procedure, Dr. Ginsberg said.

Studies suggest that not following the pre-screening guidelines results in more missed polyps.

info For more on colonoscopies, visit the Web site of the American Society for Gastrointestinal Endoscopy at *www.screen4coloncancer.org*

■ ■ ■ ■

Say Yes to Post-Op Chemo

Do you need chemotherapy after gastric-cancer surgery? You may, according to recent research. A meta-analysis of data from 17 randomized trials found that patients who received postoperative chemotherapy survived longer than patients treated with surgery alone. The right decision on chemotherapy and whether it should be started before or after surgery, as well as on the surgery itself, should be made by an interdisciplinary team including a medical oncologist, a surgeon and a radiation oncologist.

Tim F. Greten, MD, head of the gastro-intestinal malignancies section, National Cancer Institute, Bethesda, Maryland.

Fasting May Slow Tumor Growth

University of Southern California, news release
American Cancer Society

Fasting, especially when combined with chemotherapy, appears to slow the growth of cancerous tumors in mice, recent research suggests.

Experts note that the results of animal studies often don't hold up when tried in humans.

However, researchers have started testing whether fasting can help human patients with breast, ovarian and urinary tract cancer.

In the mouse study, researchers found that fasting slowed the growth of breast cancer, melanoma, glioma and human neuroblastoma in mice.

In some cases, fasting was as effective as chemotherapy, according to the study.

"The combination of fasting cycles plus chemotherapy was either more or much more effective than chemo alone," said senior study author Valter Longo, PhD, professor of gerontology and biological sciences at the University of Southern California.

The study was published in the journal *Science Translational Medicine*.

HOW FASTING + CHEMO FIGHTS CANCER

Researchers said that normal cells deprived of nutrients during fasting enter a dormant state, whereas when studied in the lab, a type of cancer cell attempted to keep growing and dividing.

That, in turn, led to a "cascade of events" that damaged the cancer cells' DNA and led to cell death.

"A way to beat cancer cells may not be to try to find drugs that kill them specifically but to confuse them by generating extreme environments, such as fasting, that only normal cells can quickly respond to," Dr. Longo concluded.

HUMAN TRIALS

The study authors noted that results from the initial phase of a clinical trial, which involved patients with breast, urinary tract and ovarian cancer conducted at the USC Norris Comprehensive Cancer Center, were submitted for presentation at the annual meeting of the American Society of Cancer Oncologists. This trial tested the safety of short-term fasts two days before and one day after chemotherapy.

"We don't know whether in humans it's effective," Dr. Longo said. "But a patient should be able to go to his or her oncologist and say, 'What about fasting with chemotherapy?' or fasting without chemo, if chemotherapy was not recommended or considered."

FASTING NOT FOR EVERYONE

The researchers warned that fasting may not be safe for all cancer patients, particularly those who have already lost a significant amount of weight or have other conditions, such as diabetes. They added that fasting can cause headaches and a drop in blood pressure. The study also pointed out that cancer-free survival resulting from fasting may not extend to large tumors.

According to the American Cancer Society, "available scientific evidence does not support claims that fasting is effective for preventing or treating cancer. Even a short-term fast can have negative health effects, while fasting for a longer time could cause serious health problems."

info The American Cancer Society provides more information on fasting and cancer. Visit its Web site at *www.cancer.org* (search "fasting and chemotherapy").

■ ■ ■ ■

Tai Chi Improves Memory in Chemotherapy Patients

Cancer patients who undergo chemotherapy often suffer from memory loss and decreased verbal skills. University of Missouri psychologists found that women who had received chemotherapy had significant improvement in their cognitive abilities after participating in a one-hour tai chi class (held twice weekly for 10 weeks) compared with before taking the classes. It's likely that men would have a similar benefit.

Mark A. Stengler, NMD, naturopathic medical doctor in private practice, Encinitas, California...adjunct associate clinical professor at the National College of Natural Medicine, Portland, Oregon...author of *The Natural Physicians Healing Therapies* and coauthor of *Prescription for Natural Cures* (both from Bottom Line Books).

Cancer Survivors Need To Pay Attention to Overall Health

American Association for Cancer Research, news release

Cancer survivors need to pay close attention to other aspects of their health as they age, researchers urge.

A recent study finds that nearly half of cancer survivors die of something other than cancer, such as heart disease or diabetes. And the further from the initial cancer diagnosis they get, the more likely it is that their cause of death will be something other than cancer.

"After the detection of cancer, clinicians and cancer survivors pay less attention to the prevention and treatment of other diseases and complications," said lead researcher Yi Ning, MD, assistant professor in the department of epidemiology and community health at Virginia Commonwealth University in Richmond, in an association news release. "We shouldn't neglect other aspects of health because we are focused on cancer and overlook other chronic conditions."

STUDY DETAILS

In following 1,800 cancer survivors over the course of more than 18 years, researchers found that 776 of the patients died—51% eventually died from cancer and 49% died from other conditions.

"We realized that the mortality rates for some types of cancer, such as breast cancer, had declined," said Dr. Ning, also an associate research member at VCU Massey Cancer Center. "Cancer survivors live much longer than they did several decades ago. So with this large group of cancer survivors, we need to pay more attention to cancer survivors' overall health."

The patients followed in the study survived some of the most common forms of cancer, including breast, prostate, cervical, lung and colorectal. A large percentage of patients were also diagnosed with conditions other than cancer, including high blood pressure and diabetes.

MORE TIME, LESS HEALTHY

The more time that passed after the initial cancer diagnosis, the more likely cancer survivors were to die from another illness. Among those who died from a condition other than cancer during the study period, 33% had been diagnosed with cancer within the previous five years and 63% had been diagnosed 20 years earlier.

info The American Cancer Society provides tips for cancer survivors on how to stay active and healthy. Visit *www.cancer.org/treatment/survivorshipduringandaftertreatment/index* for more information.

Citrus Supplement Helps Stop Cancer From Spreading

Mark A. Stengler, NMD, naturopathic medical doctor in private practice, Encinitas, California...adjunct associate clinical professor at the National College of Natural Medicine, Portland, Oregon...author of *The Natural Physicians Healing Therapies* and coauthor of *Prescription for Natural Cures* (both from Bottom Line Books).

We usually think of the peels of oranges and grapefruit as good for compost heaps and garnish on foods and not much else. But research has found another use for a substance found in peels that is known as *pectin*—and it is at the root of a cancer therapy.

WHERE IT COMES FROM

Pectin is a compound found in the peel and pith (the white strands attached to the peel) of citrus fruits. It also is found in the peel and core of other fruits, such as apples. Even if you were to eat an orange peel, you wouldn't get any pectin that your body could use because in its natural state, its molecules are too large for us to digest. But researchers have found that when they break down pectin molecules into smaller sizes, it can be absorbed into the bloodstream.

Modified citrus pectin (MCP), which is what the over-the-counter supplement is called, has been found to stop the spread of cancer. (The word "modified" in this case means that the substance has been changed so that it can be absorbed by humans.) MCP is not meant to be used on its own as a cancer treatment, but it provides anticancer effects when used in conjunction with conventional cancer treatments such as chemotherapy. Its benefit is impressive because the spread (metastasis) of cancer from the original site to other parts of the body is the main cause of cancer-related death. MCP has been widely studied as a treatment for prostate and breast cancers and could help many other cancers.

HOW MCP WORKS

MCP prevents tumors from metastasizing by binding with a protein called galectin-3, a receptor molecule on the surface of cancer cells that usually carries out a number of cancer-promoting activities. One of galectin-3's most important functions involves helping cancer cells adhere to blood vessel walls and to other cancer cells, allowing the cells to colonize healthy body tissues. By binding with galectin-3, MCP blocks this adhesion process. MCP also blocks galectin-3's ability to stimulate the formation of blood vessels in new tumors, a process called angiogenesis that is essential to tumor growth...and it appears to encourage cancer-cell death (apoptosis) by interfering with signaling pathways related to cancer-cell proliferation and survival.

Galectin-3 also helps cancer cells survive chemotherapy treatment. MCP disrupts this, enabling chemotherapy to be more effective.

WHAT THE STUDIES SHOW

In a study published in *Integrative Cancer Therapies*, Columbia University researchers found that when prostate cancer cells were exposed to MCP in the laboratory, they died off. Its effect on androgen-independent prostate cancer (a prostate cancer in which cells do not depend on the androgen hormone for growth) is especially exciting, because there are not many effective treatments for this form of cancer, which tends to be aggressive.

A study conducted at Miami Children's Hospital (and funded by a supplement company that makes MCP) and published in *BMC Complementary and Alternative Medicine* found that MCP had a powerful effect on the immune system's ability to fight cancer, inducing a dose-dependent increase in cytotoxic T-cells and natural killer (NK) cells—two immune system components that attack and kill tumor cells. The study also found that the highest dose of MCP tested (800 micrograms per milliliter of blood in a lab sample, which has no exact equivalent in terms of an oral dose) increased NK cells' ability to destroy leukemia cancer cells by more than 50%. Some forms of chemotherapy fight galectin-3 molecules, too, but they also kill healthy cells. MCP is the first natural substance shown to fight galectin-3—and the hope is that with MCP the body's normal NK cell activity will work overtime to kill cancer cells while leaving healthy cells alone.

WHO SHOULD TAKE MCP

There's growing interest among holistic practitioners and some oncologists in MCP. One of MCP's most important features is that it is nontoxic. The only side effect is mild digestive upset. People can take MCP with other drugs—two hours apart is best, since MCP's fiber may hinder absorption of the other drugs. It also is safe for children.

MCP is a particularly good adjunct therapy for prostate and breast cancers, which have been the most studied. MCP's cancer-fighting ability also provides a protective benefit to cancer survivors and people with a family member (parent or sibling) who has had cancer.

One brand I like: PectaSol-C, a proprietary formulation developed and manufactured by EcoNugenics. PectaSol-C MCP can be purchased online at *www.econugenics.com*. Follow directions on the label.

■ **More from Dr. Mark A. Stengler...**

Boost Broccoli's Cancer Fighting Power

When you eat broccoli with certain other vegetables, such as broccoli sprouts, arugula or radishes, you get twice the cancer-fighting power of broccoli consumed on its own, say University of Illinois researchers. These additional vegetables contain the enzyme *myrosinase*, which boosts the effectiveness of broccoli's cancer-preventive component, sulforaphane. To protect the nutrients and the enzyme, steam broccoli and vegetables for only two to four minutes.

■ ■ ■ ■

Bladder Cancer Patients Often Don't Get the Right Care

For patients with high-grade bladder cancer that has not invaded the muscle of the bladder, guidelines call for injecting a cancer-killing drug directly into the bladder and then launching an intense follow-up protocol. But many doctors don't follow these guidelines.

info Learn more about the disease and its treatment from the Bladder Cancer Advocacy Network, *www.bcan.org*.

Karim Chamie, MD, urologist in the UCLA Health System, Los Angeles, and leader of a study of 4,545 bladder-cancer patients, published in the online edition of *Cancer*.

■ ■ ■ ■

Can Selenium Protect You From Bladder Cancer?

Women are less likely than men to get bladder cancer—but are less likely to survive if they do get it, according to the National Institutes of Health.

Encouraging news from a recent study: Compared with women who had the lowest blood levels of the mineral selenium, those with the highest levels were 34% less likely to get bladder cancer.

Bottom line: Further research is needed before selenium supplements can be recommended for bladder cancer prevention, but results of several studies are promising. Meanwhile, selenium-rich foods—including nuts, seafood and whole wheat—can be a healthful part of your diet.

Margaret Karagas, PhD, professor of community and family medicine at Dartmouth Medical School in Hanover, New Hampshire, and leader of a study of 1,875 people.

■ ■ ■ ■

Chinese Cancer-Fighter

A Chinese herbal remedy, Dang Gui Long Hui Wan, appears to inhibit the growth and spread of *glioblastoma multiforme*, a deadly brain cancer.

Cancer Research

■ ■ ■ ■

Coffee Cancer Cure

Recent research shows that coffee protects against aggressive cancers of the prostate and breast.

Study results: Women who drank more than five cups of coffee a day had a 57% lower risk for ER-negative breast cancer—the most aggressive subtype—than women who drank less than one cup a day. Men who consumed six or more cups of coffee daily had a 60% lower risk for lethal prostate cancer. The coffee in the women's study was caffeinated…in the men's study, both regular and decaffeinated coffee reduced the risk for cancer.

Michael F. Roizen, MD, chief wellness officer and chair, Wellness Institute, Cleveland Clinic.

Strawberries Join the Fight Against Cancer

Tong Chen, MD, PhD, assistant professor in medical oncology, The Ohio State University Comprehensive Cancer Center, Columbus.

Strawberries are high on a select list of super-healthy foods that virtually everyone likes. Now comes news that they are much more important to our health than previously thought. A recent study done at The Ohio State University Comprehensive Cancer Center on freeze-dried strawberries found that the berries were extremely effective in slowing the development of precancerous esophageal lesions.

Anything that helps the fight against esophageal cancer is very welcome news. Not only have the number of cases been growing, it's also a very deadly cancer.

BERRIES BRING REVERSALS

The research (which was sponsored by the California Strawberry Commission) was done in China, where the incidence of esophageal cancer—the type known as squamous cell carcinoma—is extremely high. Americans more typically suffer from a different type of esophageal cancer, known as *adenocarcinoma*. Lead researcher Tong Chen, MD, PhD, assistant professor in medical oncology at Ohio State, said that strawberries may similarly affect the type of cancer common in the West because they impact some genes common to both types.

In Dr. Chen's study, in which each participant ate about two ounces of freeze-dried strawberries a day, 29 of the 36 participants—about 80%—experienced at least some reversal of lesion progress, with some moderate lesions becoming mild and some mild ones reverting to normal. Dr. Chen said, "Our study is important because it shows that strawberries may be an alternative to—or may work together with chemopreventive drugs to help stop esophageal cancer. But we will need to test this in randomized placebo-controlled trials in the future."

BIG POWER IN A LITTLE BERRY

As a cancer fighter, strawberries have a powerful combination of molecular components, said Dr. Chen. They contain antioxidant polyphenols, of course, and also vitamins A, C and E, folic acid, calcium, selenium and zinc. She pointed out that you can buy all of these in supplemental form, but in strawberries there seems to be a synergistic effect among the components that makes them more potent than the individual components are on their own. Freeze-drying the fruit takes it to an even more impressive level as a nutrient powerhouse—this process removes water from the fruit, leaving a much denser nutritional content within. In the case of strawberries, which are 90% water, when freeze-dried, the end product is 10 times more nutritious than the equivalent weight of fresh berries.

Freeze-dried strawberries are widely available now in supermarkets and health-food stores. This is one rare case in which a processed version of a food might be more healthful than the natural version—probably because freeze-drying takes out only water and adds no flavorings or sugar.

■ ■ ■ ■

Aspirin Cuts Cancer Deaths Up to 54%

According to recent research, taking low-dose aspirin daily for five years decreased gastrointestinal cancer deaths by up to 54% and overall cancer mortality by 34%. The longer aspirin is used, the greater the benefit. The mechanism by which aspirin helps prevent cancer deaths is not yet fully understood.

Peter Rothwell, MD, PhD, professor of clinical neurology, Oxford University, England, and senior author of an analysis of studies of 25,570 patients, published in *The Lancet*.

■ ■ ■ ■

Stop Pancreatic Cancer Before It Starts

Pancreatic cancer can sometimes be stopped before it starts. Most pancreatic cysts are benign—but up to 20% become malignant. The cysts usually are detected when CT or other scans are performed for other reasons. Additional testing can help determine whether surgery is indicated. Patients who have a cyst and/or a strong family history of pancreatic cancer—for example, a parent or sibling who has or had the disease—should have regular imaging tests.

Christopher Wolfgang, MD, PhD, director of pancreatic surgery at The Johns Hopkins Hospital and associate professor of surgery and oncology at The Johns Hopkins University School of Medicine, both in Baltimore.

The Risk Every Cancer Patient Needs to Know

Gary Lyman, MD, MPH, professor of medicine and director of the Comparative Effectiveness and Outcomes Research Program in Oncology at Duke University School of Medicine in Durham, North Carolina. Dr. Lyman also chairs the Venous Thromboembolism Expert Panel that draws up guidelines for clot prevention in cancer patients for the American Society of Clinical Oncology.

If you have cancer and you're being treated for it with surgery and/or chemotherapy, you may have heard that you're at high risk for life-threatening blood clots. To make bad news even worse, a recent study reveals that the risk may be even higher than scientists previously thought.

ASSESSING YOUR RISK

Gary H. Lyman, MD, MPH, a professor of medicine and an expert in cancer treatment at Duke University School of Medicine in Durham, North Carolina, explained that researchers looked at the records of 30,552 female patients, average age 64, receiving chemotherapy or surgery for cancers of the bladder, colon, lung, ovaries, pancreas, rectum or stomach. Patients who were already at a higher risk for blood clots were excluded from the study.

The results of the study are concerning. Within one year of surgery or chemo, a specific kind of clot called a *venous thromboembolism* (VTE) developed in 9.9% to 21.5% of the cancer patients either while they were in the hospital or after they had returned home—bladder cancer patients had the lowest occurrence rate, while pancreatic cancer patients had the highest.

A VTE, said Dr. Lyman, is a clot that first forms in a vein anywhere in the body (though it usually occurs in the leg or the pelvis), and without treatment, it may travel to the lungs and block an artery. This type of clot is serious and can cause anything from breathing difficulty to heart failure to sudden death. In fact, of the 300,000 to 600,000 Americans who develop severe blood clots like this each year, the Centers for Disease Control and Prevention estimates that 60,000 to 100,000 die.

The study, presented at the recent European Multidisciplinary Cancer Congress in Stockholm, Sweden, was funded by the pharmaceutical company Sanofi-Aventis which, it should be noted, markets a drug specifically aimed at solving this problem—an anticoagulant called *enoxaparin* (Lovenox).

WHAT CAUSES THE CLOTS?

Is it the cancer, the surgery or the chemotherapy? "All of the above," Dr. Lyman said. It's partly the cancer, he explained, because tumors naturally secrete inflammatory substances that are blood-clotting agents—though scientists aren't sure why. It's also partly the surgery, said Dr. Lyman, because surgery increases the risk for infections (a risk factor for blood clots), as does being sedentary in bed recovering from surgery. And finally, chemotherapy plays a role, too, because both intravenous catheters and the chemical irritation of the chemotherapy on the blood vessel walls may increase risk for clots. Researchers don't fully understand why patients with some types of cancer get more clots than others, Dr. Lyman said, but he added that those questions will be the subject of studies in the near future.

HOW TO STAY SAFE

The recent study is expected to get considerable attention from oncologists, Dr. Lyman said. The American Society of Clinical Oncology and the National Comprehensive Cancer Network are both updating guidelines that encourage doctors to be on the lookout for clots and, when appropriate, to give patients anticoagulant drugs early on to reduce the possibility of clots. Dr. Lyman also advises doctors to tell cancer patients about safer interventions, such as standing up every hour at work or on long car or plane rides and not crossing your legs for long stretches.

Cancer patients themselves, he said, should be vigilant. Tell your doctor immediately about any swelling in the leg or pain in the calf, which can be signs that you have a potentially dangerous VTE. Also report any unexplained shortness of breath, coughing, an irregular heartbeat or coughing up blood, all of which can be signs that a life-threatening clot has reached the heart or lungs. And, by all means, let all of your doctors know if you have a personal or family history of blood clots.

■ ■ ■ ■

Marriage Can Help You Survive Cancer

Did you know married people are more likely to survive cancer than people who have never married? Never-married men were 35% more likely to die from their cancer between 2005 and 2007 (latest data available) than men who were married, divorced or widowed. Never-married women were 22% more likely to die from their cancer. The findings apply to 13 common cancers, including breast and prostate.

Astri Syse, PhD, researcher, Cancer Registry of Norway, Oslo, and leader of a study of more than 440,000 people from 1970 to 2007, published online in *BMC Public Health*.

Consumer Health Alerts

Don't Drink the Water

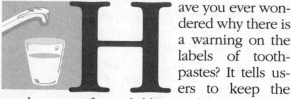

Have you ever wondered why there is a warning on the labels of toothpastes? It tells users to keep the product away from children and to seek medical attention if more than the recommended amount for brushing is swallowed.

Reason: Toothpaste contains fluoride.

For years, this chemical has been added to our water to reduce the occurrence of dental cavities—but unbelievably, the newest evidence shows that fluoridated water does not protect against cavities. In fact, it turns out that we don't need fluoride to protect our teeth at all.

Dentists advise that children use toothpaste that contains fluoride—and yet we keep all kinds of other medications and dangerous products away from children. But is toothpaste as dangerous? Yes. The average tube of toothpaste contains enough fluoride to kill a child. And how safe is a glass of fluoridated tap water?

Fluoride occurs naturally in soil, water and some plants. It also is a by-product of phosphate fertilizer production and is an industrial waste product of the aluminum smelting industry. The FDA maintains that fluoride is a drug. It's also known to be a highly toxic substance, even more toxic than lead. Once used as rat poison, it can cause serious health problems when ingested in unsafe amounts, including weak bones, hormone disruption and neurological damage.

And the truth is—fluoride is everywhere. It's not only in dental-hygiene products but also still in our water supply. It's been there since the 1940s, when extensive tooth decay was common across the US. In 1999, the Centers for Disease Control and Prevention (CDC) called water fluoridation one of the 10 greatest public health achievements of the 20th century.

Mark A. Stengler, NMD, licensed naturopathic medical doctor in private practice, Encinitas, California...adjunct associate clinical professor at the National College of Natural Medicine, Portland, Oregon...author of *The Natural Physician's Healing Therapies* and coauthor of *Prescription for Natural Cures* (both from Bottom Line Books).

Fast forward to 2013…and we are at risk for health problems because we are overexposed to fluoride. It is even in a number of products that our families consume (either when we add in fluoridated water or when the products themselves are made with fluoridated water), such as baby formula, processed cereals, juice, soda, tea, wine and beer. *What you need to know to protect yourself…*

FLUORIDE IN TAP WATER

It's not only the natural medicine community that is alarmed. In 2011, for the first time in about 50 years, the US Department of Health and Human Services (HHS) announced that there was too much fluoride in the US water supply and recommended reducing the amount of fluoride added to water to 0.7 parts per million (ppm) everywhere. The limit had previously been 0.7 ppm in warm climates where people drink a lot of water to 1.2 ppm in cooler climates (where people presumably drink less).

FLUORIDE CAUSES HEALTH PROBLEMS

When you ingest fluoride, about half is excreted by the kidneys. The rest is stored in your bones and teeth, where it does the opposite of what it is supposed to do—it causes damage. According to the CDC, 41% of American adolescents now have dental *fluorosis,* an increase from 23% in 1987. This disfigurement of tooth enamel in teeth, which can range from white patches to brown mottling, typically occurs before age eight (when permanent teeth are all formed). This very high rate of fluorosis is thought to be caused by fluoride intake during childhood, from drinking fluoridated water (including commercial drinks made with fluoridated water) and swallowing toothpaste with fluoride.

In addition to fluorosis, fluoride causes other health problems…

•**Fluoride decreases bone strength.** A 2010 *Journal of Dental Research* study found that bone strength in animals decreases with increased levels of fluoride in bones. HHS also has noted that excess fluoride can result in bone fractures and skeletal fluorosis, a crippling condition.

•**Fluoride impairs brain function in children.** A 2008 systematic review published in *Biological Trace Element Research* found that children in China who live in an area with fluoridated water have five times greater risk for a lower IQ than children who live in a nonfluoridated or slightly fluoridated area. The water was fluoridated at a level of 2.47 milligrams per liter (mg/L), three times the US safe level. (Note that 1 ppm equals 1 mg/L.)

•**Fluoride upsets cardiac function.** Increased fluoride can result in abnormal calcification of cardiac tissue. This can impair cardiac function in animals, say researchers from Agricultural University Wageningen in the Netherlands, whose study was published in *Biological Trace Element Research.*

•**Fluoride interferes with cell metabolism.** Research published in *Toxicology Letters* in 2010 points to chronic fluoride exposure as a possible cause of oxidative stress, which results in inflammation throughout the body.

In addition, in 2006, the National Research Council (NRC) reviewed EPA water-safety standards. The NRC found that excessive fluoride intake was associated with hormone disruption, impaired thyroid function, increased free radical activity in the brain (potentially contributing to dementia) and abnormal insulin response.

Population studies show that people who live in communities that fluoridate their water have no fewer cavities, on average, than people in communities without fluoridated water. While it's true that the US has experienced dramatic declines in cavities and tooth decay over the past 50 years, the same holds true for people in Europe, where many countries discontinued the practice of water fluoridation starting in the 1970s. It is believed that cavities have decreased despite water fluoridation cessation because of better oral hygiene.

MINIMIZE YOUR FLUORIDE INTAKE

Water fluoridation is an unsafe practice that should be stopped. If you live in the US, there's a 70% chance that your tap water is fluoridated. Since water fluoridation is left up to individual states and municipalities, practices vary from town to town.

Examples: New York City, Minneapolis and Chicago currently maintain a water fluoride content of 1 mg/L. To check the fluoride content of your water, contact your local water utility or visit *http://apps.nccd.cdc.gov/mwf/index.asp*. You can join the growing number of people who are letting their local government agencies know about the health concerns of fluoridated water.

To further protect yourself...

• **Drink spring water.** It usually contains less than 0.1 ppm of fluoride.

• **Use a water filter.** One of the best types of filters for removing fluoride is the reverse-osmosis filter, available at appliance stores for $300 to $400. Many household filters, such as Brita and Pur, do not eliminate fluoride.

AVOIDING FLUORIDE IN DENTAL PRODUCTS

The concentration of fluoride in many commercially made toothpastes is high—about 1,000 ppm to 1,500 ppm. Even when you don't swallow fluoridated toothpaste, some fluoride is absorbed by the body and goes into the bloodstream. I'm convinced that there is no benefit from any kind of topical application of fluoride—whether it's toothpaste, mouthwash or even a onetime fluoride treatment from the dentist. Both children and adults should not use fluoride treatment or supplements of any kind.

Switch to a toothpaste that doesn't include fluoride—and that does contain only natural ingredients. Make sure these include xylitol, a compound derived from plant fibers that is known to prevent cavities. Many such toothpastes are available at health-food stores. Also, work with a holistic dentist to ensure dental health.

■ ■ ■ ■

Carcinogen in Tap Water

The EPA is planning to tighten drinking-water standards to eliminate the carcinogen *hexavalent chromium*. In the meantime, a reverse-osmosis filter will remove hexavalent chromium from household water systems. However, it can cost anywhere from $170 to $500, more if you have it installed professionally.

Alternative: Any filter using activated carbon can remove 40% to 90% of hexavalent chromium, depending on the levels of hexavalent chromium present in your water. Unfortunately, there is no sure way to know your levels. A recent

study found that water samples from 31 out of 35 cities across the country had detectable levels of hexavalent chromium. Unless your water supply comes from a protected watershed or is one of the four cities in the study with safe levels, a reverse-osmosis filter is recommended.

 For the cities studied, go to *www.ewg. org/chromium6-in-tap-water*.

Robert Morris, MD, adjunct professor at University of Washington School of Engineering, Seattle, and author of *The Blue Death: The Intriguing Past and Present of the Water You Drink* (Harper).

Are Your Appliances Killing You?

David O. Carpenter, MD, director of the Institute for Health and the Environment and a professor of environmental health and toxicology at the University at Albany, New York.

You've probably heard about the scientific studies linking cell phones to a variety of tumors, including brain cancer (see page 72). The World Health Organization has now classified cell phones as a "possible carcinogen."*

What's being largely overlooked: Electromagnetic radiation—from electrical appliances, such as hair dryers, microwave ovens and washing machines...as well as that from wireless signals for computers—also may contribute to cancer risk independent of cell-phone use.

What you need to know...

INVISIBLE POLLUTION

Every electrical appliance in your home emits electric and magnetic fields (EMFs) of energy. An appliance that is plugged in has an electric field even when it is turned off. The appliance produces a magnetic field when it is turned on and the electrical current is flowing. However, the EMFs from appliances are considered extremely low frequency (ELF), meaning that the radiation flows at very low levels.

*A team of 31 scientists from 14 countries analyzed peer-reviewed studies before classifying radiofrequency electromagnetic fields from wireless cell phones as "possibly carcinogenic to humans" based on an increased risk for glioma, a type of brain cancer.

Still, some studies show that regular exposure to even low levels of ELF electromagnetic radiation, such as 3 milligauss (mG), may increase the risk for leukemia in children—and possibly, to a lesser degree, in adults. Preliminary research has also linked this form of energy to Alzheimer's disease and Lou Gehrig's disease, but this association is still being debated.

Some experts maintain that the electromagnetic radiation from cell phones and electrical appliances is too weak to cause the types of cell damage that can lead to cancer. But evidence is emerging that even weak forms of energy may interfere with normal cell functions, perhaps contributing to the development of cancer and other diseases.

SAFER POWER

Appliances that use the most electrical current, such as handheld hair dryers, emit the highest levels of ELF radiation. But even small appliances, such as coffeemakers, produce some.

Important: ELF fields are strongest at the point where the electrical wires enter the device. The fields diminish to almost nothing within a foot or two.

To test electromagnetic radiation around your appliances: Use a gauss meter—available online for about $150 to $500.

Important: ELF fields are *directional*—if you hold the meter to the right of a washing machine, for example, the reading might be zero, but it may be much higher a foot to the left. For accurate readings, test in different locations around the electrical appliance within a radius of a few feet.

Electrical wiring in the walls also can be an issue.

What I've found: In my son's bedroom, most of the wiring that carries electricity to lights and electrical outlets is in one of the walls. When we tested with a gauss meter, the EMFs were highest near his bed, so we moved his bed to the other side of the room.

In general, electrical wiring in walls generates high ELF only when the current is flowing or there is a ground current created by faulty wiring. However, the ELF exposure from wiring adds to the total exposure from appliances.

To reduce exposure…

•**Don't linger near appliances when they're running.** Even though the ELF levels are typically highest at the back of an appliance where the electrical cord plugs in, the magnetic field directly in front of a typical washing machine can reach 20 mG. You'll be exposed to only normal background levels by moving a foot or two away.

Important: Even the best microwave ovens leak some of the radiation they use to heat the food, so stand at least four feet away from the front of the oven when it's running. Microwave ovens also produce high levels of ELF electromagnetic radiation from the electricity used to power the oven, so there's a double risk.

•**Towel-dry your hair.** Hair dryers are among the most dangerous sources of magnetic fields because they use a lot of power and the motor/heater is held close to the head. Although using a low-fan and/or low-heat setting helps some, it's better to avoid hair dryers altogether.

If towel-drying is not convenient, consider using a low EMF hair dryer such as the Chi Ceramic Low EMF Ionic Hair Dryer available for about $100 online…or a low-EMF wall-mounted hair dryer for $89.95 from the EMF Safety Superstore, *www.lessemf.com.*

•**Use the electric blanket before you get into bed.** Electric blankets don't draw a lot of electrical current, but they expose your entire body to ELF radiation for the entire night if you leave them on. If you want a warm bed, turn on the blanket half an hour before bedtime, then turn it off when you get into bed.

•**Get a new bedside clock.** Old-style alarm clocks—analog clocks with lighted dials—produce surprisingly high levels of electromagnetic radiation.

My advice: Get a digital bedside clock, which emits almost no ELF.

•**Throw out your cordless phones.** Cordless phones emit electromagnetic radiation whether or not they are being used. That's why I recommend replacing cordless phones with corded phones.

SAFER COMPUTER USE

Most computers give off electromagnetic radiation. If you use a desktop model, position it toward the back of your desk. Most monitors, which produce lower levels of electromagnetic radiation than computers, have conductive screens to block the ELF exposure. But it's still wise to position your monitor as far away from you as possible.

What I've found: I once measured the fields near my secretary's desk. The reading was about 10 mG, which is extremely high. I realized that the high-powered electrical wiring used by the computer was behind the wall closest to her. We moved her desk 10 feet to get out of range.

Also, virtually every modern computer (including laptops) is designed to receive wireless signals. If you have a wireless router, which connects to a cable and wirelessly "routes" this connection to one or more computers in your home, your exposure to electromagnetic radiation is constant. *To be safer...*

•**Hardwire the computer to the modem.** Use cables to connect computers to your modem rather than using a wireless signal, so you can forgo the router. If more than one person uses a computer at home, however, this approach may not be practical.

•**Turn off the router when it's not in use.** If you do use a router, turn it on only when you need the signal for using the Internet, streaming video to the TV, etc.

•**Disable Wi-Fi settings on your computer if you don't use a router.** Otherwise, the computer—or any device that operates wirelessly, such as some printers—will constantly emit electromagnetic radiation as it tries to find the nearest wireless source. Shut down your computer when it's not in use to reduce ELF radiation in your home.

■ **More from Dr. David O. Carpenter...**

iPad, Laptop Safety

It is advised that you do not hold e-tablet or portable computer devices in your lap. No one has studied cancers of the abdomen from iPads or laptops. But an iPad is a wireless device, and there is some evidence, though not definitive, that holding a cell phone to your head may increase risk for brain cancer on the side of the head where it is used intensely for many years (see below). But if the iPad or the cell phone is held away from your body, it will not give significant exposure.

Yes, Cell Phones Do Cause Brain Tumors! How to Protect Yourself

Magda Havas, PhD, associate professor of environmental and resource studies at Trent University in Peterborough, Ontario, Canada. She is a leading expert in radiofrequency radiation, electromagnetic fields, dirty electricity and ground current. She is coauthor, with Camilla Rees, of *Public Health SOS: The Shadow Side of the Wireless Revolution* (CreateSpace). *www.magda havas.com*

About nine out of 10 US households now have at least one cell phone—and that doesn't include other wireless devices, such as cordless phones, iPads, baby monitors and computers.

Result: The average adult (and child) is flooded with nonionizing radiation, a form of energy that—for the first time—has been officially linked to cancer. In May 2011, a panel of the World Health Organization (WHO) listed cell phones as a class 2b carcinogen, which means that it's "possible" that cell phones, like some industrial chemicals, increase the risk for cancer.

This conclusion has been disputed by many scientists. But careful analysis of the best studies to date indicate that people who log the most cell-phone minutes are more likely to develop tumors on the same side of the head that they hold the cell phone, compared with those who use cell phones less often.

DISTURBING RESEARCH

The largest study of cell-phone use, known as INTERPHONE, was conducted in 13 countries over a 10-year period. The study, published in the *International Journal of Epidemiology*, found that people who used cell phones for at least 1,640 hours over the 10-year period—that comes to about 30 minutes a day—had a 40% higher risk of developing a *glioma*, a deadly type of brain tumor.

Disturbing: The development of a brain tumor to the point that it can be detected often takes 20 to 30 years. The fact that these tumors are showing up after 10 years of exposure is disturbing because it is much faster than expected.

Previous studies have linked frequent or prolonged cell-phone use to an increase in parotid (salivary gland) and auditory nerve tumors.

The actual risk probably is higher than the studies indicate. The INTERPHONE study defined "heavy use" as using a cell phone for about 30 minutes a day. That's a fraction of the time that many people currently spend on their cell phones.

Also, the study looked only at adults, even though young people are frequent users of cell phones and the ones who face the highest cancer risks from decades of radiation exposure.

In addition, the study "diluted" the data by identifying people as regular cell-phone users who may have used their phones only once a week for at least six months. These light users were obviously exposed to far less radiation than heavy users. Including them in the study caused the cancer percentages to appear artificially low. For example, we would not expect someone who smoked one cigarette a week for at least six months to develop lung cancer.

SAFER USE

Skeptics of cell-phone dangers argue that nonionizing radiation is too weak to heat tissues or break chemical bonds, factors that are known to increase cancer risks. But recent studies indicate damage to DNA in rat brains exposed to cell-phone radiation, and this type of damage can lead to cancer.

Ways to stay safe…

•**Hold the phone away from your ear.** The fine print in cell-phone manuals usually advises users to hold the phone at least ⅞ of an inch away from the ear. Farther is better. Use speakerphone mode.

•**Wait for good reception.** Cell phones emit much higher levels of radiation when the antenna is sending out signals to search for a tower or satellite. These signals can travel hundreds of miles—and the poorer the reception, the greater the radiation emitted by your cell phone.

•**Use a hollow-tube headset.** This is the safest type of headset because the last few inches, those closest to the ear, consist of a hollow tube. This hollow tube transmits sound like a stethoscope. Wired headsets need to be kept away from the body because the continuous wire that runs from the phone to the earpiece will expose you to some unnecessary radiation. Hollow-tube headsets (Blue Tube) can be purchased at *www.mercola.com.*

•**Use "airplane mode."** Even when you're not talking on a cell phone, the phone is sending out signals every few minutes to search for the nearest tower. Turn off the phone when you're not using it. Or switch it to airplane mode so that it can't send or receive signals, but you still can use the phone to listen to music, watch videos and check your calendar.

•**Keep the phone on your desk when working.** When the phone is switched on, don't keep it in your pocket or attached to your belt. This is particularly important for men. Preliminary research indicates that men who keep their phones close to their bodies (often in holsters or pockets) have lower sperm counts and poorer sperm quality than those without this exposure.

Caution: The worst way to use a Bluetooth wireless headset is to place it on your ear with the cell phone in your pocket. This way, your head and lower body are both being irradiated. A better way to use a Bluetooth is to keep the cell phone on a table several feet away from all body parts and to periodically move the earpiece from one ear to the other to minimize one-side radiation exposure.

•**Text instead of talk.** There's a burst of radiation when you send or receive a text message, but the intensity and duration of the radiation are lower than when you talk. Texting is a better alternative to talking on your cell phone, but keep the phone as far away from your body as possible. Normal clothing, including leather, will not reduce your exposure.

•**Don't use your phone in a car, train or bus.** Using a cell phone inside a metal vehicle can increase levels of radiation due to reflection and the fact that your cell-phone signal has to be higher to exit the vehicle. The best practice is to keep the phone off or in airplane mode and to check it periodically for messages. Then return messages by text or use a landline phone later.

■ ■ ■ ■

Cell-Phone Radiation Bad for Bones

Researchers examined the bones of 48 healthy men who carried cell phones.

Result: Men who carried cell phones on their hips were more likely to have lower mineral content and density in the upper thigh bones where the phones were placed.

Theory: Over time, the low levels of electromagnetic radiation emitted by cell phones appear to degrade the bone in the hip.

Self-defense: Avoid carrying your cell phone against any part of your body.

Fernando D. Saravi, MD, PhD, professor, department of morphology and physiology, National University of Cuyo, Mendoza, Argentina.

How Safe Are Full-Body Airport Scanners?

Mahadevappa Mahesh, PhD, associate professor of radiology and medicine, Johns Hopkins University School of Medicine, and chief physicist, Johns Hopkins Hospital, both in Baltimore.

The full-body scanners in airports are safe for everyone, including children and pregnant women. *Different airports use different scanner types…*

•**Millimeter radio wave scanners,** which look like glass booths, bombard travelers with radio waves and collect the reflected waves to generate images. The radio energy projected is tens of thousands of times lower than the energy of radio waves generated by cell phones.

•**Backscatter scanners, which resemble two refrigerators, are the source of most people's concern.** They use X-rays, but of a type that does not penetrate the body—the X-rays bounce off the body and are captured by detectors. This is fundamentally different from transmission X-rays, which are used in medical diagnosis. The radiation from backscatter systems is very low—a single scan is equal to about four to five minutes of air travel. An annual limit set by the Nuclear Regulatory Commission would be reached if a person undergoes 2,500 or 5,000 scans per year, which is highly improbable.

Bottom line: Both of the new scanning systems are safe for everyone, but passengers who remain worried are entitled to refuse a scan and have a thorough pat-down instead.

■ ■ ■ ■

Hospitals Make Misleading Claims About Robotic Surgery

Researchers studied 400 randomly chosen hospital Web sites to scrutinize their claims about robotic procedures, typically used in minimally invasive gynecological, heart and prostate surgeries.

Result: Most sites (89%) that made claims about robotic surgery cited clinical superiority over traditional surgery even though there is no scientific evidence that robotic surgery is always better than conventional surgery. No sites mentioned any risks. Most (73%) used promotions from the robots' manufacturers.

Marty Makary, MD, associate professor of surgery, Johns Hopkins University School of Medicine, Baltimore.

■ ■ ■ ■

Do You Need That MRI?

Did you know doctors who own or lease MRI equipment order more scans for low-back pain? The scan rate is 13% higher for patients of orthopedists and 32% higher for patients of primary care doctors who own the machines, compared with the rate for patients of doctors who don't own or lease the equipment.

Caution: There is no strong evidence that an MRI for nonspecific low-back pain improves long-term patient outcomes.

Jacqueline Baras Shreibati, MD, resident physician, Stanford University School of Medicine, California, and leader of a study published in *Health Services Research.*

■ ■ ■ ■

Where to Get the Best Care

States with the best hospital care at reasonable cost—North and South Dakota, followed by Pennsylvania, Nebraska and Iowa. At the bottom of the list are Texas, New Mexico, Arizona, California and Nevada. Rankings were based on the number of hospital beds per 1,000 people, medical staffing levels, average daily cost of inpatient care and average annual spending on health-care services.

Data analysis by Bundle.com, TheStreet.com and the Kaiser Family Health Foundation, published online at *www.bundle.com.*

America's Top Hospitals

Carey Gold, founder of The Health Advisory, a New York City–based medical consulting service that provides personalized medical advocacy to individuals faced with serious diagnoses, as well as undiagnosed symptoms. *www.thehealthadvisory.com*

If you or a loved one has been diagnosed with a serious medical condition, finding the right care can be a matter of life and death.

To identify the leading medical institutions in the country for various conditions, ranging from cancer and heart disease to Parkinson's disease and degenerative joint disease, we recently spoke with Carey Gold, a medical advocate who has provided expert guidance to individuals and families faced with serious medical diagnoses for the past 20 years.

Before traveling, obtain copies of all your pertinent medical records to take with you (or double-check to make sure that they have been forwarded). Also check with your insurance carrier about coverage and precertifications. If you are unable to travel, many of the institutions offer second opinions by mail and/or telephone.

Mr. Gold's recommendations for four key medical specialties (institutions are listed alphabetically)…

ONCOLOGY*

• **Dana-Farber/Brigham and Women's Cancer Center,** Boston, 877-332-4294, *www. dfbwcc.org.*

• **Johns Hopkins Medicine,** The Sidney Kimmel Comprehensive Cancer Center, Baltimore, 410-955-5000, *www.hopkinsmedicine.org/ kimmel_cancer_center/*

• **MD Anderson Cancer Center,** The University of Texas, Houston, 877-632-6789, *www. mdanderson.org.*

• **Memorial Sloan-Kettering Cancer Center,** New York City, 212-639-2000, *www.mskcc. org.*

Other excellent options: Mayo Clinic Cancer Center, Rochester, Minnesota…Duke Cancer Institute, Durham, North Carolina…University of California, Los Angeles, Jonsson Comprehensive Cancer Center…University of Pittsburgh Cancer Institute.

CARDIOLOGY AND CARDIOTHORACIC SURGERY

• **Cleveland Clinic,** The Heart & Vascular Institute, Cleveland, 800-659-7822, *www.mycleve landclinic.org/heart.*

• **Johns Hopkins Medicine,** The Heart and Vascular Institute, Baltimore, 410-955-5000, *www.hopkinsmedicine.org/heart_vascular_in stitute.*

• **Mayo Clinic,** Cardiovascular Diseases, Rochester, Minnesota, 507-284-2511, *www.mayo clinic.org/cardiovascular-disease-rst.*

• **St. Luke's Episcopal Hospital,** The Texas Heart Institute, Houston, 832-355-4011, *www. texasheartinstitute.org.*

Other excellent options: Massachusetts General Hospital Heart Center, Boston…New York–Presbyterian Hospital's Vivian and Seymour Milstein Family Heart Center and Ronald O. Perelman Heart Institute, New York City…Stanford Heart Center, Palo Alto, California…Duke Heart Center, Durham, North Carolina.

*When seeking cancer care, whenever possible, it's wise to look for one of the 40 institutions (such as those listed here) that have been designated by the National Cancer Institute as a Comprehensive Cancer Center.

NEUROLOGY AND NEUROSURGERY

•**Johns Hopkins Medicine,** Neurology and Neurosurgery, Baltimore, 410-955-5000, *www. hopkinsmedicine.org/neurology_neurosurgery.*

•**Massachusetts General Hospital,** Neurology and Neurosurgery, Boston, 617-726-5533, *www.massgeneral.org/neurology.*

•**New York–Presbyterian,** The Neurological Institute and Neuroscience Center, New York City, 212-305-2500, *www.nyp.org/services/neurology.html.*

•**University of California,** San Francisco, Neurological Disorders, San Francisco, 888-689-8273, *www.ucsfhealth.org/conditions/neurological_disorders.*

Other excellent options: Ken & Ruth Davee Department of Neurology at Northwestern University's Feinberg School of Medicine, Chicago...departments of neurology and neurosurgery at Duke University, Durham, North Carolina...Mayo Clinic, Rochester, Minnesota... University of Pittsburgh.

ORTHOPEDIC SURGERY

•**Cleveland Clinic,** The Orthopedic & Rheumatologic Institute, Cleveland, 800-223-2273, *www.myclevelandclinic.org/ortho.*

•**Hospital for Special Surgery,** New York City, 212-606-1000, *www.hss.edu.*

•**Johns Hopkins Medicine,** Orthopedic Surgery, Baltimore, 410-955-3870, *www.hopkinsortho.org.*

•**Mayo Clinic,** Orthopedic Surgery, Rochester, Minnesota, 507-284-2511, *www.mayoclinic.org/orthopedic-surgery.*

Other excellent options: Washington University Orthopedics in the Center for Advanced Medicine at Barnes–Jewish Hospital, St. Louis... departments of orthopedic surgery at Duke University, Durham, North Carolina...The University of Iowa, Iowa City...University of Pittsburgh... Massachusetts General Hospital, Boston.

How to Find the Best Hospital in Your Area

E. Wesley Ely, MD, MPH, professor of medicine and critical care, Vanderbilt University Medical Center, Nashville. Dr. Ely is the founder of Vanderbilt's ICU Delirium and Cognitive Impairment Study Group and associate director of aging research for the VA Tennessee Valley Geriatric Research and Education Clinical Center (GRECC).

You research the pros and cons and shop around before you buy a car—so why not compare local hospitals in case you, or someone close to you, becomes ill or has an accident? The Centers for Medicare & Medicaid Services (CMS) now reports hospital error rates on its Web site. The information is right there at *www.hospitalcompare.hhs.gov*, making it easy to see how the various medical centers in your area stack up against each other.

The above list shows that it's a good idea to track hospital error rates. E. Wesley Ely, MD, MPH, a professor and specialist in pulmonary and critical care medicine at Vanderbilt University Medical Center agrees—but, he adds, it's something that needs to be done very carefully for the benefit of both patients and the hospitals themselves.

For example: It's reasonable and helpful to hold hospitals responsible for mistakes such as transfusing the wrong blood type or leaving a foreign object in a patient during a surgical procedure—but it's not helpful to automatically blame hospitals when patients develop delirium after surgery, as the CMS originally proposed, because delirium is not always preventable. Fortunately, the CMS reversed its position on this condition, says Dr. Ely.

WHAT YOU NEED TO KNOW BEFORE YOU GO

To increase your odds of a safe and successful hospital stay, become an educated consumer...

•**Check hospital ratings.** Visit CMS's Web site and read about hospital errors. At *www.hospitalcompare.hhs.gov*, you can learn how satisfied other people were with their hospital stays...how closely hospitals followed best practices of care...how many people died within 30 days of hospitalization for a heart attack, heart failure or pneumonia…and 30-day readmission rates for these conditions.

●**Don't pay for their mistakes.** Medicare does not pay for treatment of conditions that result from hospitals' mistakes, and you don't have to either. If you develop any of the eight "Hospital Acquired Conditions" (as defined by CMS—visit *www.cms.gov* and search "hospital-acquired condition"), you can't be charged for the resulting necessary treatment, according to the Deficit Reduction Act of 2005.

●**Work with caregivers as a team.** For best results, Dr. Ely urges families to communicate closely with doctors, nurses and other health-care professionals. Provide caregivers with a complete list of all prescription and over-the-counter medications and supplements that the patient takes. Ask questions about the risks and potential benefits of treatment options, and speak up about any other concerns, such as a patient being sedated too deeply or for too many days. As well-meaning as most health-care professionals are, the demands of their jobs mean that a patient's quality of care isn't necessarily automatic.

Doctors Think Patients Get Over-Treated

Brenda Sirovich, MD, MS, staff physician and research associate, VA Outcomes Group, White River Junction, Vermont, and assistant professor, medicine, Dartmouth Medical School.

Calvin Chou, MD, PhD, professor of medicine, University of California, San Francisco, and general internist, San Francisco Veterans Affairs Medical Center.

Archives of Internal Medicine

When it comes to medical care, nearly half of US primary care physicians believe their own patients are over-treated.

A national mail survey of 627 doctors randomly selected from the American Medical Association Physician Masterfile showed that 42% believe patients in their own practice get too much medical care, while 52% think the amount of care is just right.

But only 6% believe their patients receive too little care, the survey found.

WHAT DOCTORS ARE SAYING ABOUT THEIR OWN PATIENTS

"Remember, these are patients in their own practice—that's an important part of the way we chose to ask the question," said study author Brenda Sirovich, MD, MS, a staff physician and research associate at the VA Outcomes Group in White River Junction, Vermont, and an assistant professor of community and family medicine at the Dartmouth Institute for Health Policy and Clinical Practice.

"Presumably these physicians have a hand in overseeing their patients' care," Dr. Sirovich added. "We believe that's a provocative finding. The most important thing we found is that primary care physicians see there's a problem with the excesses of the health care system, and successful reform would be much harder if successful physicians didn't see that and weren't engaged in the solution."

The study was published in the *Archives of Internal Medicine*.

STUDY DETAILS

Dr. Sirovich and her colleagues said several measures, including malpractice reforms or having more time with patients, could reduce pressure on doctors to offer more care than they feel is needed. Many health care epidemiologists and economists have suggested that a good amount of US health care is actually unnecessary, the study authors said.

The survey, conducted between June and December 2009, also found that 28% of respondents said they were practicing more aggressively—such as ordering more tests—than they would like, while 29% felt other primary care physicians in their community were practicing too aggressively.

Almost all said they believed that primary care physicians vary in patient testing and treatment, and three-quarters were interested in learning how their own practice compared with others.

Malpractice concerns drive many decisions to treat aggressively, the doctors said. More than 80% felt they could easily be sued for failing to order a test that was indicated, while 21% felt they could be sued for ordering a test that wasn't. Having too little time with patients was cited by 40% as another reason for aggressive treatment.

"The whole survey is based on their opinions and perceptions, and that's really what we were going after," Dr. Sirovich said. "Of course, there are limitations inherent in asking physicians what they themselves do…among them may be the natural desire to be viewed favorably, which is why we also asked about other physicians—which of course is speculative. That's the nature of the design of the study."

While few doctors said they order expensive treatments to boost their own income, nearly two-thirds suggested that other doctors might do so.

EXPERT COMMENTARY

In a commentary published with the study, Calvin Chou, MD, PhD, a professor of medicine at the University of California, San Francisco, said the findings imply a "trained helplessness" among physicians since they know they are practicing aggressively but feel they have no recourse.

"I would say most doctors probably feel somewhat helpless when they're expected to practice defensive medicine and check off a whole bunch of boxes," said Dr. Chou, also a general internist at San Francisco Veterans Affairs Medical Center. More and more, doctors feel like they're under the gun and are less likely to be able to meet the challenge it presents, he said. "I think it's possible, but it requires perspective."

"We were very intrigued that a large majority of physicians are interested in where they stand in relation to other physicians," Dr. Sirovich said. "We think that means they're open to feedback and to practicing differently."

Four Medical Tests and Treatments You Really Don't Need

Stephen R. Smith, MD, MPH, professor emeritus of family medicine and former associate dean of The Warren Alpert Medical School of Brown University in Providence.

If you're like most people, you assume that you need the tests and treatments that your doctor orders.

But that's not always true. According to a report from the National Physicians Alliance, some of the most frequently used tests and treatments often are unnecessary—and may be harmful. Even the common PSA test to detect prostate cancer has come under scrutiny recently (see page 243).

The excessive use of tests and treatments adds billions of dollars to the nation's spiraling health-care costs. And these can lead to further—and also unnecessary—testing if there's a false-positive, a reading that indicates an abnormality when everything actually is normal.

Why do doctors order questionable tests and treatments? One reason is habit. Doctors tend to do things the way they were taught in medical school even though new evidence shows that something isn't helpful. Also, many doctors practice "defensive medicine" to reduce the risk for lawsuits, assuming that a physician is unlikely to get sued for giving too much care.

If your doctor recommends any of the following tests and treatments, ask him/her whether they are really necessary and why…

UNNECESSARY TESTS

1. Imaging for low-back pain. Pain in the lower back is the fifth-most-common reason for doctor visits. Doctors routinely order MRIs of the lumbar spine when patients complain about back pain.

The problem: In the vast majority of cases, imaging tests are unnecessary. Low-back pain typically clears up without treatment in six weeks or less.

Exceptions: MRIs or other imaging tests may be needed for severe low-back pain or pain that lasts longer than six weeks…or when the symptoms include fever, incontinence, numbness and tingling.

2. Blood tests/urinalysis. When you have an annual exam, your doctor might order urine and/or blood tests. A urine test typically is used to check for diabetes. Blood chemistry panels are used to screen for diseases of the kidneys, liver and parathyroid gland, among many other things.

The problem: These tests rarely reveal anything in patients without symptoms who generally are healthy—and they often lead to false-positives.

Exceptions: Patients with specific symptoms—such as a persistent fever or tenderness in the abdomen—probably will need to have blood tests to determine the cause. A blood test also is recommended for checking cholesterol levels.

Urinalysis can be used to identify diabetes in patients who already have symptoms, such as frequent urination and/or increased thirst.

There may be other good reasons your doctor wants to order blood and/or urine tests, but he should be willing to explain to you exactly what those reasons are.

3. Cardiovascular screening. You don't need an annual electrocardiogram (EKG) if you don't have symptoms of, or risk factors for, heart disease (such as smoking, diabetes or a family history of cardiovascular disease).

The problem: Many doctors advise patients to have an EKG every year. My doctor used to recommend it for me, but in patients without symptoms, an EKG rarely reveals useful information. It may show a minor abnormality in the heartbeat that will lead to further tests, such as an echocardiogram or a stress test, even though these abnormalities rarely are important.

Exceptions: Patients who have been diagnosed with heart disease or who have significant risk factors for it probably will need an annual EKG or other cardiac tests.

4. Bone-density scan. More than 28 million Americans have osteoporosis, the leading cause of weak bones and fractures. A test called dual energy X-ray absorptiometry (DEXA) can detect bone weakness before a fracture occurs. This gives patients time to increase bone strength with exercise and vitamin D/calcium supplements.

The problem: The test doesn't make sense for younger patients with a low risk for osteoporosis. If you're a woman under age 65, you routinely should be taking calcium and vitamin D supplements and exercising to increase bone strength. The test itself won't change the treatment recommendations even if you test positive.

Exceptions: Women who are younger than 65 who have osteoporosis risk factors, such as smoking, a slight build, hyperthyroidism or a history of bone fractures, should have this test. So should men younger than age 70 with the same risk factors.

Women age 65 and older and men age 70 and older should have the DEXA screening even if they don't have risk factors. The DEXA test is important for these groups of people because they have a high risk for fractures and might benefit from medications.

■ ■ ■ ■

Critical Test Hospital Patients Need

All hospital patients should have their blood glucose levels checked, according to guidelines recently issued by the Endocrine Society.

Reason: Between 32% and 38% of hospitalized patients have hyperglycemia (high blood glucose), which increases risk for longer hospital stays, infections and death in those who are not critically ill.

If you are hospitalized: Be sure to get this test.

Guillermo E. Umpierrez, MD, professor of medicine, division of endocrinology, metabolism, Emory University School of Medicine, Atlanta.

■ ■ ■ ■

Compare the Cost of Your Medical Services

Compare the cost of medical services through state-sponsored Web sites that collect payment information and make it available online. A few states, including Maine and New Hampshire, have Web sites showing medical costs based on actual claims. Other states are expected to set up similar sites. You can see if your state has a Web site on the site of the All-Payer Claims Database Council (*www.apcdcouncil.org*).

If your state does not have a site yet: Try *fairhealthconsumer.org*, which offers typical figures for various locations…or Healthcare-BlueBook.com, which provides what it calls a fair price for services in a given area.

Also helpful: The American Medical Association's Medicare-reimbursement information (*www.amacodingonline.com*) shows what Medicare pays for services. You then can call providers in your area to find out how their charges compare.

The Wall Street Journal.

Community Hospitals Safe for Angioplasty

American College of Cardiology, news release

Angioplasty, a procedure to open blocked arteries, can be performed safely and effectively at community hospitals that don't have on-site cardiac surgery units, according to a recent study.

The study included nearly 19,000 patients who had elective angioplasty either at a facility with a cardiac surgery unit or at one of 60 community hospitals that didn't have on-site cardiac surgery but met certain requirements.

The centers had to complete a formal angioplasty development program to prepare their staffs and establish policies and protocols, and also had to demonstrate a capacity to perform at least 200 angioplasties a year.

The researchers followed the patients for nine months after their procedures. There was no difference in death rates between patients who underwent angioplasty at facilities with cardiac surgery units or at community hospitals, and no significant differences in rates of complications including bleeding, kidney failure and stroke.

"The study shows that under certain circumstances, non-primary angioplasty can be performed safely and effectively at hospitals without on-site cardiac surgery," lead investigator Thomas Aversano, MD, associate professor of medicine at Johns Hopkins University, said in an American College of Cardiology (ACC) news release.

Until recently, community hospitals without cardiac surgery units performed only emergency angioplasties. Patients who required elective surgery were transferred to facilities with cardiac surgery units. That changed when the ACC and the American Heart Association introduced new guidelines.

"The study supports and reinforces the [new] guidelines," Dr. Aversano said.

The study was presented at the ACC annual meeting in Chicago. Research presented at medical meetings should be viewed as preliminary until published in a peer-reviewed journal.

info The Radiological Society of North America/American College of Radiology has more information about angioplasty at its Web site, *http://www.radiologyinfo.org/en/info. cfm?pg=angioplasty.*

■ ■ ■ ■

Home Health Care Patients Over-Medicated!

Home health care is linked to unsafe medication use.

Recent study: A review of 3,124 adults ages 65 and older receiving home health care (from visiting nurses, for example) found that nearly 40% were taking at least one drug considered inappropriate for seniors—twice as high as older adults who did not receive home health care.

Possible reason: Home-health-care patients tend to take more drugs than similarly aged adults. These drugs are often prescribed by a variety of doctors, with little coordination regarding the drugs taken by a patient.

Yuhua Bao, PhD, assistant professor of public health, Weill Cornell Medical College, New York City.

....

Don't Let the Bedbugs Kill You

More than 100 people were sickened by the insecticides between 2003 and 2010—and one person died.

Reasons for the illnesses: Overuse of the insecticides…failing to wash or change bedding that had been treated with the insecticides.

Self-defense: Call in a certified professional to handle a bedbug problem.

Naomi L. Hudson, DrPH, Epidemic Intelligence Service Office, Centers for Disease Control and Prevention, Atlanta, and coauthor of a study published in *Morbidity and Mortality Weekly Report.*

E. Coli in Chicken Linked to Urinary Tract Infections

Amee Manges, PhD, MPH, department of epidemiology, biostatistics and occupational health, McGill University, Montreal.
Philip Tierno, PhD, director, clinical microbiology and immunology, NYU Langone Medical Center, New York City.
Elizabeth Kavaler, MD, urologist, Lenox Hill Hospital, New York City.
Emerging Infectious Diseases, online

Scientists have long believed that urinary tract infections are typically caused by a person's own E. coli bacteria, but a recent Canadian study suggests the bacteria may more often than not come from chickens.

Yes, chickens.

As many as 85% of urinary tract infections are caused by *Escherichia coli* (E. coli). Researchers compared the genetic fingerprints of E. coli from these infections with that of E. coli from chicken, beef and pork. And they found a match: chicken. What's more, they report that the infections probably came directly from the chickens, not from human contamination during food processing.

The Canadian study was published in *Emerging Infectious Diseases*, a publication of the US Centers for Disease Control and Prevention.

FOOD ANIMAL PRODUCTION UNDER FIRE

"Chicken may be a reservoir for the E. coli that cause infections like urinary tract infections," said study author Amee Manges, PhD, MPH, department of epidemiology, biostatistics and occupational health at McGill University in Montreal.

"We are also concerned about the selection and amplification of drug-resistant E. coli on the farms because of improper or overuse of antimicrobials during food animal production. It may be possible to reduce the level of drug-resistant infections in humans by encouraging rational and judicious use of antimicrobials on farms," Dr. Manges said.

"We just want to emphasize that it isn't just inappropriate use of antibiotics in human medicine that matters, but also the use of antibiotics in veterinary medicine and food production that leads to greater drug-resistant bugs," the study author added.

The US Food and Drug Administration already advises against the overuse of antibiotics in livestock because it can lead to resistant strains of bacteria.

EXPERT REPLY AND RECOMMENDATIONS

Philip Tierno, PhD, director of clinical microbiology and immunology at NYU Langone Medical Center in New York City, said it is not surprising that the food supply, especially chicken, may play a role in causing urinary tract and other infections. He said the best protection begins with proper hygiene.

"If you practice good personal hygiene, good food hygiene and good home hygiene, we can reduce the number of infections," he suggested.

Proper hand washing should last for 20 seconds. "Wash in between your [fingers] and under your nails," Dr. Tierno said. "When dealing with counter surfaces, use a product that can disinfect surfaces and prevent cross-contamination."

Cooking also helps kill disease-causing bugs. "Eat nothing raw. Cook it well, and if you are eating vegetables, make sure to soak them and wash them well," he said.

The solution is definitely not to throw more antibiotics at livestock, Dr. Tierno agreed. As far as preventing E. coli in chicken coops, "we need to develop a better system to raise chickens so they are not in crowded conditions and prone to diseases like E. coli," he explained.

Good hygiene is never a bad idea, but the truth is that E. coli is everywhere, said Elizabeth Kavaler, MD, urologist at Lenox Hill Hospital in New York City.

"The best defense against urinary tract infections is to exercise, eat well and get proper sleep so your immune system is strong and can fend off what you can't see, including E. coli," she said. "Be healthy, wash your hands, take care of yourself and when you have a urinary tract infection, see your doctor for an antibiotic to treat it."

info For more information about food safety, visit the Web site of the US Department of Agriculture (*http://www.fsis.usda.gov/food_safety_education/index.asp*).

Poison Found in Some Organic Foods

Brian Jackson, PhD, director, Trace Element Analysis Core Facility, Dartmouth College, Hanover, New Hampshire.

Connie Diekman, director, university nutrition, Washington University, St. Louis.

Environmental Health Perspectives

A sweetener used in many organic foods may be a hidden source of arsenic, a recent study suggests.

Researchers at Dartmouth College also noted that the sweetener, organic brown rice syrup, is found in some infant formulas. Their report appears in the journal *Environmental Health Perspectives*.

Arsenic is a natural element that can contaminate groundwater. As the Dartmouth team explained, rice may be particularly prone to contamination because it pulls in arsenic from soil. There are no federal limits currently set for arsenic levels in food, although there are limits set for arsenic levels in water.

STUDY DETAILS

Study author Brian Jackson, PhD, director of the Trace Element Analysis Core Facility at Dartmouth, set out to determine the concentrations of arsenic in commercial food products containing organic brown rice syrup, including infant formula, cereal/energy bars and high-energy foods used by athletes. Dr. Jackson and his colleagues bought commercial food products containing organic brown rice syrup and compared them with similar products that did not have rice syrup in them.

In all, 17 infant formulas, 29 cereal bars and three energy shots were all purchased from local stores in the Hanover (New Hampshire) area.

Of the 17 infant milk formulas tested, two had listed organic brown rice syrup as the primary ingredient. These two formulas, one dairy-based and one soy-based, had arsenic levels that were more than 20 times greater than the other formulas, the researchers found.

One of the infant formulas had a total arsenic concentration that was six times the US Environmental Protection Agency's safe drinking water limit of 10 parts per billion (ppb) for total arsenic. The amount of inorganic arsenic, the most toxic form, averaged 8.6 parts ppb for the dairy-based formula and 21.4 ppb for the soy formula, the study said.

Cereal bars and high-energy foods using organic brown rice syrup also had higher arsenic concentrations than those without the syrup, the study showed.

"The baby formula findings are concerning," Dr. Jackson said. Infants and people who eat gluten-free diets, which are largely rice-based, are most at risk for consuming too much arsenic via food, he explained, while "the risk for the occasional cereal bar eater is low."

INDUSTRY RESPONSE

The Organic Trade Association said that the findings "add to a growing body of evidence supporting the conclusion that arsenic dietary exposures pose a serious food safety problem… Regardless of how it is raised, rice plants growing in soils still contaminated with arsenic will extract the element from the soil, and some will be present in the grain harvested from those plants."

"The Organic Trade Association [OTA] agrees with the researchers that it is time for the US Food and Drug Administration and US Environmental Protection Agency to work together to set and enforce regulatory limits on arsenic in our food supply. Both the government and food industry must determine now whether any consumer food products containing brown rice sugar, whether conventional or organic, contain arsenic levels high enough to justify product recalls or changes in ingredients," the association said in its statement. "Any rice product destined for baby food or children's food should come only from regions known to have arsenic-free soils. Prevention is a core principle of organic farming and food processing, and will drive the response to this new challenge across the organic food industry."

ARSENIC IN THE NEWS

This isn't the first time arsenic levels in foods have made the headlines.

Mehmet Oz, MD, host of "The Dr. Oz Show," caused a public health stir in 2011 when he reported that roughly one-third of apple juice samples he'd tested had arsenic levels exceeding 10 parts per billion, the limit for drinking water. At first, Dr. Oz was criticized by the US Food and Drug Administration, but his findings were later confirmed by a *Consumer Reports* study that showed many apple and grape juice samples tested were tainted with arsenic.

IS THERE A CONCERN FOR CONSUMERS?

What exactly are the health risks with arsenic?

"All we can fall back on is what we know about exposure through drinking water—risk of certain cancers or heart disease are slightly elevated in drinking water with a certain level of arsenic," Dr. Jackson said. "Moms should know that these rice-based formulas may contain arsenic and should limit exposure. Look at the ingredients when you purchase formula."

Connie Diekman, director of university nutrition at Washington University in St. Louis, said consumers shouldn't panic over the Dartmouth findings.

"As a registered dietitian, I would encourage consumers to not worry about this study, but to use it as a reminder that foods that grow in soil are growing with a wide variety of chemicals, both those found naturally in the soil and those that may be there from use of chemicals to foster growth," she said. "Whether the amount of any one chemical is enough to worry about is still a question that needs better research. Focusing on single foods as 'dangerous' or 'harmful' ignores how those foods impact the whole diet.

"Whether organic foods contain more arsenic, or other minerals, than conventional foods is hard to estimate, but this study does remind us that 'organic' is not necessarily equal to 'healthier or better for you' or 'safe from harm'," she added. "Ask a registered dietitian to help decipher new studies, and how those studies translate to their individual eating goals."

info For more about arsenic in foods and drinks visit the Web site of the US Food and Drug Administration (*www.fda.gov*, search "arsenic").

■ ■ ■ ■

Harmful Soup Ingredient

How much BPA is in that soup can? Consuming a 12-ounce serving of canned soup daily for five days led to a 1,000% increase in the amount of the chemical bisphenol A (BPA) in urine, say researchers from Harvard School of Public Health. The study did not look at how increased BPA affected health, but other research has shown a link between BPA and reproductive problems, neurological disorders and heart disease. Look for soup sold in BPA-free, plastic-coated paper cartons, commonly used for milk and other liquids.

Mark A. Stengler, NMD, naturopathic medical doctor in private practice, Encinitas, California...adjunct associate clinical professor at the National College of Natural Medicine, Portland, Oregon...author of *The Natural Physician's Healing Therapies* and coauthor of *Prescription for Natural Cures* (both from Bottom Line Books).

■ ■ ■ ■

St. John's Wort Alert

St. John's wort may be contaminated with lead or cadmium.

Recent finding: Nearly half the bottles of St. John's wort tested contained these toxins, which can naturally accumulate in this herb. Cadmium is a carcinogen and kidney toxin, while lead can affect mental functioning. Other bottles of St. John's wort were found to have less of the active ingredient than stated on the labels. St. John's wort may help battle mild-to-moderate forms of depression by increasing levels of mood-enhancing brain chemicals.

Best brand in the study: Nature's Bounty Double Strength.

Study of 10 brands of St. John's wort by ConsumerLab, 333 Mamaroneck Ave., White Plains, New York 10605. *www.consumerlab.com*

■ ■ ■ ■

Dead Sea Salts Can Be "Deadly"

The safety of evaporated seawater depends on what was in the water before it evaporated. Water from the Dead Sea has the highest concentration of bromide of any large body of water, and bromide can be toxic in large amounts.

Recent case: After consuming three to four tablespoons daily of Dead Sea salts that he bought through a Web site, a man sought medical care because he became confused and disoriented and was slurring his speech. He was diagnosed with bromide poisoning.

The American Journal of Medicine

■ ■ ■ ■

Antibiotic Creams May Increase MRSA Resistance

Over-the-counter triple-antibiotic creams and ointments, such as Medi-Quik and Neosporin, seem to be leading to the emergence of a form of methicillin-resistant Staphylococcus aureus (MRSA) that resists bacitracin and neomycin—two of the antibiotics found in the creams.

Self-defense: Washing with soap and water is all that many scrapes and cuts require. If you do use an antibiotic cream, apply only a small amount and use it for as short a time as possible.

William Schaffner, MD, professor of preventive medicine, Vanderbilt University School of Medicine, Nashville, commenting on a study by Japanese researchers, published in *Emerging Infectious Diseases*.

An Assistance Dog May Be Just What You Need

Marcie Davis, coauthor of *Working Like Dogs: The Service Dog Guidebook* (Alpine). She is cofounder of Working Like Dogs, LLC, a Santa Fe, New Mexico–based organization dedicated to honoring and celebrating assistance dogs around the world.

For more than 35 years, I have relied on a wheelchair for mobility, because I am paralyzed from the waist down. But while a wheelchair gets me from point A to point B, I often require assistance with daily tasks, such as getting in and out of bed, answering the phone, picking up dropped items, turning light switches on and off and more.

That's where Whistle comes in. Half Labrador retriever, half golden retriever, Whistle is my service dog and companion, trained to do everything from picking up a dime off the floor, to retrieving the last sock in the dryer, to helping me roll over in the middle of the night.

While most people are familiar with guide dogs that assist individuals who are blind or have partial vision loss, there are a variety of assistance dogs trained to help those impacted by hearing loss, spinal cord injury, multiple sclerosis, epilepsy, psychiatric illness, diabetes and many more medical conditions…

•**Service dogs assist their human owners by carrying or retrieving items,** pushing buttons (for example, on an elevator), opening and closing drawers, assisting with balance while dressing, helping with household chores and more.

•**Hearing alert dogs alert individuals with hearing loss to specific sounds,** including phones, doorbells, sirens, smoke alarms, crying babies or other humans.

•**Seizure alert/seizure response dogs respond to epileptic seizures**—they may be trained to pull an emergency cord, lick their owner's face (to arouse him/her) or retrieve the phone (or push a call button) for a 911 call. Dogs can be trained to help with other chronic medical conditions as well, such as heart attacks, strokes and panic attacks. Some dogs possess the ability to predict a medical event such as a seizure or detect changes in blood sugar and will become restless or push against their partners to warn them.

COMPANIONSHIP AND SECURITY

Assistance dogs provide true companionship and an invaluable sense of security. I considered myself independent until I met my first service dog, Ramona, in 1993. Yet before that, I wasn't driving—I was too worried about dropping my keys in a parking lot and not being able to pick them up…or of falling while getting in and out of my car. Ramona empowered me to get behind the wheel.

If you have a medical condition and think an assistance dog may be for you, ask yourself, *Could having an assistance dog enable me to be more independent? If the answer might be yes,* consider whether…

•**You can physically care for a dog.**

•**You are able to care for the dog** or provide alternative care through a family member or friend.

•**You can afford the dog.** This includes food, pet insurance and veterinary care. Keep in mind that an assistance dog requires more frequent vet visits and higher-quality food than a regular pet.

Contact different assistance dog training agencies to find out their policies and which will meet your needs best. Visit my organization's site, *www.workinglikedogs.com*, for a list or try the sites of Assistance Dogs International (*www.assistancedogsinternational.org*) for certified assistance dog agencies and International Association of Assistance Dog Partners (*www.iaadp.org*), an advocacy group for people with disabilities who use assistance dogs.

What to consider: How quickly will you be able to bring home a new dog? Will you ultimately own the dog, or does the agency retain ownership? What up-front costs are involved?

Some agencies offer dogs for free, and others may charge more than $15,000.

GETTING YOUR DOG

If you decide to use an assistance dog training agency, you'll need proof of your disability (your physician can provide this) and will have to complete a written application, interview and home visit. Potential owners may need to be able to travel to and stay at the training facility, where they'll often participate in a multiweek "boot camp" with their dogs. And of course, it takes time to "learn" your dog—for example, its temperament and how it responds to commands. It took my first dog and me one year to truly feel in sync…with my second dog, the bond was instantaneous. It can take up to a year or longer to complete the entire process.

Owning any animal is a serious commitment. But the daily care and financial responsibilities pale in comparison to the new freedom, security and companionship you'll experience.

■ ■ ■ ■

Rx for Drug Shortages

A record number of drugs, including certain medications for cancer, high blood pressure and anxiety, were not available in 2010 due to manufacturing and quality problems, production delays and products being taken off the market. The trend continued in 2011. Although conditions improved in 2012, shortages still occur. Ask your doctor whether any prescriptions you take may be in short supply in the future. If so, ask if an alternative within the same class of drugs can be prescribed if needed. The FDA maintains an up-to-date listing of current shortages at *www.fda.gov/drugs/drugsafety/drugshortages*.

Unfortunately, a drug shortage could lead to a rise in drug counterfeiting.

To protect yourself: Purchase your prescriptions from reliable sources, and always examine the product, its packaging and the color of the tablets or capsules. Report any changes in the appearance, taste or drug side effects to the FDA.

Jack E. Fincham, PhD, RPh, professor, division of pharmacy practice and administration, University of Missouri–Kansas City School of Pharmacy.

Dental X-Rays May Be Linked to Brain Tumors

Elizabeth Claus, MD, PhD, neurosurgeon, Brigham & Women's Hospital, Boston, and professor, epidemiology, Yale University School of Medicine, New Haven, Connecticut.

Isabelle Germano, MD, professor, neurosurgery, and director, Comprehensive Brain Tumor Program, Mount Sinai School of Medicine, New York City.

Matthew Messina, DDS, dentist and spokesman, American Dental Association, Cleveland.

Cancer

People who underwent frequent dental X-rays in the past, before radiation doses were lowered, may be at greater risk for a usually benign form of tumor in the lining of the brain, called *meningiomas*, a recent study suggests.

Meningiomas affect the lining of the brain and the spinal cord. More than 90% are classified as benign, not malignant. But in some cases they can grow to the size of a baseball and disrupt the brain's functioning, leading to vision problems, headaches, hearing and memory loss, and seizures. Neurosurgeons often try to remove them in the most severe cases.

"They cause problems as soon as they achieve a certain size, because there is no room in the skull to accommodate growth. Any growth that is more than a couple centimeters can result in symptoms," explained Isabelle Germano, MD, director of the Comprehensive Brain Tumor Program at Mount Sinai School of Medicine in New York City.

The recent research doesn't definitively link dental X-rays to the tumors, which affect about 1% of people. It's also possible that dental X-rays, which are now given at a lower radiation dose, have nothing to do with the tumors.

Still, the study suggests that dental X-rays could be a risk factor for the tumors, said study author Elizabeth Claus, MD, PhD, a neurosurgeon at Brigham & Women's Hospital in Boston and a professor of epidemiology at Yale University School of Medicine.

STUDY DETAILS

In the study, researchers sought to determine whether dental X-rays are connected to menin-giomas that affect the lining of the brain specifically.

The researchers examined a group of more than 1,400 patients ages 20 to 79 who were treated for the tumors between 2006 and 2011, and compared them with 1,350 similar people who did not develop the tumors. The average age in both groups was about 57.

Those with tumors were more than twice as likely as the others to report having more frequent bitewing X-rays (at any time) and panorex X-rays (especially at a young age).

Bitewing X-rays allow views of the back teeth—patients bite onto a tab during the X-rays. Panorex X-rays show the whole area in and around the mouth from below the nose to the chin.

The design of the study didn't allow the researchers to specify the level of increased risk of a tumor that a person who's had dental X-rays would conceivably face. It does appear, however, that the raised risk would remain low, Dr. Claus said.

Overall, more than 92% of people in the study reported having had at least one bitewing X-ray.

The findings suggest that patients should talk to their dentists about the possible dangers of X-rays and be aware of national recommendations regarding their use, Dr. Claus pointed out.

"I do not get the feeling that people are aware of those guidelines," she said. "Many people are having them every six months or every year when the American Dental Association is saying once every two to three years." (That's the recommendation for the patient who's never had a cavity or only a small number of fillings and isn't at increased risk for a cavity.)

The study appeared in the journal *Cancer*.

EXPERT COMMENT

Matthew Messina, DDS, a Cleveland dentist and spokesman for the American Dental Association, said one weakness of the study is that people's memories about their X-rays are fuzzy.

"It's difficult to pin this down," he said, especially without dental records.

Dr. Messina added that the amount of radiation in dental X-rays has gone down significantly over the years, thanks to factors such as the improved speed of X-ray film and the advent of digital X-rays.

The study was also observational in nature, meaning it can show an association but not cause-and-effect.

So what should patients do?

Dr. Germano concurred with Dr. Claus that adult patients and parents of child patients should talk to their dentists about X-rays.

"It's always important to discuss what the X-ray is for and what the advantage is. It's not a good idea to assume that X-rays are a benign procedure," she said.

Dr. Messina also agreed. "It's always good for patients to talk to their dentists about why they're getting X-rays and what is being done to shield the patient."

Overall, dentists are trying to balance the possible dangers of radiation and the usefulness of X-rays, Dr. Messina said. "We take dental X-rays because we're trying to make sure the person is healthy or trying to diagnose what's wrong with them."

info For more about brain tumors, including meningiomas, visit the US National Library of Medicine Web site at *www.nlm.nih. gov/medlineplus/ency/article/007222.htm.*

■ ■ ■ ■

Dangerous Tooth Pain Gels And Sprays

These products containing benzocaine are sold over the counter to relieve pain from teething or canker sores, for example. They can lead to *methemo-globinemia*—a potentially fatal condition in which the amount of oxygen in the bloodstream is reduced—even after a single use. Symptoms, which include pale, gray or blue-colored skin, lips and nail beds…headache…light-headedness…rapid heart rate…fatigue…and shortness of breath, usually appear within hours of application. If affected, seek medical attention immediately.

Family Safety & Health, National Safety Council, 1121 Spring Lake Dr., Itasca, Illinois 60143. *www.nsc.org*

■ ■ ■ ■

Concerned About Mercury in Your Mouth? Ask for This Instead…

Ask your dentist about porcelain if you need to have a tooth filled but are concerned about amalgam.

Recent development: An FDA advisory committee has recommended that the agency review its 2009 ruling stating that the mercury from amalgam fillings poses no safety risk. The American Dental Association maintains that amalgam fillings are safe, but new data has raised additional concerns that mercury vapors from these fillings may harm the body—especially the brain and kidneys.

If you prefer not to receive an amalgam filling: Discuss options with your dentist. Porcelain is superior to resin because it does not degrade over time the way resin can.

Alan Winter, DDS, periodontist in private practice, New York City.

■ ■ ■ ■

Illegal Chelation Products

Over-the-counter chelation products sold online are illegal. Genuine chelation—available only with a prescription—is used to treat people who have been poisoned with heavy metals, such as lead and mercury. Sellers of online products falsely claim that their products can be used to treat autism, heart disease and other chronic diseases.

Warning: Chelation can cause dehydration, kidney failure and even death and should always be supervised by a health-care professional.

Michael Levy, MD, director, FDA division of new drugs and labeling compliance, Washington, DC. *www.fda.gov*

■ ■ ■ ■

Cancer-Causing Home-Building Material

A common home-building material may cause cancer. Formaldehyde typically is found in plywood, particleboard and other wood composites, such as medium-density fiberboard (MDF) used to make furnishings and in housing construction. It has been officially identified by the National Institutes of Health as a possible cause of cancer.

Self-defense: Buy formaldehyde-free products, such as ones made of solid wood, or products labeled ULEF (ultra-low-emitting formaldehyde). The half-life of formaldehyde emissions is about one year, so if products have been in your home for many years, current off-gassing may be negligible.

Richard J. Shaughnessy, PhD, program manager, The University of Tulsa Indoor Air Program, Oklahoma.

■ ■ ■ ■

Avoid Using Airplane Restrooms

Restrooms on airplanes are rarely sanitized during flights and often are infected with E. coli and other harmful bacteria. If you have to use the bathroom, use a paper towel to open and close the toilet lid…turn faucets off and on…and open the door. When you get back to your seat, use sanitizer to disinfect your hands.

Peter Sheldon, vice president of operations and development, Coverall Health-Based Cleaning System, franchisor of commercial cleaning businesses, Deerfield Beach, Florida. *www.coverall.com*

■ **More from Peter Sheldon…**

Items to Clean in Your Hotel Room

Clean your hotel room's TV remote, alarm clock and ice bucket before using them. These items are rarely cleaned by housekeepers.

Also likely to be covered in germs: The steering wheel and gearshift of a rental car.

■ ■ ■ ■

When "Green" Doesn't Mean Good

Avoid scented cleaning and laundry products. Even products that claim to be "green," "organic" or "natural" may emit hazardous chemicals.

Recent finding: Nearly one-quarter of chemicals emitted by scented household products, such as air fresheners, detergents, fabric softeners and disinfectants, are classified as toxic or hazardous…and more than one-third of products tested emitted at least one chemical identified as a probable carcinogen.

To avoid potentially dangerous chemicals: Clean with baking soda and/or vinegar…open windows for ventilation instead of using air fresheners…and buy products without any fragrance.

Anne Steinemann, PhD, professor of civil and environmental engineering and public affairs, University of Washington, Seattle, and lead author of study of 25 fragranced consumer products, published in *Environmental Impact Assessment Review.*

Diabetes

Say Good-Bye to Your Diabetes Medication

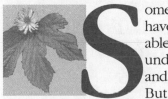

Some of my patients who have type 2 diabetes are able to keep the disease under control with diet and exercise. Lucky them! But for other diabetes patients, that's not enough and they must take pharmaceutical medications.

There is another natural treatment option for diabetes patients who currently take pharmaceutical medications. Research has found that a plant extract called *berberine* can control diabetes as well as, or better than, common medications such as *metformin* (Glucophage) and *rosiglitazone* (Avandia). And it does this with no side effects—and without damaging the liver, as some medications do. *Here's how berberine can help people with diabetes...*

A naturally occurring chemical compound, berberine is found in the roots and stems of several plants, including *Hydrastis canadensis* (goldenseal), *Coptis chinensis* (coptis or gold-thread) and *Berberis aquifolium* (Oregon grape). Long used as a remedy in Chinese and Ayurvedic medicines, berberine is known for its antimicrobial properties and as a treatment for bacterial and fungal infections. Several decades ago, berberine was used to treat diarrhea in patients in China. That was when doctors noticed that the blood sugar levels of diabetes patients were lower after taking the herbal extract—and berberine began to be investigated for this purpose.

Over the past 20 years, there has been much research on berberine and its effectiveness in treating diabetes. In 2008, Chinese researchers published a study in *Metabolism* in which adults with newly diagnosed type 2 diabetes were given 500 milligrams (mg) of either berberine or the drug metformin three times a day for

Mark A. Stengler, NMD, naturopathic medical doctor in private practice, Encinitas, California...adjunct associate clinical professor at the National College of Natural Medicine, Portland, Oregon...author of *The Natural Physician's Healing Therapies* and coauthor of *Prescription for Natural Cures* (both from Bottom Line Books).

three months. Researchers found that berberine did as good a job as metformin at regulating glucose metabolism, as indicated by hemoglobin A1C (a measure of blood glucose over several weeks)…fasting blood glucose…blood sugar after eating…and level of insulin after eating. Berberine even reduced the amount of insulin needed to turn glucose into energy by 45%! In addition, those taking berberine had noticeably lower trigylceride and total cholesterol levels than those taking metformin.

In a 2010 study in *Metabolism*, Chinese researchers compared people with type 2 diabetes who took either 1,000 mg daily of berberine or daily doses of metformin or rosiglitazone. After two months, berberine had lowered subjects' fasting blood glucose levels by an average of about 30%, an improvement over the rosiglitazone group and almost as much as people in the metformin group. Berberine also reduced subjects' hemoglobin A1C by 18%—equal to rosiglitazone and, again, almost as good as metformin. In addition, berberine lowered serum insulin levels by 28.2% (indicating increased insulin sensitivity)…lowered triglycerides by 17.5%…and actually improved liver enzyme levels. Pharmaceutical medications, on the other hand, have the potential to harm the liver.

These were remarkable findings. Here was a botanical that was holding up to scientific scrutiny—and performing as well as, or better than, some drugs that patients had been taking for diabetes for years.

HOW BERBERINE WORKS IN THE BODY

Berberine helps to lower blood glucose in several ways. One of its primary mechanisms involves stimulating the activity of the genes responsible for manufacturing and activating insulin receptors, which are critical for controlling blood glucose.

Berberine also has an effect on blood sugar regulation through activation of *incretins*, gastrointestinal hormones that affect the amount of insulin released by the body after eating.

HOW BERBERINE CAN HELP

I recommend berberine to my patients with newly diagnosed type 2 diabetes to reduce their blood sugar and prevent them from needing pharmaceutical drugs. When a diet, exercise and supplement program (including supplements such as chromium) is already helping a diabetes patient, I don't recommend that he/she switch to berberine.

Some patients are able to take berberine—and make dietary changes—and stop taking diabetes drugs altogether. People with severe diabetes can use berberine in conjunction with medication—and this combination treatment allows for fewer side effects and better blood sugar control. I don't recommend berberine for prediabetes unless diet and exercise are not effective. Berberine is sold in health-food stores and online in tablet and capsule form. The dosage I typically recommend for all diabetes patients is 500 mg twice daily.

For patients with diabetes who want to use berberine, I recommend talking to your doctor about taking this supplement. It's also important for every patient with diabetes to participate in a comprehensive diet and exercise program.

Note that berberine helps patients with type 2 diabetes, not type 1 diabetes (in which the body does not produce enough insulin).

New Stem Cell Treatment May Help Those with Type 1 Diabetes

Yong Zhao, MD, PhD, assistant professor, section of endocrinology, diabetes and metabolism, department of medicine, University of Illinois at Chicago.

Luca Inverardi, MD, deputy director of translational research at the Diabetes Research Institute, University of Miami School of Medicine.

A new type of stem cell treatment for people with type 1 diabetes appears to help re-educate rogue immune system cells, which allows cells in the pancreas to start producing insulin again.

The treatment, which combines a patient's immune system cells with stem cells from a donor's umbilical cord blood, even worked in people with long-standing diabetes who were believed to have no insulin-producing ability.

Although the treatment didn't wean anyone off insulin completely, average blood sugar levels dropped significantly, which reduces the risk of long-term complications.

"Our study brings a new hope for people with type 1 diabetes. If we can control the autoimmunity, we may reverse the diabetes. We showed that the islets [cells] can start to work again," said Yong Zhao, MD, PhD, assistant professor, endocrinology, diabetes and metabolism at the University of Illinois at Chicago.

Results of the study were published in the journal *BMC Medicine*.

This treatment could potentially be useful in other autoimmune diseases, such as lupus and rheumatoid arthritis.

HOW THE TREATMENT WORKS

Dr. Zhao's team developed a completely new approach. They take blood from a patient and separate out the immune system cells (lymphocytes). They briefly expose those cells to stem cells from umbilical cord blood from an unrelated infant and return the lymphocytes alone to the patient's body. The researchers have dubbed this "Stem Cell Educator Therapy" because while exposed to the stem cells, the lymphocytes seem to relearn how they should behave.

The study participants, who were 15 to 41 years old, had type 1 diabetes for an average of nine years. Six had some residual beta cell function and six did not. Both groups were given stem cell educator therapy. The other three people served as the control group.

The researchers measured C-peptide, a protein fragment that's a byproduct of insulin production, and found that the educator therapy group had improved levels of C-peptide at 12 weeks. These levels continued to improve until 24 weeks, and remained stable through the follow-up at 40 weeks. There were no changes in C-peptide in the control group.

EXPERT COMMENTARY: WELCOME NEWS

"It's quite remarkable that this approach, based on the re-education of immune cells, might work so well. The concept is very intriguing, and the treatment seems to be so simple and so safe," said Luca Inverardi, MD, deputy director of translational research at the Diabetes Research Institute, University of Miami School of Medicine.

But he's also "reasonably cautious," he said. "The follow-up is long, up to 40 weeks, but it's not long enough to declare victory against diabetes yet," said Dr. Inverardi.

Also, he noted that the study involved only 15 Chinese participants, and that type 1 diabetes is a bit different in that population. He said he'd like to see larger studies with a more diverse population, followed over a longer period of time.

For Dr. Zhao's study, the average daily dose of insulin dropped almost 39% after 12 weeks for the group with some beta cell function and 25% in those with no beta cell function, suggesting that the group with no beta cell function now produced insulin.

"That means if you stop the autoimmune reaction, you may see beta cell regeneration, or there might be other precursor cells in the pancreas. If these data are confirmed, this is a very provocative and remarkable finding," Dr. Inverardi said.

This was an initial clinical trial designed to test for safety. Dr. Zhao said that in future trials he hopes that with additional treatments people might get off insulin altogether.

But, even if that's not possible, the recovery of some beta cell function would be welcome news. "In the absence of complete remission, there are very sizable advantages to having some beta cell function," Dr. Inverardi noted.

Both experts said the treatment appears safe, with no risk of rejection. No significant side effects were reported during the trial, other than some arm soreness where blood was taken and returned.

info Learn more about type 1 diabetes from the American Diabetes Association. Visit its Web site at *http://www.diabetes.org/diabetes-basics/type-1/*.

Hidden Diabetes—You Can Be Healthy...But at High Risk

Mark Hyman, MD, founder and medical director of The UltraWellness Center in Lenox, Massachusetts, www. DrHyman.com. Dr. Hyman is author of several books, including The Blood Sugar Solution: The UltraHealthy Program for Losing Weight, Preventing Disease, and Feeling Great Now! (Little, Brown).

With all the devastating complications of diabetes, such as heart disease, stroke, dementia and blindness, you might assume that most doctors are doing everything possible to catch this disease in its earliest stages. Not so.

Problem: There are currently no national guidelines for screening and treating diabetes before it reaches a full-blown stage.

Research clearly shows that the damage caused by diabetes begins years—and sometimes decades—earlier, but standard medical practice has not yet caught up with the newest findings on this disease.

Fortunately, there are scientifically proven ways to identify and correct the root causes of diabetes so that you never develop the disease itself.

WHEN THE PROBLEM STARTS

Diabetes is diagnosed when blood sugar (glucose) levels reach 126 mg/dL and above. "Prediabetes" is defined as blood sugar levels that are higher than normal but not high enough to indicate diabetes. Normal levels are less than 100 mg/dL.

What most people don't know: Although most doctors routinely test blood sugar to detect diabetes, it's quite common to have a normal level and still have "diabesity," a condition typically marked by obesity and other changes in the body that can lead to the same complications (such as heart disease, stroke and cancer) as full-fledged diabetes.

Important: Even if you're not diabetic, having "belly fat"—for example, a waist circumference of more than 35 inches in women and more than 40 inches in men—often has many of the same dangerous effects on the body as diabetes.

Important finding: In a landmark study in Europe, researchers looked at 22,000 people and found that those with blood sugar levels of just 95 mg/dL—a level that's generally considered healthy—already had significant risks for heart disease and other complications.

AN EARLIER CLUE

Even though we've all been told that high blood sugar is the telltale sign of diabetes, insulin levels are, in fact, a more important hallmark that a person is in the early stages of the "diabetes continuum."

High blood sugar is typically blamed on a lack of insulin—or insulin that doesn't work efficiently. However, too much insulin is actually the best marker of the stages leading up to prediabetes and diabetes.

Why is high insulin so important? In most cases, it means that you have insulin resistance, a condition in which your body's cells aren't responding to insulin's effects. As a result, your body churns out more insulin than it normally would.

Once you have insulin resistance, you've set the stage to develop abdominal obesity, artery-damaging inflammation and other conditions that increasingly raise your risk for prediabetes and diabetes.

A BETTER APPROACH

Because doctors focus on prediabetes and diabetes—conditions detected with a blood sugar test—they tend to miss the earlier signs of diabesity. *A better approach...*

•**Test insulin as well.** The standard diabetes test is to measure blood sugar after fasting for eight or more hours. The problem with this method is that blood sugar is the last thing to rise. Insulin rises first when you have diabesity.

My advice: Ask your doctor for a two-hour glucose tolerance test. With this test, your glucose levels are measured before and after consuming a sugary drink—but ask your doctor to also measure your insulin levels before and after consuming the drink.

What to look for: Your fasting blood sugar should be less than 80 mg/dL…two hours later, it shouldn't be higher than 120 mg/dL. Your fasting insulin should be 2 IU/dL to 5 IU/dL—anything higher indicates that you might have diabesity. Two hours later, your insulin should be less than 30 IU/dL.

Cost: $50 to $100 (usually covered by insurance). I advise all patients to have this test every three to five years…and annually for a person who is trying to reverse diabetes.

STEPS TO BEAT DIABESITY

With the correct lifestyle changes, most people can naturally reduce insulin as well as risk for diabesity-related complications, such as heart disease.

Example: The well-respected Diabetes Prevention Program sponsored by the National Institutes of Health found that overweight people who improved their diets and walked just 20 to 30 minutes a day lost modest amounts of weight and were 58% less likely to develop diabetes. *You can reduce your risk even more by following these steps…*

•**Manage your glycemic load.** The glycemic index measures how quickly different foods elevate blood sugar and insulin. A high-glycemic slice of white bread, for example, triggers a very rapid insulin response, which in turn promotes abdominal weight gain and the risk for diabesity.

My advice: Look at your overall diet and try to balance higher-glycemic foods with lower-glycemic foods. In general, foods that are minimally processed—fresh vegetables, legumes, fish, etc.—are lower on the glycemic index. These foods are ideal because they cause only gradual rises in blood sugar and insulin.

•**Eat nonwheat grains.** Many people try to improve their diets by eating whole-wheat rather than processed white bread or pasta. It doesn't help.

Fact: Two slices of whole-wheat bread will raise blood sugar more than two tablespoons of white sugar. If you already have diabetes, two slices of white or whole-wheat bread will raise your blood sugar by 70 mg/dL to 120 mg/dL.

Wheat also causes inflammation…stimulates the storage of abdominal fat…and increases the risk for liver damage.

These ill effects occur because the wheat that's produced today is different from the natural grain. With selective breeding and hybridization, today's wheat is high in *amylopectin A*, which is naturally fattening. It also contains an inflammatory form of gluten along with short forms of protein, known as *exorphins*, which are literally addictive.

Best: Instead of white or whole-wheat bread and pasta, switch to nonwheat grains such as brown or black rice, quinoa, buckwheat or amaranth. They're easy to cook, taste good—and they don't have any of the negative effects. Small red russet potatoes also are acceptable.

•**Give up liquid calories.** The average American gets 175 calories a day from sugar-sweetened beverages. Because these calories are in addition to calories from solid food, they can potentially cause weight gain of 18 pounds a year. The Harvard Nurses' Health Study found that women who drank one sugar-sweetened soft drink a day had an 82% increased risk of developing diabetes within four years.

Moderation rarely works with soft drinks because sugar is addictive. It activates the same brain receptors that are stimulated by heroin.

My advice: Switch completely to water. A cup of unsweetened coffee or tea daily is acceptable, but water should be your main source of fluids.

Bonus: People who are trying to lose weight can lose 44% more in 12 weeks just by drinking a glass of water before meals.

Important: Diet soda isn't a good substitute for water—the artificial sweeteners that are used increase sugar cravings and slow metabolism. Studies have found a 67% increase in diabetes risk in people who use artificial sweeteners.

What Your Doctor May Not Tell You About Your Diabetes

Frederic J. Vagnini, MD, cardiovascular surgeon and director of the Heart, Diabetes & Weight Loss Centers of New York in Lake Success, *www.Vagnini.com*. Dr. Vagnini is author, with Lawrence D. Chilnick, of *The Weight Loss Plan for Beating Diabetes* (Fair Winds).

For most of the 19 million Americans diagnosed with type 2 diabetes, the main goal of treatment is simply to control their glucose (blood sugar) levels with diet, exercise and sometimes medication.

But there's much more that should be done to help prevent serious complications, which can shorten the life expectancy of a person with diabetes—by about 7.5 years in men and 8.2 years in women.

Sobering statistics: About 80% of people with diabetes die from cardiovascular complications, such as a heart attack. About half the patients with poor glucose control will eventually suffer from nerve damage (neuropathy). Another 20% to 30% may experience retinopathy or other eye disorders.

Whether or not you're taking medication for diabetes, virtually all of these complications can be avoided—and, in some cases, reversed—with natural approaches.

Important: Be sure to speak to your doctor before following any of the steps in this article—some may affect diabetes drugs and other types of medication.

Best ways for people with diabetes to avoid complications...

FIGHT ARTERIAL CALCIFICATION

The Rotterdam Heart Study, which looked at the dietary histories of more than 4,800 patients, found that those with low blood levels of vitamin K-2 were 57% more likely to develop heart disease, due in part to an increase in calcium in the arteries. Paradoxically, these patients had lower bone levels of calcium, which increases the risk for fractures.

Because diabetic patients have an extremely high risk for heart disease, I routinely recommend a daily supplement (45 mcg) of vitamin K-2. You can also get more of this nutrient by eating such foods as liver, eggs and certain cheeses.

Caution: Because there are different forms of vitamin K—some of which interfere with the effects of *warfarin* (Coumadin) and other blood thinners—always speak to your doctor before taking any vitamin K supplement.

OVERCOME FATIGUE

Both inflammation and elevated blood sugar increase fatigue, making it one of the most common symptoms of diabetes. *Helpful...*

•**Coenzyme Q10 (CoQ10) increases the body's production of adenosine triphosphate (ATP),** a molecule that enhances the performance of mitochondria, the energy-producing components of cells. CoQ10 is also an antioxidant that reduces inflammation.

Typical dose: 100 mg to 200 mg, twice daily.

•**Magnesium is involved in glucose and insulin reactions** and is typically lower than normal in people with diabetes who experience fatigue. Patients who eat a healthy diet, including magnesium-rich foods such as nuts and oatmeal, and supplement with magnesium often report an increase in energy. They also show improvements in blood pressure and cardiac performance. Talk to your doctor about the appropriate dosage of a magnesium supplement—especially if you have kidney disease or heart disease, both of which can be worsened by too much magnesium.

All forms of supplemental magnesium can be used, but magnesium citrate causes diarrhea in some people. If this happens to you, take a different form, such as magnesium taurate or magnesium glycinate.

AVOID DIABETIC NEUROPATHY

Excess blood sugar can damage the tiny blood vessels that carry blood and nutrients to nerves in the fingers, legs and/or feet, causing neuropathy. Neuropathy can eventually lead to tissue damage that requires amputation. *What to try...*

•**Alpha-lipoic acid makes the cells more sensitive to insulin** and can relieve symptoms of diabetic neuropathy.

Typical dose: 600 mg to 1,200 mg daily for people with diabetes who have neuropathy. To help prevent neuropathy, 100 mg to 300 mg daily is the typical dose.

•**B-complex supplement may help prevent neuropathy** or reduce symptoms in patients who already have it.

Typical dose: Two B-100 complex supplements daily for people with diabetes who have neuropathy…one B-100 complex daily to help prevent neuropathy.

PREVENT EYE DAMAGE

High blood sugar can cause diabetic retinopathy, which can lead to blindness. It can also increase eye pressure and lead to glaucoma.

Self-defense: Eat more fresh fruits and vegetables. These foods contain antioxidants such as lutein, zeaxanthin and vitamin C, which strengthen eye capillaries, fight free radicals and reduce the risk for blindness. Frozen fruits and vegetables also can be used.

Best choice: Blueberries or bilberries—both contain *anthocyanins*, antioxidants that help prevent eye damage and appear to improve glucose levels.

Type 1 Diabetes? Lower Your Risk of Kidney Damage by 50%

Ian H. de Boer, MD, assistant professor of medicine, University of Washington, Seattle.
Joel Zonszein, MD, director, clinical diabetes center, Montefiore Medical Center, New York City.
American Society of Nephrology annual meeting.
New England Journal of Medicine online.

People with type 1 diabetes who maintain tighter control of their blood sugar levels help protect their kidneys from long-term damage, finds a recent study.

Those treated early with more intensive diabetes management halved their risk of a kidney complication called impaired *glomerular filtration rate* (GFR), the researchers said. An impaired GFR can lead to end-stage renal disease,

the most serious kidney complication associated with diabetes.

"Our study shows that impaired GFR can be prevented in type 1 diabetes. This kidney complication that leads to end-stage renal disease doesn't have to happen," said the study's lead author, Ian de Boer, MD, an assistant professor of medicine at the University of Washington in Seattle.

Results of the study were presented at a meeting of the American Society of Nephrology and published online simultaneously in the *New England Journal of Medicine*.

ABOUT TYPE 1 DIABETES

Type 1 diabetes is an autoimmune disease that occurs when the body's immune system mistakenly attacks and destroys healthy cells in the pancreas that produce insulin. Insulin is a hormone involved in the metabolism of carbohydrates, including sugar.

Because their insulin-producing cells have been destroyed, people with type 1 diabetes must inject insulin to survive. If they use too little insulin, they'll have high blood sugar levels, which puts them at risk of long-term complications. But, too much insulin increases the risk of low blood sugar levels, which can be life threatening.

Kidney disease is a potential long-term complication of both type 1 and type 2 diabetes. High blood sugar levels cause "cell level toxicity and death that results in the loss of the filtering units in the kidney that are replaced with scar tissue," explained Dr. de Boer.

STUDY DETAILS

He and his colleagues reviewed data from the Diabetes Control and Complications Trial (DCCT) and the Epidemiology of Diabetes Interventions and Complications (EDIC) study. The DCCT included more than 1,400 people with type 1 diabetes who were randomly assigned to receive either intensive diabetes management or conventional diabetes therapy at the time (1980s). The average time since diagnosis with diabetes was about six years when the study started.

Intensive management was aimed at lowering hemoglobin A1C levels (HbA1C) to less than 6.05%. HbA1C is a long-term (about two to three months) measurement of blood sugar levels, and levels below 6.05% are similar to levels for people who don't have diabetes. This lower level generally translates into a lower risk of serious complications.

The DCCT lasted for 6.5 years, and the EDIC trial is an observational study that has followed the health of 1,375 participants since the DCCT ended. EDIC currently has 16 years of follow-up data.

RESULTS

During the DCCT, people in the intensive management group averaged an HbA1C of 7.3, while the conventional group had an HbA1C average of 9.1%. During EDIC, both groups had HbA1Cs around 8%, according to Dr. de Boer.

The current analysis looked specifically at the glomerular filtration rate, which is a measure of how well kidneys function.

The researchers found that 24 people in the intensive therapy group developed an impaired GFR, compared with 46 people in the conventional therapy group.

"That's a risk reduction of 50%," said Dr. de Boer.

The risk of end-stage renal disease in the intensive therapy group was also half that of the conventional therapy group—eight people versus 16.

"Getting good glucose control up front in the disease course provides benefits immediately and in preventing complications for years to come," Dr. de Boer said. "The longer you're able to maintain good glucose control, the more benefit you're likely to derive."

EXPERT REACTION

"The good news is that even in the control group, the incidence of renal failure is much lower than we used to see, and there's a further 50% reduction in the intensive group," said Joel Zonszein, MD, director of the Clinical Diabetes Center at the Montefiore Medical Center in New York City.

"Very aggressive treatment early on can make a very big difference in renal function 20 years later," he added.

info Learn more about type 1 diabetes and its management from the Juvenile Diabetes Research Foundation. Visit the Web site *www.jdrf.org* (search "type 1").

CDC Warns Against Sharing Insulin Pens

US Centers for Disease Control and Prevention news release

Due to a growing number of reports about improper use of insulin pens, the US Centers for Disease Control and Prevention issued a reminder that the devices must never be used on more than one person.

Using insulin pens on more than one person puts people at risk for infection with blood-borne pathogens such as hepatitis viruses and HIV, which causes AIDS, the agency warns. Infection can occur even if an insulin pen's needle is changed.

Insulin pens are injector devices that contain a reservoir for insulin or an insulin cartridge. They're designed to enable patients to self-inject insulin and are intended for single-person use.

Reports of improper use of insulin pens in hospitals led the US Food and Drug Administration in 2009 to issue an alert for health care professionals to remind them that insulin pens are for use on a single patient only. Despite the alert, there have been continuing reports of patients put at risk through inappropriate reuse and sharing of insulin pens, including an incident last year that required notification of more than 2,000 potentially exposed patients, the CDC said.

In the clinical reminder, the CDC says…

•**Insulin pens containing multiple doses of insulin are meant for use on a single patient only,** and should never be used for more than one person, even when the needle is changed.

•**Insulin pens should be clearly labeled with the patient's name** or other identifying information to ensure that the correct insulin pen is used only on the correct patient.

•**Hospitals and other facilities should review their policies** and educate staff regarding safe use of insulin pens and similar devices.

•**If re-use of an insulin pen occurs, exposed patients should receive immediate**

notification and be offered appropriate follow-up, including blood-borne pathogen testing.

The recommendations apply to any setting where insulin pens are used, including health care facilities, assisted living or residential care facilities, health fairs, shelters, detention centers, senior centers, schools and camps, according to the CDC.

info The American Diabetes Association offers an overview of insulin routines at its Web site, *www.diabetes.org/living-with-diabetes/treatment-and-care/medication/insulin/insulin-routines.html.*

Weight-Loss Surgeries Beat Standard Treatments For Diabetes

Francesco Rubino, MD, chief, gastrointestinal metabolic surgery, and director, Metabolic and Diabetes Surgery Center at New York-Presbyterian/Weill Cornell, and associate professor, surgery, Weill Cornell Medical College, New York City.
Loren Wissner Greene, MD, endocrinologist, NYU Langone Medical Center, and clinical associate professor, New York University School of Medicine, New York City.
New England Journal of Medicine, online

A recent international analysis comparing weight-loss procedures to standard diabetes treatments found that surgery is more effective at helping people combat type 2 diabetes.

The finding stems from two years of tracking 60 severely obese patients with type 2 diabetes who were between the ages of 30 and 60.

One-third of the patients were treated with diabetes drugs and diet–lifestyle modifications, while the rest underwent one of two surgical procedures: Roux-en-Y gastric bypass or biliopancreatic diversion surgery.

The end result: All of the surgical patients were ultimately able to stop taking their diabetes medications, while the vast majority entered into full disease remission. Neither outcome occurred in the traditional treatment group.

"We have known for many years that bariatric surgery, and specifically certain types of operations like gastric bypass, are very effective in terms of helping to control diabetes," noted senior study author Francesco Rubino, MD, chief of gastrointestinal metabolic surgery and director of the Metabolic and Diabetes Surgery Center at New York-Presbyterian/Weill Cornell in New York City.

"But what this study shows is that even when you compare surgery against standard treatment, surgery performs far better in terms of the improvement that you can get in terms of diabetes," he continued. "Surgery dramatically reduces blood sugar levels, and very often surgical patients can stop taking the medications used for diabetes."

Dr. Rubino and his colleagues from Rome's Catholic University reported their findings in the online edition of the *New England Journal of Medicine*. Cleveland Clinic researchers recently reported similar findings in the same journal.

TWO STUDIES, SIMILAR RESULTS

In their study, the Cleveland Clinic doctors followed 150 patients with type 2 diabetes for a year, and found those who had undergone one of two types of weight-loss surgeries were much more likely than those on traditional therapies to get their blood sugar lowered to the desired level and reduce their use of diabetes medications.

The Italian study authors pointed out that standard medicinal therapies, while effective, could pose their own set of problems. For one, insulin therapy can cause patients to gain weight, which itself can have a negative impact on diabetes.

To explore the comparative benefit of surgical options, the team focused on 60 diabetic patients who had a body mass index (BMI) of 35 or more (BMI is a measurement that takes into account height and weight, and over 30 is considered obese). All had a minimal five-year history of struggling with diabetes.

Undergoing treatment in Rome, the patients were randomly divided into three groups. The first was treated with conventional insulin therapy and a range of other hypoglycemic drugs, alongside what was described as "rigorous" dietary and exercise counseling. The second and third group had one of the two types of bariatric surgery, and were placed on a daily regimen of vitamin and mineral supplementation.

The research team found that all of the surgical patients were able to stop taking all diabetes medications within just 15 days.

What's more, at the two-year mark, three-quarters of those who underwent Roux-en-Y gastric bypass surgery had entered diabetes remission, meaning that for a minimum of one year they had a fasting glucose level under 100 milligrams/deciliter and a hemoglobin A1c count of less than 6.5%.

The same was true among 95% of the biliopancreatic surgery group. By contrast, none of the patients in the standard treatment group had entered remission.

The team observed that BMI levels, diabetes history, postsurgical weight loss, age and gender did not appear to play a role in the likelihood that patients would enter into diabetes remission.

"Two years is a relatively short outcome," acknowledged Dr. Rubino. "And this was a small study. But the effect of surgery was almost immediate. And I think it's clear that while patients getting medicinal therapy did improve somewhat, the chance for patients to achieve robust improvement in diabetes is much greater for those who have surgery than those who are treated with standard medications."

EXPERT COMMENTARY

Loren Wissner Greene, MD, endocrinologist at NYU Langone Medical Center in New York City, expressed little surprise at the findings.

"That's been widely reported," she noted. "Of course, how one fares does depend on the individual. One can eat around any procedure, meaning that if a patient drinks high-caloric liquids following surgery, and manages not to lose weight, that can affect the result," Dr. Greene explained.

"At the same time, there is very good evidence for diabetic remission after surgery, particularly for diverting procedures, where there could be a beneficial impact on gut hormones like leptin and ghrelin," Dr. Greene added.

"There are some risks, however," she cautioned. "And people who have presurgical problems—those with high blood pressure or

obesity-related sleep apnea—might be limited in terms of the type of obesity surgery they can get. But for those who can do it, it may really be the better way to go. And in the end, though surgery is extremely expensive, it might even be cheaper than having to take expensive diabetic medications for years to come."

Not to mention all the costs savings and relieved suffering of avoiding such diabetic complications as blindness, kidney failure and amputated limbs.

info For more information on weight-loss surgery, visit the US National Library of Medicine at its Web site, *www.nlm.nih.gov/medlineplus/weightlosssurgery.html.*

Don't Settle for Costly MRIs When Cheaper Test Works Better

Archives of Internal Medicine

Doctors are more likely to use high-cost MRI scans to diagnose peripheral neuropathy than cheaper—and more effective—glucose tolerance tests, a recent US study has found.

In people with peripheral neuropathy, the nerves that carry information to and from the brain don't work properly. Symptoms of the disorder include tingling, burning or less feeling in the arms or legs, and can range from mild to severe.

Diabetes is the most common cause of peripheral neuropathy, which affects about 15% of those over age 40.

When diagnosing peripheral neuropathy, doctors differ greatly in what tests they turn to, researchers at the University of Michigan noted in their study, published in the *Archives of Internal Medicine*.

"We spend a lot of money to work up a diagnosis of neuropathy. The question is whether the money is well spent," said study leader Brian Callaghan, MD, assistant professor of neurology at the University of Michigan Medical School.

STUDY DETAILS

Dr. Callaghan and his colleagues analyzed data from the 1996–2007 US Health and Retirement Study to identify patients diagnosed with peripheral neuropathy. The researchers focused on 15 diagnostic tests and looked at the number and patterns of tests six months before and after diagnosis.

The investigators found that nearly one-quarter of patients underwent MRIs, while very few (about 1%) had a simpler, less expensive glucose tolerance test, which is used to determine if someone has diabetes by measuring how well the body responds to sugar (glucose).

"Our findings, that MRIs were frequently ordered by physicians, but a lower-cost glucose tolerance test was rarely ordered, show that there is substantial opportunity to improve efficiency in the evaluation of peripheral neuropathy," Dr. Callaghan said.

IMPLICATIONS

"Currently no standard approach to the evaluation of peripheral neuropathy exists. We need more research to determine an optimal approach," he added.

info The US National Institute of Neurological Disorders and Stroke has more information about peripheral neuropathy at its Web site, *http://www.ninds.nih.gov/disorders/peripheral neuropathy/detail_peripheralneuropathy.htm*.

New Genes Linked to Type 2 Diabetes Could Mean New Treatments

American Journal of Human Genetics, news release

Four new genes associated with type 2 diabetes have been identified by researchers, who also pinpointed six independent diabetes-associated gene variants at previously known locations on chromosomes.

These findings, from an analysis of 50,000 genetic variants across 2,000 genes linked to heart and metabolic function, appeared in the *American Journal of Human Genetics*.

The results offer valuable insight into the genetic risk for type 2 diabetes in multiple ethnic groups and could help lead to new treatments, according to researchers.

BACKGROUND

A number of environmental and genetic factors are associated with type 2 diabetes.

"Together, known [type 2 diabetes] genetic variants explain only about 10% of the genetic variance, indicating that additional genetic factors are likely to contribute to disease risk," senior study coauthor Brendan Keating, MD, Children's Hospital of Philadelphia, said.

"Further, previous studies have been based almost exclusively on individuals of European ancestry, and genetic contributors to [type 2 diabetes] are less well understood in non-European populations," he added. "An important first step toward understanding genetic risk across populations is to establish whether known [diabetes-associated] genes span ethnicities or are population-specific."

THE ANALYSIS

Dr. Keating and an international team of colleagues analyzed 39 multiethnic studies on type 2 diabetes that included more than 17,000 people with diabetes and 70,000 people without the disease.

"As a result of our large-scale genetic analysis, we uncovered previously unknown European and multiethnic genetic variants and confirmed that, together, known genetic risk factors influence [type 2 diabetes] risk in multiethnic populations, including African-Americans, Hispanics and Asians," said senior coauthor Richa Saxena, PhD, Massachusetts General Hospital and Harvard Medical School.

WHAT RESULTS MEAN

Dr. Saxena said that identifying new genes associated with type 2 diabetes in diverse ethnic groups could eventually guide strategies for developing treatments.

■ ■ ■ ■

Vitamin D Lowers Risk for Diabetes

Researchers in Germany have found that people with adequate blood levels of vitamin D had a lower risk for type 2 diabetes than those with low levels of vitamin D. Protection against diabetes, which is a chronic inflammatory condition, is believed to come from vitamin D's anti-inflammatory effect. People should have their vitamin D levels checked annually and ensure that they have blood levels of between 50 ng/ml and 80 ng/ml.

C. Herder, et al., "Effect of Serum 25-Hydroxy-vitamin D on Risk for Type 2 Diabetes May Be Partially Mediated by Subclinical Inflammation: Results from the MONICA/KORA Augsburg Study," *Diabetes Care* (2011).

■ ■ ■ ■

Diabetes Medication Raises Bladder Cancer Risk by 40%

The Food and Drug Administration has found that people with diabetes who take *pioglitazone* (Actos) for one year or longer have a 40% increased risk for bladder cancer. If you are taking pioglitazone, speak to your doctor about changing medications…or work with a holistic doctor to treat diabetes naturally.

The FDA Safety Information and Adverse Event Reporting Program.

■ ■ ■ ■

One in Three US Adults Could Have Diabetes by 2050

Currently one in nine people has the disease. The predicted increase in cases is attributable to aging of the population, obesity, sedentary lifestyle, people with diabetes living longer and an increase in the population of minority groups that are at higher risk for type 2 diabetes.

Ann Albright, PhD, RD, director, Division of Diabetes Translation, Centers for Disease Control and Prevention, Atlanta. *www.cdc.gov*

■ ■ ■ ■

Proteins That Reduce Diabetes Risk

Replacing one daily serving of red meat with nuts, whole grains or a low-fat dairy product reduced risk for type 2 diabetes by 16% to 35% according to a recent study. Consuming about four ounces of red meat per day increased diabetes risk by 19%. Processed meats such as bacon and hot dogs increased risk the most.

Possible reasons: Red meat is high in "heme" iron, which can contribute to diabetes. Processed meat has a high sodium content and contains chemical preservatives, such as nitrates, that can damage insulin-producing cells in the pancreas.

Self-defense: Limit unprocessed red meat to two or three servings per week and processed meat to one serving a week.

Frank B. Hu, MD, PhD, professor of nutrition and epidemiology, Harvard School of Public Health, Boston, and leader of a study of 203,157 people, published in *American Journal of Clinical Nutrition*.

■ ■ ■ ■

Diabetes and Cancer Risk

People with diabetes have about a 10% greater likelihood of all cancers combined and a much higher likelihood of certain other cancers, including cancers of the pancreas, bladder and kidney.

Possible reason: High blood levels of glucose and insulin, plus chronic inflammation.

Chaoyang Li, MD, epidemiologist at the Centers for Disease Control and Prevention, Atlanta, and lead author of a study of nearly 400,000 people, published in *Diabetes Care*.

■ ■ ■ ■

Insulin Resistance Causes More Than Diabetes

High blood pressure, memory problems and fatigue can be linked to insulin-resistance. People who are insulin-resistant have an impaired ability to control their bodies' blood glucose levels. In addition to diabetes, the condition can lead to cardiovascular disease, decreased immunity, depression, increased inflammation, weight gain and breast and colon cancers.

Self-defense: Ask your doctor about getting tested for insulin-resistance.

Allan Magaziner, DO, founder and director of Magaziner Center for Wellness, Cherry Hill, New Jersey, and author of *The All-Natural Cardio Cure* (Avery). *www.dr magaziner.com*

■ ■ ■ ■

Extreme Heat Is More Dangerous for Diabetics

People who have type 1 or type 2 diabetes often have difficulty adjusting to rises in temperature. Also, due to nerve damage associated with diabetes, their sweat glands may not produce enough perspiration to cool them down. This may explain why people with diabetes have higher rates of hospitalization, dehydration and death in warmer months. Winter also can be a problem for diabetics because poor circulation increases the likelihood of skin damage in the cold weather.

Jerrold S. Petrofsky, PhD, professor of physical therapy, School of Allied Health Professions, Loma Linda University, Loma Linda, California, and coauthor of a study published in *The Journal of Applied Research.*

Exercise Routine for Diabetes That Lowers Need for Medications

Timothy S. Church, MD, PhD, MPH, director of preventive medicine research at the Pennington Biomedical Research Center at Louisiana State University System in Baton Rouge, and leader of a study of the effects of various exercise regimens on diabetes patients.

Exercise is essential for everybody, of course. But people with diabetes stand to benefit particularly—provided that their workouts include the right variety of physical activity. This finding, from a recent study published in the *Journal of the American Medical Association*, addresses questions that had not previously been well studied.

Researchers recruited 262 sedentary patients with type 2 diabetes, 63% of whom were women, with an average age of 56. Participants had an average blood test score of 7.7% for hemoglobin A1C, an indicator of how well blood sugar concentration has been controlled in the previous eight to 12 weeks (for comparison, levels under 6% generally are considered normal in people without diabetes). One group of participants did aerobic exercise, walking at a moderate pace for two-and-a-half hours per week...a second group did resistance training, performing a full-body routine (primarily with weight-lifting machines) three times per week...a third group combined the aerobic workout and resistance training, doing a shortened version of both routines so that the total exercise time was the same for the three groups. A fourth group, which did not exercise, served as a control.

After nine months: Participants in all three exercise groups showed improvement in several areas, including reduced waist size, as compared with the nonexercisers—but improvement was greatest in the combination aerobics/resistance training group. Combination exercisers were the only ones who lowered the amount of diabetes medication they needed, lost weight and showed significant improvement in hemoglobin A1C levels...they also lost the most fat mass—about four pounds' worth, on average.

Bottom line: If you have diabetes, work with your doctor to develop an appropriate exercise regimen that includes both aerobics and resistance training.

Diet, Fitness & Nutrition

How to Lose 12 Pounds...in Just 17 Days

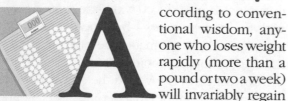

According to conventional wisdom, anyone who loses weight rapidly (more than a pound or two a week) will invariably regain the lost pounds because the diet will be too strict to maintain. But some researchers are now finding evidence that slow isn't necessarily better when it comes to weight loss.

Recent research: A study in the *International Journal of Behavioral Medicine* analyzed data from 262 middle-aged obese women.

Result: The fast weight losers dropped more pounds overall and maintained their weight loss longer than the gradual weight losers.

Good news: With rapid weight loss, most people can boost their metabolism, combat fat storage and help prevent obesity-related diseases, such as diabetes and certain types of cancer—all without feeling deprived of satisfying food.

Sound impossible? I've seen thousands of people lose weight by following what I call the 17 Day Diet.*

Why 17 days? This is roughly the amount of time it takes for your body's metabolism to adapt to a change in calories. By varying your diet at 17-day intervals, you "trick" your metabolism into functioning at its maximum efficiency to help you reach your target weight. *Four simple cycles to follow...*

Cycle 1: Cleanse Your System. For the first 17 days, the goal is to "cleanse" your system by eating lots of lean protein, such as poultry and fish. Lean protein requires more energy to digest than carbohydrates, so it burns additional calories and helps control your blood sugar. Because it's satisfying, protein also fights food cravings.

*Be sure to check with your doctor before you start this or any other weight-loss program.

Mike Moreno, MD, physician in charge of primary care and coordinator for new physician education at Kaiser Permanente in San Diego. Dr. Moreno is author of *The 17 Day Diet* (Free Press).

During this cycle, you're also allowed as many vegetables as you like. You will need to temporarily cut out all grains, potatoes, pasta and desserts. Doing this helps you avoid the dramatic fluctuations in blood sugar that fuel binge eating.

Note: Use olive oil for cooking during this cycle.

Fruit is allowed but only before 2 pm—when sugar (including natural sugar from fruit) is less likely to be stored as fat.

Good fruit choices: Apples, berries, oranges, pears, plums and red grapes. These fruits are relatively low in sugar and high in fiber, which slows digestion and helps you feel full. Avoid bananas and pineapple—both contain too much natural sugar.

During this 17-day cycle, people lose an average of 10 to 12 pounds (depending on their starting weights) while eating three to four meals daily plus snacks (for a total of 1,300 calories per day for men and women). Some of this weight loss will be due to water loss—but this is also beneficial because fluid retention can contribute to fatigue.

Sample day's meals: Breakfast—two scrambled egg whites...one-half grapefruit or other fresh fruit...one cup green tea. Lunch—fish, poultry or eggs...vegetables...one cup green tea. Dinner—fish or chicken...vegetables...one cup green tea. Snack—raw, cut-up veggies.

Cycle 2: **Reset Your Metabolism.** During the second 17-day cycle, the goal is to reset the metabolism by alternating higher calorie intake (1,500 to 1,700) on even days with lower calorie intake (1,300) on odd days. Switching back and forth stimulates fat burning because it prevents your body from adapting to a certain level of daily calories.

Slow-digesting complex carbs, such as oatmeal, sweet potatoes and brown rice, are reintroduced during this cycle.

Cycle 3: **Good Eating Habits.** By now, a little more than a month since you started, your body has undergone a significant metabolic shift that will allow you to reintroduce moderate portions—and no more than two to three servings per day before 2 pm—of carbohydrates such as whole-grain breads and pastas that may have made you feel sluggish or heavy before.

If you've reached your target weight, you may proceed to cycle 4, the maintenance cycle. If not, be sure to focus on portion control and continue to emphasize lean protein and non-starchy vegetables, limiting carbohydrates after 2 pm until you reach cycle 4.

Cycle 4: **Weight Maintenance.** During this cycle, which is followed indefinitely to maintain your weight loss, you are more strict with yourself throughout the workweek but relax your eating habits on the weekends. From 6 pm Friday to 6 pm Sunday, you can enjoy your favorite indulgences, such as pizza or hamburgers, as long as you maintain portion control and enjoy no more than three indulgences over a single weekend. This approach allows you to eat some favorite foods in moderation while also giving your metabolism the variety it needs to function efficiently.

Rule of thumb: Weigh yourself on weekends. If you gain five pounds or more over a week's time, return to any of the earlier cycles.

OTHER SECRETS TO WEIGHT LOSS

In addition to following the cycles described earlier...

•**Get more probiotics.** New research suggests that people who have an overabundance of "bad" bacteria in the intestinal tract are more susceptible to weight gain. But healthful bacteria, known as probiotics (found in such foods as certain yogurts, sauerkraut and miso soup), control the proliferation of bad bacteria and help fight infection—and ensure that your metabolism functions effectively.

My advice: Aim to consume two daily servings of foods containing probiotics. *Examples of one probiotic serving*: Six ounces of fat-free plain yogurt or one-half cup of Breakstone Live-Active cottage cheese (which includes added probiotics).

Or: Take probiotic supplements, following label instructions.

•**Don't forget to exercise.** To avoid getting run down while you're scaling back on calories (especially the first few days of cycle 1), do only 15 to 20 minutes of walking a day.

Thereafter, aim for at least 30 minutes of aerobic exercise five days a week. Walking is a good choice, as is jogging, swimming or using a stationary bicycle or an elliptical machine. For strength training, make the exercises as aerobic as possible using lighter weights and more repetitions.

Mid-Morning Snacks Can Block Your Diet

Anne McTiernan, MD, PhD, member, Public Health Sciences Division, and director, Hutchinson Prevention Center, Fred Hutchinson Cancer Research Center, Seattle.

Dieters may want to reconsider that mid-morning snack. In a 12-month study of 123 overweight or obese women, those who snacked between breakfast and lunch lost less weight than those who skipped a mid-morning nosh.

The finding may not relate to time of day as much as the short interval between breakfast and lunch for these snackers, explained study author Anne McTiernan, MD, PhD, director of the Prevention Center at the Fred Hutchinson Cancer Research Center in Seattle.

The women may have been eating out of boredom, or for reasons other than hunger, she said. The net result is too many calories in a given day.

"Snacking, per se, isn't bad, it's more what you eat and when you are snacking," she said. "If you start snacking in the morning, you might be eating more throughout the day and taking more food in."

Smart snacking can be part of a sound weight-loss plan, Dr. McTiernan noted. The timing of snacks, frequency of eating them and quality of snacks all have to be considered, she added.

STUDY DETAILS

Dr. McTiernan assigned the women, ages 50 to 75, to either a diet-alone program or a diet plus exercise program. Those in the diet-alone group ate 1,200 to 2,000 calories a day, depending on their starting weight. Those in the diet and exercise group also reduced calories but, in addition, put in 45-minute workouts five times a week.

The participants were given counseling on nutrition but no special instructions about snacking.

The women recorded the time, type and frequency of meals on a normal day. The researchers evaluated calories from fat and fiber, fruit and vegetable intake, and other information.

At the study start, the average body mass index (BMI) was 31.3. (A BMI of 30 is termed obese.) Weight loss in the two groups was similar. Those in the diet-only group lost about 10% of their body weight and those in the diet and exercise group lost 11.6% after one year.

However, snacking patterns were linked with the amount of weight loss. The mid-morning snackers lost about 7% of their total body weight, but those who didn't snack mid-morning lost 11.5%, according to the report.

More women snacked in the afternoon than the morning. Snacks might be appropriate if the interval between meals is long, such as five hours or more, Dr. McTiernan said.

The study was published in the *Journal of the American Dietetic Association*. The US National Cancer Institute and US National Institutes of Health funded the research.

EXPERT ADVICE

Until more research is in, Dr. McTiernan encourages dieters to limit a snack to no more than 200 calories. Healthier snacks include low-fat yogurt, string cheese or a handful of nuts, she suggested. Other good choices are non-starchy vegetables (avoid potatoes and corn), fresh fruits and whole grain crackers.

The study included only women, so the researchers can't say for sure if it applies to men. "But studies have shown calorie intake is equally important in men and women," Dr. McTiernan noted.

info To learn more about smart snacking, visit the Web site of the American Heart Association, *www.heart.org,* and search "healthy snacking."

Win at Weight Loss
With hCG

Mark A. Stengler, NMD, naturopathic medical doctor in private practice, Encinitas, California...adjunct associate clinical professor at the National College of Natural Medicine, Portland, Oregon...author of *The Natural Physician's Healing Therapies* and coauthor of *Prescription for Natural Cures* (both from Bottom Line Books).

It's no secret that the hCG diet I'm about to describe is controversial. How could it not be when it involves using a hormone produced during pregnancy while following an extremely low-calorie diet?

I also was skeptical about this diet when I first heard about it. In fact, several patients asked me a few years ago to put them on this diet and I refused.

What changed my mind: I spoke with other physicians who were prescribing the diet and came to understand that they were able to help patients lose weight—patients who hadn't been able to lose weight any other way. That convinced me. Because of the way that hCG functions in the body, it makes a very restricted diet much easier for patients. Individuals who benefit most are those who are obese—and anyone who is having difficulty losing 15 pounds or more. *Find out how it can help...*

HOW hCG WORKS

The compound hCG, which stands for *human chorionic gonadotropin,* should not be confused with human growth hormone (HGH). Instead, hCG is a hormone produced during pregnancy. Its main function is to enrich the uterus so that it can sustain the fetus. In this role, hCG functions as a release mechanism for stored fat and nutrients from the mother to the fetus. It also is produced in the pituitary glands of males and females of all ages. For weight loss, the hCG that I prescribe is bioidentical and comes from the urine of pregnant women.

It was discovered that when the hormone was given to women who were not pregnant (and to men), it promoted the movement of excessive fat deposits. The discovery of hCG for weight loss is credited to British endocrinologist A.T.W. Simeons, who found that obese patients were able to get rid of hard-to-lose fat when injected with small amounts of the hormone daily. The patients lost weight when the injections were accompanied by an extremely low-calorie diet (500 calories daily). Dr. Simeons found that hCG helped patients cope with a low-calorie diet without the side effects that usually accompany it, such as fatigue, headache and irritability. Also, hCG encourages the body to use fat as fuel—and this helps people feel less hungry when on a low-calorie diet. Dr. Simeons' work was published in the 1950s and 1960s in respected medical journals, such as *The Lancet.*

There is no doubt that hCG diet studies show mixed results in terms of effectiveness. But like many doctors who provide hCG treatments, I offer this treatment not because of the studies that I see on it, but because of the results that I have seen in my practice. It is a nontoxic way for people to lose weight that they would not otherwise lose.

MY PROTOCOL

I check my patients' overall health before they begin this diet. I do blood tests to confirm there is no hormone imbalance or a nutritional deficiency. If patients need hormone treatment or a detoxification program, I make sure that they have these before beginning weight loss with hCG. I also perform a physical exam and an EKG if it looks as though these are needed.

MODIFIED DIET

I have modified Dr. Simeons' original hCG diet because some of the requirements were quite difficult for patients.

Instead of a diet of 500 calories per day, my patients consume a restricted 660-calorie-per-day diet for 30 days. You might think that a difference of 160 calories is not all that much, but when you are eating this few calories, it's a significant amount.

On the Simeons plan, people ate a high-fat diet for two days before cutting out all fats. My plan does not include a two-day fat binge. Instead, my patients consume about 35% of calories from carbohydrates...18% from fat...and 47% from protein throughout the month. A typical day for a patient following my hCG diet might include a protein shake for breakfast...an apple or a few strawberries as a snack…and chicken or fish (three ounces per serving) with a generous amount of vegetables for lunch and dinner.

If this diet is so restricted that it causes low blood sugar or weakness, I increase the number of calories with similar food choices until the patient feels better. My patients eat healthful fats such as omega-3 fatty acids from salmon. They drink lots of water—80 to 100 ounces daily—which keeps nutrients moving through the body. At the end of 30 days, calorie intake is increased over a few days to between 1,100 and 1,300 calories. This calorie count forms the basis of the maintenance diet. Patients are able to keep the weight off indefinitely when they stay on the maintenance diet.

SUPPLEMENTS

During treatment, I have my patients see a nutritionist once a week to review their diet and help with specific food choices. My patients take a multivitamin to prevent general nutritional deficiency as well as additional calcium and magnesium because they are not getting enough of these from food. If patients feel particularly tired, I prescribe vitamin B-12 injections. They also take low-dose fish oil.

If a patient on the diet is constipated, which happens with about 10% of patients, I recommend extra fiber, water and/or laxative herbs. If he/she is struggling with hunger, I often recommend the appetite suppressant Caralluma fimbriata and/or increase his hCG amount.

My patients have a choice between sublingual (under-the-tongue) hCG or a self-administered injection. Most patients choose the sublingual form simply because it's easier. I never recommend that hCG be purchased anywhere but at a compounding pharmacy to ensure that it is as fresh as possible. I don't advise buying hCG on the Internet.

RESULTS

About 90% of my patients following the diet lose about 15 to 20 pounds, and about two to three inches around their waists, in 30 days. For some patients, this is enough to kick-start their weight loss if they have more to lose.

For other patients who need to lose more weight after the first 30 days, the program can be repeated after 30 days on the maintenance diet. The hCG diet can be repeated several times, if needed.

Besides the side effects of constipation and fatigue already mentioned, hCG temporarily can increase the length of a woman's menstrual cycle and increase her fertility since it enhances ovulation, so precautions against pregnancy need to be taken if women are of childbearing age and pregnancy is not desired. There's little worry of hormone-related cancer. A study in *Cancer, Epidemiology, Biomarkers and Prevention* found that women younger than 40 years old who had used hCG for weight loss or fertility had significantly less breast cancer than the group that did not use hCG. In men, hCG can stimulate testosterone production, but this does not generally cause problems.

In addition to weight-loss success, other conditions such as diabetes or arthritis also improve.

The diet changes patients' lives—it gives them energy…makes them feel healthy…and changes their outlook on eating.

Caution: This diet should be followed only while supervised by a doctor. If you haven't been able to lose weight despite trying, ask your holistic doctor about it.

More from Dr. Mark A. Stengler…

Protein Curbs Overeating

University of Sydney, Australia, researchers gave lean volunteers a low-protein diet (10%)…an intermediate-protein diet (15%)…and a high-protein diet (25%). Each participant spent four days on each diet. Those who ate the 10%-protein diet consumed 12% more calories over the four days than those who ate the other menus. The additional calories were attributed to snacking because the participants did not feel full. Consuming 15% or more of your calories from protein can help curb your appetite and control weight. This confirms findings from a 2011 study published in *Obesity*.

Finally…a Detox Diet That's Tasty

Keri Glassman, RD, a New York City–based registered dietitian who is president and founder of NutritiousLifeMeals.com. She is author of *The O2 Diet* and *Slim Calm Sexy Diet* (both from Rodale).

To flush toxins out of the body, "detoxification" enthusiasts recommend following extreme dietary restrictions for a few days to several weeks and/or using colon-cleansing products, including laxatives, teas, powders, capsules and/or enemas.

What you need to know: While many detox methods can help some people drop a few unwanted pounds (likely due to a loss of "water weight") or leave them feeling psychologically refreshed, the risks include dehydration, electrolyte imbalances and damage to the colon lining. In a review of 20 studies on colon cleansing published in the last decade, researchers found that products sold for this use often cause cramping, nausea, vomiting and even kidney failure.

Good news: You don't need to take extreme, potentially dangerous measures to "detoxify" yourself and give yourself more energy. There is a better, safer way.

THE POWER OF ANTIOXIDANTS

Organs such as the liver and kidneys are well designed to filter toxins. But that doesn't mean you shouldn't give your body a detoxing boost every month or so.

A short-term nutritional cleanse that emphasizes antioxidants is the best way to give yourself a fresh start if you've been eating poorly and/or not taking good care of yourself by getting regular exercise and adequate sleep.*

The four-day cleanse described in this article is based on the Oxygen Radical Absorbance Capacity (ORAC) scale, developed by the USDA to measure how well a food protects against free radicals that contribute to heart disease, cancer and other chronic health problems. The cleans-

*The nutritional cleanse described in this article is designed primarily for healthy adults. It should not be followed by people with diabetes. Consult your doctor before trying the cleanse.

ing regimen contains 50,000 ORAC points per day (significantly higher than the points contained in the typical American adult's diet) and roughly 1,200 calories—enough calories for most people to eat during a cleansing regimen so that the body's metabolism does not slow.

Important finding: Research from the Agricultural Research Service demonstrates that eating a high-ORAC diet increases the antioxidant power of human blood 10% to 25%, strengthening memory, helping prevent cancer and heart disease and aiding in weight loss.

The cleanse is high in fiber and has enough protein to keep you feeling satisfied. Rather than severely restricting food, which can leave some people feeling weak and dizzy, this cleanse includes three meals a day plus two snacks.

It also includes omega-3–rich foods such as eggs, fish and pecans…a Granny Smith apple (higher in antioxidants than most other apples) and cinnamon to help stabilize blood sugar… and other fruits, vegetables and spices (such as oregano and basil) that have the highest possible antioxidant levels.

FOUR-DAY CLEANSE

What to eat for four days…

Breakfast…

- **Scrambled eggs** (1 whole omega-3–fortified egg plus three egg whites) with 1 teaspoon dried basil
- **1 8-ounce cup green tea**
- **1 8-ounce glass water with 1 ounce lemon juice**

Mid-morning snack…

- **Sliced Granny Smith apple sprinkled with 1 teaspoon cinnamon**

Lunch…

- **Spinach** (cooked or raw) seasoned with flavored vinegar, such as fig, raspberry or orange
- **3 to 4 ounces fresh or canned salmon with 1 teaspoon dried spices,** such as oregano
- **8 pecan halves**
- **1 8-ounce glass of water with 1 ounce lemon juice**

Mid-afternoon snack…

- **Steamed artichoke or ½ cup artichoke hearts in water**
- **1 8-ounce cup green tea**

Dinner…

• **Large salad—mix romaine lettuce** (which is high in antioxidants and widely available) with carrots, tomatoes and red bell peppers…dress with 1 teaspoon extra-virgin olive oil and lemon juice to taste

• **Steamed asparagus**

• **3 to 4 ounces any lean protein,** such as chicken, shrimp or cod (grilled, baked or broiled), seasoned with 1 teaspoon oregano

• **1 8-ounce glass of water with 1 ounce lemon juice**

• **1 cup blueberries (fresh or frozen)**

In addition to the water and antioxidant-rich green tea included in the cleanse, drink five more glasses of water daily to keep your energy and metabolism up and ensure that you don't mistake thirst for hunger. Also, for best results, get around eight hours of sleep per night, exercise for 45 minutes daily and stretch for five minutes in the morning and evening.

■ ■ ■ ■

Scent Helps You Eat Less

Curb your appetite by smelling vanilla before a meal. The aroma is satisfyingly rich and tricks your brain into thinking you are eating more than you actually are, so your body feels content sooner and needs less food.

Alan Hirsch, MD, founder, Smell & Taste Treatment and Research Foundation, Chicago. *www.smellandtaste.org*

Could Two Words Help You Resist Temptation?

Journal of Consumer Research, news release

When it comes to weight loss, the words you choose when refusing something tasty can make the difference in whether you are able to resist temptation, recent research suggests.

For instance, when offered a slice of pie, responding with the words "I don't" increases the likelihood you will stick to your diet, rather than saying "I can't."

"Whether it's buffalo wings at a tailgate or heaping plates of calories at the Thanksgiving day dinner table that is your downfall, help is merely a couple of words away," wrote coauthors Vanessa Patrick, PhD, an associate professor at the University of Houston and Henrik Hagtvedt, PhD, assistant professor of marketing at Boston College.

STUDY DETAILS

In conducting the study, the researchers assigned 30 women to one of three groups and followed them for 10 days. Each group received a single strategy for refusing foods: "I don't," "I can't" or "Just say no."

The study, published online in the *Journal of Consumer Research,* revealed the 'I don't' strategy boosted people's feelings of autonomy, control and self-awareness. This strategy also created a positive change in their long-term behavior, such as renewed dedication to weight loss.

"This insight is based on the notion that saying 'I can't' to temptation inherently signals deprivation and the loss from giving up something desirable," the researchers explained.

On the other hand, they said, the "I don't" strategy shows a sense of determination and empowerment.

CONCLUSION

"What's great about this research is that it suggests a strategy that is simple, straightforward and easy to implement. And most importantly…it works," the authors concluded.

info For more information about healthy eating habits, visit the Web site of the US National Institute of Diabetes and Digestive and Kidney Diseases, *http://win.niddk.nih.gov,* and search "Changing your habits."

■ ■ ■ ■

Wield a Big Fork

Researchers have discovered that taking big bites with large forks may help people to eat less when dining out.

Journal of Consumer Research

■ ■ ■ ■

Keep Trying

Did you know that yo-yo dieting is better than no dieting? Mice that repeatedly lost then gained weight lived more than 30% longer than those that remained obese.

Edward List, PhD, scientist, Ohio University, Athens, and principal investigator of a dieting study of mice presented at The Endocrine Society's annual meeting.

Eat Late—Gain Weight

Deanna Arble, a doctoral candidate at the Center for Sleep and Circadian Biology of Northwestern University in Evanston, Illinois, and lead author of an animal study.

Isn't it just calories consumed and energy expended that count when it comes to weight? Nope. As it turns out, people with a penchant for middle-of-the-night snacking may pay for that habit with added pounds, even if they consume the same number of calories overall as people who don't eat during the night, a recent study suggests.

For six weeks, researchers fed two groups of mice an identical high-fat diet. One group was fed during times of day when mice normally are sleeping…the other group was fed during their usual active time. Overall calorie consumption and physical activity levels were equal in both groups.

Results: Compared with mice that ate during their usual waking hours, those that ate when they ought to have been asleep gained 2.4 times more weight, on average…and wound up with 8% more body fat.

Theory: The body's internal clock regulates energy use, programming itself to more effectively burn calories consumed during active times.

Lesson: Even when you stay up very late or wake up hungry at 2 am, resist the urge to make a middle-of-the-night foray to the fridge.

Best Energy Bars for Health and Good Taste

Carolyn Brown, RD, a nutritionist and registered dietician with Foodtrainers, a private nutrition consulting company based in New York City. She holds a masters degree in clinical nutrition. www.foodtrainers.net

Energy bars are supposed to provide a quick-yet-nutritious boost. But while certain bars are tasty and good for you, others are unpleasant to eat or not healthful.

Some contain more calories than we really need—often upward of 300. Many have excessive sugars—anything above 15 grams is too much.

You'll find heavily processed and artificial ingredients in some, including aspartame, soy protein isolates, whey concentrate, isoflavones, hydrolyzed collagen and hydrolyzed gelatin, which don't deliver as much nutritional value as unprocessed and natural ingredients.

The most healthful and delicious energy bars, all of which generally cost between $1.40 and $3 per bar…

Best high-fiber bar: **Gnu Bar.** One bar has 12 grams of fiber—almost half of our daily fiber needs. Unlike many high-fiber snacks, it doesn't have a "cardboardy" consistency. Gnu is among the lowest-calorie full-sized energy bars on the market—130 to 140 calories per bar. *www.gnu foods.com.*

Drawbacks: Going from a low-fiber diet directly to a high-fiber diet can cause digestive distress. Start with just half a Gnu Bar a day if you do not currently eat many high-fiber foods.

Best meal-replacement bar: **ProBar.** These taste great, and they're made from healthful ingredients such as dried fruits, nuts, seeds and rolled grains. At 370 to 390 calories, they're much too filling for a snack, but they occasionally can replace part of breakfast or lunch when you are in a hurry. *www.theprobar.com.*

Downside: ProBar's eight to 12 grams of protein are low for a full meal. If possible, supplement a ProBar with a few spoonfuls of Greek yogurt.

***Best pre- or postworkout bar:* Picky Bar.** This has the ideal ratio of carbs to protein—4:1—to prepare the body for a strenuous workout or help it recover. *www.pickybars.com.*

Downside: Picky Bar's 22 to 23 grams of sugar are acceptable before or after a workout—our bodies consume simple sugars when we exercise—but excessive at other times.

***Best energy bar that tastes like dessert:* Kookie Karma.** A cross between a cookie and a bar, this round-shaped snack is made from healthful ingredients such as nuts, seeds and fruit. *www.kookiekarma.com.*

Downside: Some varieties contain xylitol, a natural sugar alcohol that can cause gastrointestinal distress.

***Best savory energy bar:* Savory Bar.** While most bars strive to taste like dessert, Savory Bar comes in grown-up flavors such as Rosemary, Sesame, Spicy and Everything (which features sesame, poppy, onion and garlic flavors). Savory Bars have a crunchy, crackerlike consistency. *www.sheffafoods.com.*

Downside: With just four grams of protein and only 140 to 150 calories, a Savory Bar might not be sufficient to tide you over until mealtime. Consider pairing one with a healthful protein such as cottage cheese.

***Best energy bar that's very widely available:* Kind Bar.** This simple, healthful, nut-based bar can be found in many convenience stores, supermarkets and Starbucks. With as much as seven grams of protein and five grams of fiber, and 10 to 13 grams of sugar for most varieties, it's a healthier choice than other very widely distributed bars, including PowerBars, which have as much as 30 grams of sugar, and Luna Bars, which feature heavily processed ingredients such as soy protein isolates. *www.kindsnacks.com.*

■ ■ ■ ■

Build More Muscle with Chocolate Milk

Best drink after a workout—chocolate milk. When consumed immediately after a workout, low-fat chocolate milk helps athletes build more muscle than a comparable high-carbohydrate sports drink. Drinking chocolate milk also leads to faster muscle recovery and better subsequent workouts.

Also: Individuals who drank chocolate milk immediately after cycling five days a week over four weeks had twice as much improvement in their maximum oxygen uptake—an indicator of cardiovascular fitness—as individuals who drank calorie-free beverages or a carbohydrate sports drink.

John Ivy, PhD, professor of kinesiology and health education, University of Texas at Austin and leader of a study published in *Journal of Nutrition and Metabolism.*

Cool Way to Boost Your Workout

Stacy T. Sims, PhD, research scientist and exercise physiologist, Stanford University School of Medicine.

Duck-chul Lee, PhD, physical activity epidemiologist, Arnold School of Public Health, University of South Carolina, Columbia.

Looking for an exercise edge, a way to stay faithful to regular workouts? Try chilling out—literally.

Cooling the palms of the hands while working out helped obese women exercise longer, reports researcher Stacy T. Sims, PhD, a research scientist and exercise physiologist at Stanford University School of Medicine.

EXERCISE CHALLENGES FOR OBESE PEOPLE

"If you think about adipose [fat] tissue, it's a great insulator," Dr. Sims said. For people who are obese, that means they often get too hot while exercising.

"It would be like a bike racer wearing a wet suit for the entire Tour de France," she said. "We're trying to address those barriers."

Sims wanted to see if cooling off the hands of the women she studied might help them overcome fatigue and overheating while exercising.

The device she used is already in use by some professional athletes, according to Dr. Sims. She decided to test it on obese women, who she finds often abandon working out due to overheating and fatigue.

The research was not funded by the company that makes the device.

STUDY DETAILS

In the study, Dr. Sims evaluated 24 healthy women, ages 30 to 45. None had exercised long-term in the past. They were obese, with a body-mass index (BMI) of between 30 and nearly 35. BMI is a measure of body weight in proportion to height, and obesity begins at a BMI of 30.

One group of women was assigned to hold the cooling device with cool water (60.8 degrees Fahrenheit). The other group also held the device in their palms but it contained water that was body temperature (98.6 degrees Fahrenheit).

Both groups participated in three exercise sessions a week for 12 weeks. Each session included 10 minutes of body weight exercises, 25 minutes to 45 minutes of treadmill walking with the cooling device and 10 minutes of core-strengthening exercise. They worked up to the time they could handle on the treadmill.

On the first day and last day of the study, the women did a 1.5-mile walk that was timed.

The cooling group shaved more than five minutes off their time for the 1.5-mile treadmill test. They averaged 31.6 minutes at the start and 24.6 minutes at the end.

Their exercising heart rate went up, too, 136 beats per minute to 154 beats per minute—a good sign, showing they were working out more intensely.

The cooling group also took more than two inches off their waist by end of the 12-week study. Their blood pressure also went down, from 139/84 to 124/70. (Below 120/80 is the goal.)

In contrast, the comparison group didn't show any substantial differences in any of the measures, Dr. Sims found.

The cooling group also stuck with it more, Dr. Sims said. "The controls dropped out early, and skipped a lot of sessions," Dr. Sims noted.

The cooling group seemed to get into the regimen, she said. "At the end, some women were running [on the treadmill]," she said.

Dr. Sims presented her findings at the American Heart Association's Epidemiology and Prevention/Nutrition, Physical Activity and Metabolism scientific sessions in San Diego.

HOW IT WORKS

"If you reduce the heat stress, you reduce fatigue, sweating and discomfort," she explained. "You reduce a lot of the physiological barriers that [make] people say, 'I don't want to continue.'"

EXPERT COMMENTARY

The finding that the comparison group had no substantial effects "is a bit strange," said Duck-chul Lee, PhD, a physical activity epidemiologist at the Arnold School of Public Health at the University of South Carolina, in Columbia. He said he would have expected some effects after 12 weeks.

He added that "the results may not apply to people exercising in a cold condition, for example, outside in winter."

ADVICE

Dr. Sims wants to do a study of the device with more people.

Meanwhile, she says, it won't hurt to try recreating the effect at home: "Take a water bottle, freeze it and take that with you in your bare palm [as you work out]. As it melts you drink the cool water. It's worth a try."

info To learn more about getting started on a workout regimen, visit the American Council on Exercise Web site, *www.acefitness.org,* and search "Before you start an exercise program."

■ ■ ■ ■

Work Out Before Breakfast and Burn More Fat

People who exercised before eating breakfast did not gain weight despite a high-fat, high-calorie diet according to a recent study. Those on the same diet who exercised after eating breakfast did gain weight.

Karen Van Proeyen, PhD, researcher, department of biomedical kinesiology, K.U. Lueven University, Belgium, and leader of a study published in *Journal of Physiology.*

■ ■ ■ ■

"Stayin' Alive" Secret

Is there an easy way to measure moderate intensity on a 30-minute walk?

Yes, there are a few ways to tell how fast you are walking. Recent research conducted at the University of California, San Diego, defines "moderate intensity" as 100 steps per minute. An easy way to count this is to listen to (or hum) the song "Stayin' Alive" by the Bee Gees as you walk—the song's tempo is 100 beats per minute.

Of course, you can also simply apply the "talk test." With this approach, you should be able to hold a conversation without having to stop for a breath between sentences. In general, you want to walk at the speed you would if you were late for a meeting or walking to catch a bus. At least 150 minutes of moderate-intensity aerobic exercise per week is recommended to keep your heart healthy.

Simon Marshall, PhD, associate professor, department of family and preventive medicine, University of California, San Diego.

■ ■ ■ ■

Don't Fall for This Corn Syrup Alias

Did you know corn sugar is the same as high-fructose corn syrup (HFCS)? The Corn Refiners Association has asked the FDA to approve corn .sugar for use on food labels instead of HFCS. Used in soft drinks, bread and other commercially prepared products, HFCS is perceived as being likely to cause obesity.

Reality: People should consume less sugar of all types.

Karen Collins, RD, registered dietitian, American Institute for Cancer Research, Washington, DC. *www.aicr.org*

■ ■ ■ ■

Live Longer by Eating Alpha-Carotene

People with the highest blood levels of alpha-carotene were 39% less likely to die from all causes over 14 years.

Foods with the most alpha-carotene: Pumpkin, carrots, winter squash, plantains, vegetable juice cocktail, tangerines, collard greens, snap beans, tomatoes, cornmeal and corn, peas, raspberries, sweet potatoes, bell peppers and mangoes.

Chaoyang Li, MD, PhD, epidemiologist, division of behavioral surveillance, Centers for Disease Control and Prevention, Atlanta, and leader of a study of 15,318 people, published in *Archives of Internal Medicine*.

■ ■ ■ ■

Freeze-Dried Fruit Nearly as Healthful as Fresh

The antioxidant levels of freeze-dried fruit actually are higher than those of fresh fruit because the water in fresh fruit is removed by freeze-drying.

But: Some fragile nutrients are damaged by freeze-drying.

Gary Stoner, PhD, professor emeritus, College of Medicine, The Ohio State University Comprehensive Cancer Center, Columbus.

■ ■ ■ ■

Chia Seeds Are Good for You

They provide healthful omega-3 fats, fiber, protein, calcium, iron, zinc and other minerals. They may slow the absorption of sugar and help reduce cholesterol. Add the seeds to cereal, oatmeal or yogurt. You can buy them at health-food stores and online.

University of California, Berkeley Wellness Letter, 500 Fifth Avenue, New York City 10110. *www.wellnessletter.com*

Coconut Oil: The Good-for-You Fat

Mark A. Stengler, NMD, naturopathic medical doctor in private practice, Encinitas, California…adjunct associate clinical professor at the National College of Natural Medicine, Portland, Oregon…author of *The Natural Physicians Healing Therapies* and coauthor of *Prescription for Natural Cures* (both from Bottom Line Books).

Coconut oil may be one of the most misunderstood oils around. For years, we were cautioned against using it because of its high saturated fat content, but it turns out that the type of saturated fat in coconut oil actually is good for us. Coconut oil is primarily composed of *medium-chain triglycerides* (MCTs), which don't contribute to heart disease the way that *long-chain triglycerides* (LCTs) do (think beef fat). *Here are some of the ways coconut oil can help…*

•**Weight management.** Before European colonization, people from the tropical coastal areas of the Pacific were not overweight despite a diet rich in coconut. A study published in *Lipids* found that coconut oil supplementation reduced waist circumference and did not raise total cholesterol levels as did soybean oil supplementation.

•**Immune boost.** Coconut oil contains lauric acid, a powerful anti-microbial that combats infections from both fungi and viruses. It also helps to combat pathogens in the digestive tract.

•**Skin conditions.** Studies have shown that coconut oil can reduce the symptoms of dermatitis and dry skin—and it can help with psoriasis and eczema.

How to use it: Coconut oil can be substituted for most other oils. Look for virgin or extra-virgin coconut oil that is not processed with chemicals and contains no trans fat. Spread it on crackers …use it in stir-fries or to sauté…or substitute it for butter or shortening in baking. Place it in a tub of warm water to liquefy it and drizzle it over salads. You can add it when cooking rice or pasta. It has a mild coconut flavor. You also can rub it into your skin to relieve dryness.

Foods That Make Your Mouth Healthy

Marvin A. Fier, DDS, executive vice president of the American Society for Dental Aesthetics and an adjunct professor of dentistry at Loma Linda University, California, and University of Medicine and Dentistry of New Jersey, Newark. *www.rocklandnydentist.com*

Within seconds after we eat, bacteria in the mouth convert sugars into acids that can damage tooth enamel, leading to decay and cavities. We all know that we need to brush and floss to keep our teeth and gums healthy, but certain foods also can dilute acids, cleanse the teeth and reduce inflammation—the underlying cause of periodontal (gum) disease.

Important: By reducing gum disease, you also reduce your risk for other diseases that are linked to inflammation. These include heart disease, diabetes and even cancer.

Here are the best foods and beverages to keep your teeth and gums healthy…

•**Crunchy clean.** Celery, apples and carrots are ideal for dental health. These and other crisp fruits and vegetables act like mini-toothbrushes. They scour off plaque, the bacteria-laden film that accumulates on teeth and beneath the gums. These foods also have a high water content, which dilutes oral acids.

•**Cheese after meals.** The European tradition of serving cheese after meals is healthier for the mouth than after-meal desserts. Cheese neutralizes oral acids and helps remove bacteria. It stimulates the flow of saliva, which also has acid-neutralizing properties.

The calcium and phosphorus in cheese and other dairy foods remineralizes tooth enamel, making it stronger and more impervious to acids.

Bonus: The ratio of phosphorus and calcium in cheese is optimal for the absorption of fluoride, which helps prevent decay.

If you don't eat dairy: Use MI Paste (a 40-gram tube is available online for $29). It binds calcium and phosphate to tooth surfaces and makes teeth stronger. Apply twice daily after brushing with your regular toothpaste.

•**Tea.** Both green and black teas contain *polyphenols*, antioxidants that reduce inflammation and may decrease the risk for periodontal disease.

Researchers in Japan found that people who drank one cup of green tea daily were less likely to develop periodontal disease than those who didn't drink tea.

•**Vitamin C–rich foods.** The body uses vitamin C for the growth and repair of tissues. It's a necessary component of collagen, a protein that is one of the building blocks of cartilage, teeth and bones.

Why it matters: Patients with even mild periodontal disease can experience a weakening of tissues that support the teeth. In more advanced cases, periodontal disease can lead to tooth loss. A diet high in vitamin C can help repair and rebuild these tissues.

Vitamin C also is a potent antioxidant that can help counter the damaging effects of inflammation.

Foods rich in vitamin C include citrus fruits, peaches, papayas, strawberries, tomatoes, turnip greens, red and green peppers and broccoli.

If you are not getting enough vitamin C from food, consider taking a supplement. I recommend 500 milligrams (mg) daily.

Warning: Wait an hour after eating acidic foods to brush your teeth. If you brush after consuming acidic foods, such as tomato products, citrus fruits or vinegar—or after taking a chewable vitamin C tablet—the toothbrush can wear away small amounts of enamel as it rubs the acid against your teeth. If you are drinking something acidic, such as fruit juice or soda, drink through a straw so the liquid bypasses tooth surfaces.

- **Garlic.** Garlic contains *diallyl sulfide,* an antimicrobial compound that can reduce the development of tartar and plaque. A laboratory study published in *The Journal of Food and Drug Analysis* found that garlic extracts almost completely suppressed the growth of S. mutans, an acid-producing organism that is the main cause of cavities.

Other foods that contain diallyl sulfide include onions, chives, leeks and shallots.

- **Sugarless gum.** Most people think that chewing gum is bad for the teeth. Not true. It's actually one of the most effective ways to prevent tooth decay and gum disease, particularly when you chew after meals.

Chewing gum greatly increases the flow of saliva, which washes away and neutralizes bacteria. Of course, it should always be sugarless.

- **Water.** Americans consume enormous quantities of sugar, particularly in soft drinks, sports drinks and juices. We've seen an increase in eroded tooth enamel in recent years because of high sugar intake. Even diet soft drinks cause problems because, like all carbonated beverages, they're acidic.

Better: Drink plain water or water with a little added fresh lemon juice or orange juice. When you do drink sweetened beverages, rinse your mouth with water when you're finished.

Avoid candy, cookies, cakes, crackers, muffins, potato chips, french fries, pretzels, bananas and dried fruits. These provide a source of sugar that bacteria can use to produce acid.

Listen Up! These Vitamins Can Prevent Hearing Loss

Josef M. Miller, PhD, professor of otolaryngology at University of Michigan Medical School, Ann Arbor, and Karolinska Institute in Stockholm. He is director of the Cochlear Signaling and Tissue Engineering Laboratory at Kresge Hearing Research Institute, also in Ann Arbor.

If you're middle-aged or older, you've probably heard about—or experienced for yourself—"age-related" hearing loss. Many people do lose some of their hearing with advancing age. That's the bad news.

The good news is that recent research has shown that much of this hearing loss can be prevented with certain nutrients. The right foods and supplements actually can help you hear better.

SILENT DAMAGE

Exposure to loud noises over a lifetime is a major cause of *presbycusis*, hearing loss that is associated with age and heredity. A structure in the inner ear called the *cochlea* is lined with thousands of tiny hairs that translate sound vibrations into electrical signals. Noise can damage these hairs and, over time, may result in hearing loss.

Why this happens: Loud noises trigger the production of free radicals, molecules produced in the inner ear that damage the cochlear hairs. Prolonged exposure to noise also causes a constriction of blood vessels and reduces circulation to the inner ear.

In laboratory studies at the University of Michigan, animals were exposed to sounds measuring 120 decibels, about the volume of a rock concert.

During this research, some animals were given the antioxidant-rich nutrients magnesium, beta-carotene (the body converts beta-carotene to vitamin A) and vitamins C and E one hour prior to the noise exposure and then once daily for five days. The test animals had 75% to 80% less hearing loss than animals given their normal food.

WHY NUTRITION HELPS

The antioxidants in fruits, vegetables, whole grains and other plant foods help fight free radicals and inflammation throughout the body, including in the inner ear. People who consume a lot of these nutrients on a regular basis get the most protection because free radical damage persists even when the noise is gone.

The largest spike in free radicals occurs while the noise is present. After that, free radicals intermittently decline and spike again. This cycle continues for five to seven days after the initial exposure, probably because free radicals are produced by the body as it attempts to heal noise-related damage within the inner ear. *Recommended nutrients...*

BEST COMBO

Taken together, the combination of nutrients beta-carotene, magnesium and vitamins C and E seems to be most effective at preventing cell damage. Each one inhibits the formation of free radicals in cells in different parts of the body. Vitamin E and beta-carotene reduce free radicals that are formed in the lipid (fatty) portions of cells, while vitamin C acts in the watery compartments. Magnesium dilates blood vessels, improves inner-ear circulation and prevents a noise-induced reduction in blood flow followed by a rebound increase (which would lead to an additional increase in free radicals).

Recommended doses: 18 milligrams (mg) beta-carotene...500 mg vitamin C...267 mg vitamin E (in the form of alpha-tocopherol)... and 312 mg magnesium. These doses are the equivalents of those used in the studies and are only slightly different from the minimum recommended levels.

Studies have shown that the best time to take nutritional supplements to protect your hearing is about 24 hours before an anticipated noise exposure, such as a concert or a car race.

When you're exposed to loud noises that you didn't anticipate, you can gain protection by increasing your antioxidant intake afterward. Antioxidants have been shown to reduce noise damage in animals when taken as much as three days following noise exposure—although protection was greater when taken one day after the noise.

FOLATE

The Blue Mountains Hearing Study (a survey of age-related hearing loss) collected data on dietary habits and measured levels of hearing loss in nearly 3,000 participants. Those with the lowest blood levels of folate were 39% more likely to experience hearing loss than those with the highest levels. Folate—the supplemental form is folic acid—is an antioxidant that also lowers levels of *homocysteine*, an amino acid that indicates the presence of inflammation in the body. Reducing homocysteine with folate or folic acid may reduce inflammatory damage and possibly improve circulation to the inner ear.

Recommended dose: I advise patients to get 400 micrograms (mcg) daily. You can get this much in one or two servings of many fortified breakfast cereals. Most multinutrient supplements also include folic acid. Foods rich in folate include spinach (100 mcg in one-half cup cooked) and asparagus (85 mcg in four spears).

OMEGA-3 FATTY ACIDS

In the Blue Mountains Hearing Study, those who ate fish two or more times a week were 42% less likely to suffer from age-related hearing loss than those who ate less than one weekly serving of fish.

Recommended: The omega-3 fatty acids in fish are among the healthiest nutrients you can eat. Two or more fish servings a week are probably ideal.

ZINC

This mineral is a chelator that binds to iron and helps remove it from the body. This process is important for hearing because iron plays a role in the formation of free radicals.

Recommended dose: The recommended daily allowance (RDA) is 11 mg zinc for men and 8 mg for women. A serving of beef can supply nearly 9 mg of zinc. Oysters, the richest source, provide 76.7 mg in a half-dozen.

Lower Risk of Kidney Disease Up to 150%

Alexander Chang, MD, a nephrology fellow in the department of nephrology and hypertension at Loyola University Medical Center in Maywood, Illinois. Dr. Chang led the group of researchers who recently presented their findings on diet and kidney disease prevention at the National Kidney Foundation's Spring Clinical Meetings.

We hear a great deal about the best dietary strategies to help prevent heart disease and diabetes. But what about kidney disease?

Recent development: For the first time, researchers have identified some of the key eating habits that help prevent the onset of kidney disease.

Why this is important: Kidney disease, which affects all the body's main physiological functions, significantly increases one's risk for serious medical conditions such as cardiovascular disease, including heart attack and stroke…sexual dysfunction…and bone fractures. *What you need to know…*

KEY FACTS ABOUT THE KIDNEYS

The kidneys are fist-sized organs that remove waste (about two quarts) from the approximately 200 quarts of blood that are processed daily. Each kidney contains about one million filtering units—tiny, delicate networks of blood vessels and tubes that are easily damaged by diabetes, high blood pressure and other chronic diseases.

KIDNEY DAMAGE OCCURS SLOWLY

Like hypertension and diabetes, kidney disease can progress over decades. Patients can lose up to 75% of their kidney function without experiencing kidney disease's eventual symptoms, which include fatigue and loss of appetite, difficulty concentrating, muscle cramps, swelling in the feet and/or ankles and/or low urine output. Increased risk for heart attack and stroke begins when kidney function has declined by about 50%—further declines usually require medication, dialysis or a kidney transplant.

Losing weight if you're overweight and following very specific dietary strategies are among the best ways to prevent kidney disease—and to minimize further damage if you are one of the 26 million Americans who already have it. Obesity increases the risk for hypertension and diabetes, which are the two most common causes of kidney disease.

Key dietary approaches recently identified by researchers…

• **Drink fewer sugar-sweetened drinks.** In a recent unpublished analysis of data from a 25-year study of young adults, Loyola researchers found that those who drank just 3.5 soft drinks or other sweetened beverages, such as energy drinks or fruit drinks, per week were 150% more likely to develop kidney disease than those who didn't drink them.

It's possible that the sweet beverages' high concentration of fructose, in particular (in refined sugar and high-fructose corn syrup) is responsible for the increased risk.

My advice: In general, Americans consume too much sugar. Switch to diet soft drinks.

Even better: Choose unsweetened beverages, such as water with a lemon slice.

• **Eat less animal protein.** In our analysis, people who ate an average of more than 1.5 servings a day of red meat or processed meat were 139% more likely to develop kidney disease than those who ate less than that. In patients with kidney disease, reducing overall protein intake lessens stress on the kidneys and can delay disease progression and the need for dialysis.

My advice: If you have kidney disease, consider working with a nutritionist to find healthful ways to limit daily protein to 40 g to 50 g. Fish (salmon, herring, mackerel and sardines) and lean meats provide high-quality protein with less saturated fat than you would get from typical red meat. Some research suggests vegetarian diets are especially beneficial for people with kidney disease.

For prevention: Include the most healthful protein sources. For example, beans and whole grains provide not only high-quality protein but also antioxidants, vitamins and minerals.

• **Consume much less salt.** For many people, a high-salt diet is a main cause of high blood pressure—a leading risk factor for kidney disease.

My advice: Even though some recent research raises questions about universal sodium restrictions, most health organizations recommend limiting daily sodium intake to 2,300 mg.

For some people with hypertension, reducing salt to 1,500 mg daily can lower systolic (top number) and diastolic (bottom number) pressure by about 11 points. That's comparable to the reduction that typically occurs with the use of antihypertensive medications.

•**Drink low-fat milk.** A study published in the *American Journal of Clinical Nutrition* that looked at 2,245 participants found that those who consumed the most low-fat milk, along with other low-fat dairy products, reduced their risk of developing hypertension by about 7%. Keeping one's blood pressure under control also contributes to healthy kidneys.

It's possible that the proteins and minerals (such as calcium) in dairy foods are responsible. Even though full-fat dairy contains the same minerals and proteins, the higher level of saturated fat may offset the benefits.

My advice: Check the USDA's Web site, *www.choosemyplate.gov,* for general guidelines regarding daily intake of low-fat or nonfat dairy.

•**Limit phosphorus intake.** The RDA for phosphorus in adults is 700 mg daily. However, the average adult consumes about twice as much because phosphorus is found in nearly every food—and it's added to processed foods to preserve colors and improve taste and/or texture.

Healthy adults excrete excess phosphorus. But in those with impaired kidney function, phosphorus can accumulate and cause conditions such as *hyperphosphatemia*, a buildup of this naturally occurring element that can lead to accelerated bone loss.

My advice: If you have kidney disease, ask your doctor if you need to lower your phosphorus levels—and work with a nutritionist to find the best ways to stay within healthy limits. It's wise for everyone to stay away from processed foods. In general, foods that are high in protein, such as meats, are also high in phosphorus. So are cola soft drinks, starchy vegetables and hard cheeses.

Important: To avoid high-phosphorus processed foods, look for "phos" on food labels. High-phosphorus additives include phosphoric acid, calcium phosphate and monopotassium phosphate.

info For more information on kidney disease, consult the National Kidney Foundation's Web site, *www.kidney.org.*

Drugs

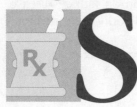

Six Surprisingly Dangerous Medicines

Some medicines are obviously risky. Most people know that codeine and driving don't mix…and that you might bleed too much when taking a blood thinner such as *warfarin*.

What people don't realize is that every drug, including over-the-counter medications, potentially can cause serious side effects. A study in *The Journal of the American Medical Association* reported that adverse drug reactions were responsible for 700,000 emergency room visits in just one year.

Here, medicines that seem safe but have unexpected risks…

MINERAL OIL

It's been used for generations for treating constipation. It's inexpensive, effective and available in supermarkets and pharmacies.

The danger: Lipoid pneumonia, a type of lung inflammation caused by inhaling an oil-based substance.

It's common to inhale (aspirate) substances into the lungs. This often happens when we eat or drink. The natural response is to cough—but mineral oil soothes the throat and calms the cough reflex.

Result: Particles of oil stay in the lungs and cause irritation that can lead to pneumonia. The symptoms include a persistent cough or difficulty breathing…and the irritation can increase your risk for a bacterial infection in addition to pneumonia.

To be safe: Don't exceed the recommended dose of one to three tablespoons daily. The more you take, the more you increase your risk for aspirating some of the oil.

Robert Steven Gold, RPh, hospital pharmacist and affiliate instructor of clinical pharmacy at Purdue University, West Lafayette, Indiana. He is author of *Are Your Meds Making You Sick? A Pharmacist's Guide to Avoiding Dangerous Drug Interactions, Reactions and Side Effects* (Hunter House). *www.areyourmedsmaking yousick.com*

Also important: Don't swallow mineral oil when you're lying down—it's more likely to get into the lungs. Consuming mineral oil after you've been drinking alcohol also is risky because alcohol impairs the body's ability to swallow normally.

Robert Steven Gold, RPh, hospital pharmacist at Purdue University, advises patients who need a laxative to use newer, safer products, such as Metamucil or Colace.

CALCIUM CARBONATE ANTACIDS (ROLAIDS, TUMS)

Antacids can be risky. Up to 10% of patients who frequently use calcium-based antacids to relieve heartburn or increase calcium intake experience side effects.

The danger: High doses of calcium carbonate can lead to *hypercalcemia*, elevated blood calcium, which can cause heart problems.

Warning signs: Nausea, abdominal and/or lower back pain, increased urination and/or impaired thinking.

To be safe: Follow the dosing instructions on the label, and don't take the tablets for more than two weeks without a doctor's supervision.

Also, ask yourself if you really need an antacid. People who frequently use aspirin or *naproxen* (Aleve), for example, may experience gastrointestinal (GI) irritation that feels like heartburn. *Acetaminophen* (Tylenol) may be less likely to cause GI problems.

Alternative: For relief from heartburn, you occasionally can substitute other, noncalcium types of antacids, such as Alka-Seltzer.

THE DIURETIC *FUROSEMIDE* (LASIX)

It's among the most frequently prescribed diuretics—"water pills" that remove excess fluid from patients with cardiovascular problems such as hypertension and heart failure.

The danger: Hearing loss. Drugs in this class, known as *loop diuretics* (others include *bumetanide* and *ethacrynic acid*), affect the concentration of potassium and other electrolytes in the inner ear. When given at high doses, usually in intravenous treatment, they're estimated to cause hearing loss in up to 100,000 patients a year.

To be safe: Talk to your doctor if you notice hearing loss in both ears soon after starting the medication. You might need to take a lower dose...or your doctor might switch you to a different medication that doesn't affect hearing.

Hearing usually returns once the dose and/or medication is changed—but the risk for permanent damage increases the longer you take the medication.

THE DIURETIC *SPIRONOLACTONE* (ALDACTONE)

This drug is used to reduce *edema* (fluid retention) in patients with heart, liver or kidney disease. It also can be used to treat hypertension.

The danger: It sometimes causes a dangerous increase in blood potassium, a condition known as hyperkalemia, which can cause an irregular heartbeat that is potentially deadly.

To be safe: Patients who take this drug must undergo frequent testing for blood potassium. When you are first prescribed it, you will need to have an electrolyte panel two to four weeks later...a follow-up test after three months...and regular tests about every six months.

If your potassium is elevated, your doctor might advise you to stop taking the drug.

Also helpful: Don't combine this medication with supplements—such as energy drinks or multinutrients—that contain potassium.

METFORMIN (SUCH AS GLUCOPHAGE) FOR DIABETES

One of the main drugs for type 2 diabetes, metformin improves the body's sensitivity to insulin and decreases production of glucose (blood sugar) in the liver.

The danger: It can cause *lactic acidosis*, a rare but potentially deadly complication that occurs when a metabolic by-product, known as lactate, accumulates in the body. Only about five in 100,000 patients who take metformin will develop lactic acidosis, but it's fatal in up to 50% of cases.

To be safe: Know the signs. The onset of lactic acidosis often is subtle and accompanied by symptoms such as fatigue, muscle pain and respiratory distress.

Patients with kidney or liver disease usually are advised not to take metformin—or, if they do take it, to undergo frequent (every three to six months) blood and urine tests.

Also, don't combine metformin with *cimetidine* (Tagamet), a medication used for heartburn and ulcers. It can increase the amount of metformin in the body by up to 40%. Other GI-protecting drugs, such as *famotidine* (Pepcid), don't have this effect.

SEROTONIN FOR DEPRESSION

Millions of Americans take *selective serotonin reuptake inhibitors* (SSRIs), the most frequently used medications for depression. SSRIs such as *escitalopram* (Lexapro) and *paroxetine* (Paxil) increase brain levels of serotonin, a neurotransmitter that affects mood.

The danger: Some people retain too much serotonin, a condition known as *medication-induced serotonin syndrome*. It can cause muscle twitches, loss of coordination, agitation, heavy sweating and other symptoms, including shivering or diarrhea. It is fatal in rare cases.

To be safe: Ask your doctor to review all your medications before starting treatment with an SSRI antidepressant. The risk for serotonin syndrome increases when SSRIs are combined with other medications, including *dextromethorphan* (an ingredient in cough medications), the antibiotics *linezolid* (Zyvox) and *ritonavir* (Norvir), and narcotic painkillers such as codeine.

Important: Don't take the herbal supplement St. John's wort if you're also taking an SSRI. St. John's wort increases serotonin.

■ ■ ■ ■

Drugs Cause Nightmares

These include antibiotics, antidepressants, beta-blockers, statins and drugs for such conditions as Alzheimer's, anxiety, epilepsy, hypertension, Parkinson's and smoking cessation. Nightmares also may occur in people who have recently stopped taking medications, such as *chlordiazepoxide* (Librium) and other benzodiazepines...and phenobarbital and other barbiturates.

Naresh Dewan, MD, director of the sleep medicine program at Creighton University, Omaha, and coauthor of a review of drug-induced sleep disorders, published in *The Consultant Pharmacist*.

Are Your Osteoporosis Meds Doing More Harm Than Good?

Harris H. McIlwain, MD, founder of the Tampa Medical Group and adjunct professor at the University of South Florida College of Public Health, both in Tampa. He is coauthor of *Reversing Osteopenia* (Henry Holt) and *The Osteoporosis Cure* (Avon).

When bone-building medications known as bisphosphonates were introduced 18 years ago, they were hailed as near-miracle drugs for people with thinning bones. Studies showed that these drugs—first, *aldendronate* (Fosamax) and later, *risedronate* (Actonel), *ibandronate* (Boniva) and *zoledronic acid* (Reclast)—significantly reduced the incidence of hip and spine fractures in people with osteoporosis and osteopenia (bone loss that is less severe than osteoporosis).

Now: Despite the established benefits of bisphosphonates, the medications are increasingly coming under fire for having potentially serious side effects. For example, studies have shown that the drugs may increase risk for various conditions, such as breakage of the femur (thigh bone), osteonecrosis (death of bone tissue) in the jaw and even esophageal cancer.

Two FDA advisory panels recently wrote in a report that due to the potential risks associated with long-term use of bisphosphonates, bisphosphonate therapy could be safely discontinued in some cases—but did not specify when or for how long to discontinue the drug.

Studies on the safety of bisphosphonates are ongoing. Thus far, the research is mixed on the benefits of taking the drug for more than five years. For example, research has shown that women who took Fosamax for another five years (for a total of 10 years) had the same rate of femur fractures as those who took a placebo. The risk for spine fracture, however, was higher in the group taking a placebo.

FINDING THE BEST TREATMENT

The decision to take bisphosphonates (or any medication) requires balancing benefits against risks. People at high risk for fractures should not stop taking these medications but instead work with their doctors to determine the duration of treatment. This includes people who have had previous fractures or a family history of fractures...and those with rheumatoid arthritis, which can increase bone loss. Other high-risk individuals include those who take the corticosteroid *prednisone* for a chronic condition... women who weigh under 127 pounds....people who lead a sedentary lifestyle (weight-bearing exercise strengthens bones)...and smokers (their risk for bone loss is twice that of a nonsmoker).

Women and men who have a high risk for fracture but who have other health concerns may want to talk to their doctors about taking a nonbisphosphonate bone-strengthening medication. *Examples*...

•*Denosumab* (Prolia), a monoclonal antibody that reduces the body's bone-breakdown mechanism. If you have gastroesophageal reflux disease, this drug, which is delivered via an injection, may help you avoid the gastrointestinal side effects common with bisphosphonates. However, in a few rare cases, osteonecrosis of the jaw has been reported.

•*Teriparatide* (Forteo), a type of parathyroid hormone that builds bone. This injectable drug increases bone thickness, so if you have a history of periodontal disease, you may be better off with this drug.

The Bone Drug That Battles Breast Cancer Too

Michael Gnant, MD, professor, surgery, Medical University of Vienna, Austria.

Jane Carleton, MD, oncologist, Monter Cancer Center, Lake Success, New York, North Shore-Long Island Jewish Health System.

A drug developed to treat osteoporosis appears to boost survival in women with certain types of breast cancer, according to two studies.

These preliminary findings regarding the bone-building drug *zoledronic acid* potentially give scores of women more options to battle their tumors. The studies were presented at the San Antonio Breast Cancer Symposium.

DETAILS OF ONE STUDY

The first study looked at premenopausal women with estrogen receptor-positive breast cancer receiving either the bone drug plus hormone therapy or a placebo plus hormone therapy for three years.

Earlier data from this study were encouraging, and this update—84 months after the trial's start—provides further evidence of improved disease-free survival and recurrence rates among women receiving zoledronic acid. The drug is known by the brand names Reclast and Zometa.

RESULTS

The recent research shows that women receiving zoledronic acid had a 28% reduced risk for recurrence and a 36% reduced risk for dying.

Women over the age of 40 received the most benefit, the researchers said.

"In general, the overall survival is excellent, which demonstrates that treating these patients without adjuvant chemotherapy is a very good approach," said study author Michael Gnant, MD, a professor of surgery at the Medical University of Vienna, Austria. He said the study received academic and not pharmaceutical funding.

Many women were still seeing the benefit four and five years after their treatment stopped. "This means we've changed something in the beginning in terms of the disease," Dr. Gnant said.

Cancer patients often take bone-building drugs, commonly referred to as bisphosphonates, to prevent fractures related to the spread of cancer to the bone. But zoledronic acid is not an approved treatment for breast cancer in many countries, including the United States, which makes its availability uncertain, Dr. Gnant noted.

THE SECOND STUDY

In another study, postmenopausal women who received zoledronic acid plus an *aromatase inhibitor* (drugs that block estrogen synthesis in the body) had a 29% lower risk for a recurrence and a 35% improvement in survival versus women receiving zoledronic acid plus a placebo.

The drug also appeared to increase bone density.

"We've been waiting for these data," said Jane Carleton, MD, an oncologist with Monter Cancer Center in Lake Success, New York. "Not only did it just prevent bone loss, it decreases the chances of the cancer coming back. That's powerful."

RESEARCH ON CLODRONATE

A third study of bisphosphonates found that the drug *clodronate* reduced the likelihood of cancer spreading in postmenopausal women by about 9%, less than was hoped for.

Slightly more encouraging were reductions in mortality (16%). Clodronate is known by the brand name Bonefos.

The trial was partially supported by Bayer Schering Pharma Oy, which makes Bonefos.

DISAPPOINTING RESULTS

A final study had disappointing results for patients receiving high-dose chemotherapy and another bisphosphonate, *ibandronate* (Boniva).

The drug did not improve either time to a recurrence or overall survival in women already treated with chemotherapy.

Other trials had shown more positive results.

info The Web site of the National Cancer Institute, *http://www.cancer.gov/cancertopics/treatment/breast*, has more information about treatments for breast cancer.

■ ■ ■ ■

Make Pills Easy to Swallow

Before putting the pill in your mouth, take a deep breath and exhale to help you relax and reduce your gag reflex. Swallow some water, then place the pill far back on your tongue, and swallow it with another sip of water. Don't throw your head back when swallowing—it is better to tilt it forward and toward your chest. If you still have trouble—and if your doctor and pharmacist say it is OK—open capsules or crush pills and add to applesauce, chocolate pudding or other foods that go down easily. Or ask if there are easier-to-swallow versions available, such as liquids, powders or chewables.

UC Berkeley Wellness Letter, www.wellnessletter.com

Beware Cancer Drugs With Fatal Side Effects

Dana-Farber Cancer Institute, news release

Treatment with three relatively new cancer drugs may be linked to a slightly increased risk of death, a recent analysis suggests.

While the risk is low, it should be taken into account by doctors and patients, according to Dana-Farber Cancer Institute scientists and colleagues.

The investigators analyzed the findings of 10 clinical trials that included nearly 4,700 patients treated with *sorafenib* (Nexavar) for kidney and liver cancer, *sunitinib* (Sutent) for kidney cancer and gastrointestinal stromal tumor or *pazopanib* (Votrient) for kidney cancer.

These so-called "targeted" drugs are used to stop the growth or spread of cancer by blocking the vascular endothelial growth factor tyrosine kinase receptors in cancer cells, the researchers explained in a Dana-Farber news release.

The analysis of the clinical trials revealed that the incidence of fatal complications was 1.5% in patients who received any of the three drugs, compared with 0.7% in patients who received standard treatments or placebos.

Bleeding, heart attack and heart failure were the most common fatal side effects noted in the clinical trials. In addition, liver failure was also reported, according to the report published in *Journal of Clinical Oncology*.

"There is no doubt for the average patient, these drugs have benefits and are [US Food and Drug Administration]-approved for these indications," said study leader Toni Choueiri, MD, assistant professor, department of medicine, Harvard Medical School. "While the absolute incidence of these fatal side effects is very small, the relative risks are higher and patients and practitioners need to be aware of it."

info The US National Cancer Institute has more information about targeted cancer therapies. Visit its Web site at *www.cancer.gov/cancertopics/factsheet/therapy/targeted*.

Drug Helps Control Dangerous Side Effect of Stem Cell Transplants

Gary Schiller, MD, director, Hematological Malignancies/Stem Cell Transplantation Unit, Jonsson Comprehensive Cancer Center, University of California, Los Angeles.
The New England Journal of Medicine
Dana-Farber Cancer Institute, news release

Preliminary research suggests that a drug typically used to kickstart the immune system may help cancer patients who receive stem cell transplants and then develop a potentially deadly side effect.

Researchers found that daily low-dose injections of *interleukin-2* appeared to help some patients by treating the side effect, known as *graft-versus-host disease* (GVHD). The drug appears to work by preventing the donor's immune system cells from overreacting to their new home and causing systemic inflammation.

BACKGROUND

Stem cell transplants can treat blood cancers such as leukemia. "More than half of patients who successfully undergo hematopoietic stem cell transplants [in which the blood-making tissue in the bone marrow is wiped out with chemotherapy and replaced with blood-forming stem cells from a donor] develop chronic GVHD," study author John Koreth, MD, PhD, of Dana-Farber Cancer Institute in Boston, said in an institute news release. "The conventional treatment, glucocorticoids, are limited in their effectiveness and can produce significant side effects."

EXPERT COMMENTARY

GVHD is "a big problem," said Gary Schiller, MD, director of the Hematological Malignancies/Stem Cell Transplantation Unit at the Jonsson Comprehensive Cancer Center at the University of California, Los Angeles. Dr. Schiller was not involved with the study.

STUDY DETAILS

In the study, 12 of 23 patients who took the drug for eight weeks showed improvement in symptoms related to GVHD, including skin rash and other skin problems, hepatitis and inflamed lungs. The condition didn't worsen while the patients took the drug.

The study is the first phase of three stages of research that drug treatments must undergo before the federal government approves them to treat specific conditions. That means the findings are preliminary and may not be replicated in future research.

TREATS THE COMPLICATIONS, BUT NOT THE CANCER

Dr. Schiller said the findings make sense. However, the treatment "has no impact, to my knowledge, on curing cancer. It only has an impact on decreasing the complications of the cancer cure."

The study, published in *The New England Journal of Medicine*, was funded by several research grants and awards.

info The US National Library of Medicine has more information on stem cells at its Web site *http://www.nlm.nih.gov/*.

■ ■ ■ ■

Cancer Drug Shows Promise for Alzheimer's

The skin cancer drug *bexarotene* (Targretin) was shown in animal studies to promptly stimulate the removal of amyloid plaques that can lead to the cognitive and memory deficits of Alzheimer's disease. Research to confirm these findings in humans is under way.

Science

■ ■ ■ ■

Sleeping Pills Increase Cancer Risk Up to 35%

In a recent study, researchers compared health outcomes of 10,529 people who had been prescribed sleeping pills, such as *zolpidem* (Ambien) and *temazepam* (Restoril), with those of 23,676 people not taking the pills.

Results: After 2.5 years, study participants prescribed 18 or more doses per year were more than 3.5 times more likely to die than those taking none and had a 20% increased risk for cancer. Study participants taking 132 or more annual doses had a fivefold risk for death and were 35% more likely to be diagnosed with cancer than people taking none.

Daniel Kripke, MD, codirector of research, Scripps Clinic Viterbi Family Sleep Center, La Jolla, California.

New Study Warns About Common Respiratory Drug

The Lancet news release

A study assessing intravenous infusion of the drug *salbutamol* in patients with acute respiratory distress syndrome was halted because the treatment did not improve patient outcomes and was associated with an increased risk of death, researchers say.

BACKGROUND

Acute respiratory distress syndrome (ARDS) occurs in about 14% of patients who require being placed on mechanical ventilation. The death rate among patients with ARDS is high—40% to 60%—and survivors have a substantial decrease in their quality of life.

However, "routine use of [beta-2] agonist therapy in mechanically ventilated patients with ARDS cannot be recommended," the researchers wrote in an article published in the online edition of *The Lancet*.

The British study included 326 patients who received either *salbutamol* (also known as *albuterol*) or a placebo within 72 hours of developing ARDS, and the treatment continued for up to seven days. But the study was stopped after 55 (34%) of the 161 patients in the salbutamol group died, compared with 38 (23%) of the 163 patients in the placebo group.

Overall, the death rate was 47% higher in the salbutamol group than in the placebo group, the report indicated.

In addition, patients in the salbutamol group had fewer ventilator-free days and organ failure-free days than those in the placebo group.

CONCLUSIONS

"Our findings show that intravenous salbutamol given to patients with early ARDS significantly increased 28-day mortality, and reduced ventilator-free days and duration of organ support compared with those given placebo," explained Fang Gao Smith, MD, and her colleagues from the University of Warwick.

The authors added that the therapy was "poorly tolerated" by patients because it was linked to heart rhythm abnormalities and lactic acidosis (a dangerous buildup of lactic acid in the blood). "These findings were unexpected," the researchers noted.

EXPERT COMMENTARY

The findings of the cancelled study may be sufficient to change treatment of patients with ARDS, B. Taylor Thompson, MD, of Massachusetts General Hospital and Harvard Medical School, wrote in an accompanying editorial.

"[Beta-2] agonist treatment in patients with ARDS should be limited to the treatment of clinically important reversible airway obstruction and should not be part of routine care," Dr. Thompson recommended.

info For more information on acute respiratory distress syndrome, visit the Web site of The US National Heart, Lung, and Blood Institute at *http://www.nhlbi.nih.gov/health/health-topics/topics/ards/*.

■ ■ ■ ■

Use Nicotine Patches Safely for More Than 12 Weeks

Quit-smoking aids can be used for longer than 12 weeks. The Food and Drug Administration is considering eliminating the current warning on most nicotine-replacement gum, lozenges and patches recommending that people stop using them after 12 weeks. Use of these medications beyond 12 weeks may help some people abstain from smoking. And nicotine itself is not believed to raise the risk for cancer, though it can elevate heart rate, raise blood pressure and may cause adverse skin reactions.

K. Michael Cummings, PhD, chair, department of health behavior, division of cancer prevention and population sciences, Roswell Park Cancer Institute, Buffalo.

Stop-Smoking Drug May Also Curb Problem Drinking

Ihsan Salloum, MD, MPH, professor, psychiatry, and director, alcohol and drug abuse treatment program, University of Miami Miller School of Medicine.

Emma Childs, PhD, research associate, University of Chicago.

Alcoholism: Clinical & Experimental Research, online.

The quit-smoking drug Chantix may also help problem drinkers cut their alcohol consumption, a small study suggests.

Exactly how this drug curbs drinking is not fully understood, but its use may increase blood pressure, heart rate and feelings of sadness and nausea, thereby blunting the pleasurable effects of alcohol, the researchers said.

"Chantix might reduce alcohol consumption by reducing overall enjoyment of the alcohol drinking experience," said study author Emma Childs, PhD, research associate at the University of Chicago.

"Chantix increased the unpleasant effects of alcohol, for example feeling drowsy and irritable, [and] participants also reported that they didn't like the alcohol effects as much," Dr. Childs said.

BACKGROUND ON CHANTIX

Approved to help smokers quit in 2006, Chantix (*varenicline*) has its share of potential side effects. In July 2009, the US Food and Drug Administration mandated that Chantix carry a "black box" warning about the potential risks of depression and suicidal thoughts. Recently, the drug was linked to a small but significant risk of heart attack and stroke among people with pre-existing heart disease. Chantix costs roughly $3 per pill.

STUDY DETAILS

The study included 15 healthy participants who took part in six sessions. They received a 2-mg dose of Chantix and an inactive placebo, followed three hours later by a beverage containing a placebo, a low dose of alcohol or a high dose of alcohol.

Before and after the sessions, the researchers asked the participants about their mood, tested visual ability and measured physiological responses such as blood pressure and heart rate.

The participants found the Chantix-booze combination increased the unpleasant effects of alcohol and reduced the rewarding aspects of drinking.

The results of the new study were published in *Alcoholism: Clinical & Experimental Research*.

IMPLICATIONS

Whether the drug might someday be approved to help problem drinkers cut back remains to be seen, said the researchers, who acknowledged that the study's small size is a limitation.

"We are not currently performing any studies with Chantix, although other groups are actively pursuing this line of research with a view to developing Chantix as an aid to people wanting to quit or cut down their drinking," Dr. Childs said.

EXPERT COMMENTARY

Ihsan Salloum, MD, professor of psychiatry and director of the alcohol and drug abuse treatment program at the University of Miami Miller School of Medicine, termed the study encouraging.

Noting that new ways of treating alcoholism are much needed, Dr. Salloum said that Chantix may have a niche among smokers with alcohol-dependence issues. "We need a lot more options in terms of medicines to help curb drinking," he said. "We have many options for depression and need more for alcoholism—considering it is one of the most common diseases around the world."

More research is needed, he noted, but "this medication may be helpful for people with a drinking problem who are also smokers."

The study was funded by the US National Institute on Drug Abuse and the US National Institute on Alcohol Abuse and Alcoholism.

info Learn more about alcoholism and how it is treated at the Web site of the US National Institute on Alcohol Abuse and Alcoholism, *http://www.niaaa.nih.gov.*

■ ■ ■ ■

New Macular Degeneration Medicine Costs Less and Works Well

New medication for macular degeneration costs less and works as well as Lucentis (*ranibizumab*). The medication Eylea (*aflibercept*) treats the wet form of age-related macular degeneration—the major cause of blindness in those over age 55. Eylea can be given once every two months after an initial series of three monthly doses. Eylea costs about $1,850 per dose, compared with about $2,000 per dose for Lucentis (which is administered monthly). Both drugs are injected into the eye with a tiny needle.

Abdhish R. Bhavsar, MD, retina surgeon and director of clinical research, Retina Center of Minnesota, Minneapolis, and a clinical correspondent for the American Academy of Ophthalmology.

■ ■ ■ ■

Common Antinausea Drug Linked to Heart Problems

Andrew Rubman, ND, founder and director, Southbury Clinic for Traditional Medicines, Southbury, Connecticut. *www.southburyclinic.org*
Kerry S. Russell, MD, PhD, associate professor of medicine in the section of cardiovascular medicine at Yale University School of Medicine, New Haven, Connecticut.

The good news is that patients don't tend to get as sick to their stomachs after treatment or surgery as they used to thanks to a drug called Zofran (*ondansetron*), which has turned out to be very good at quelling nausea—especially the kind caused by chemotherapy. All kinds of patients (not just cancer patients) are given Zofran postoperatively to prevent nausea after general anesthesia.

The bad news is that this drug has now been linked with a health problem that is far more dangerous than transitory nausea—a potentially fatal heart condition. The number of drugs that link to this specific heart condition is well over a dozen, and now Zofran has been added to the list.

Does this mean a return to the times when cancer patients were vomiting for days and days following each chemotherapy treatment? Well, no—not yet, anyway.

The FDA hasn't banned Zofran, but after reviewing all available information on Zofran and its potential link to this heart condition, the FDA has ordered GlaxoSmithKline, the maker of Zofran, to conduct more thorough research on the drug's potential impact on the heart. In the meantime, the FDA has issued warnings to clinicians that certain types of patients require extra-careful monitoring if they take this drug.

According to the FDA, the people most at risk include…

•**People with underlying heart conditions.**

•**People predisposed to low levels of potassium, magnesium and calcium.**

•**Patients who are taking other medications that might also trigger high risk of heart failure (prolonged QT intervals).** The medication list is surprisingly long and includes drugs in a number of categories such as antihypertensives, antibiotics, antidepressants, antihistamines, gastrointestinal agents and more. Your doctor can work with you on how best to handle drugs on the list that you are taking. (For detailed drug information see *http://www.uspharmacist.com/content/c/26648/*.)

OTHER OPTIONS FOR NAUSEA

According to Andrew L. Rubman, ND, founder and director of Southbury Clinic for Traditional Medicines in Southbury, Connecticut, nausea is actually a healthy reaction that our bodies produce when a toxin, be it residue from a chemo drug, spoiled food or something else, gets into the digestive system. This reaction, intended to rid your body of the toxin, is triggered when the toxin passes into the *duodenum*, the upper part of the small intestine that uses enzymes to break down food for digestion.

Zofran stops nausea by interfering with normal digestive processes. In so doing, however, it also disrupts the balance of some important minerals, such as calcium, potassium and magnesium. This is the root of why it may cause the heart problem—calcium, potassium and magnesium in balanced, proper amounts are crucial to the heart's electrical stability.

This heart condition may also be caused by the generic equivalents of Zofran, said Dr. Rubman, and the antinausea drug Kytril (*granisetron*). Dr. Rubman said he'd like to see doctors—especially those at cancer centers who work with patients after chemotherapy—add a natural approach for helping patients avoid nausea. This natural approach works by binding the chemo residue to get it out of the body quickly without causing mischief in the duodenum.

NATURAL WAYS
TO COMBAT NAUSEA

Here are some natural ways from Dr. Rubman that chemo patients might be able to prevent nausea. He suggests printing this out, talking with your naturopathic physician about the appropriate regimens and then bringing it with you to discuss with your oncologist…

•**B-complex vitamins give the liver additional support** in breaking down chemo drugs after they have done their work. Generally, B-12 and B-6 are the most important to take, but they need to be supported by others in the group.

•**Dietary fiber supplements bind and limit the reabsorption of the chemo drug's residue.**

•**Ginger supplements may also help.** Studies have shown that taking ginger on a specific schedule—including the day before treatment—reduces chemo-induced nausea.

■ ■ ■ ■

Ease Angina With This Gout Drug

In a recent study of 65 adults with heart disease and stable angina (chest pain that occurs with activity or stress), those who took 600 mg of the gout medication *allopurinol* (Aloprim) daily for six weeks could exercise longer before chest pain occurred than those who took a placebo.

Theory: Allopurinol blocks a crucial enzyme, reducing oxygen demand during exercise.

If you have stable angina: Ask your doctor about allupurinol. Side effects may include upset stomach, diarrhea and drowsiness.

Allan D. Struthers, MD, professor of cardiovascular medicine, Centre for Cardiovascular & Lung Biology, University of Dundee School of Medicine, Dundee, UK.

■ ■ ■ ■

90% of OTC Thyroid Pills Can Be Dangerous

Thyroid-support pills can be dangerous. People who feel tired or have unexplained weight gain sometimes turn to over-the-counter (OTC) thyroid supplements.

But: Nine of the 10 OTC products tested contained the hormone T3…and five contained the hormone T4. These hormones should be used only under a doctor's guidance. Overdoses can lead to heart palpitations, blood pressure abnormalities and other problems.

Victor J. Bernet, MD, endocrinologist at Mayo Clinic, Jacksonville, Florida, and senior investigator of a study of OTC thyroid supplements, presented at a recent meeting of the American Thyroid Association.

Newer Blood Thinner Dangerous for Trauma Patients

Bryan Cotton, MD, trauma surgeon and intensivist, Memorial Hermann Hospital and University of Texas Health Science Center, Houston.

Lisandro Irizarry, MD, chair of emergency medicine, Brooklyn Hospital Center, New York City.

Jack Ansell, MD, chairman, department of medicine, Lenox Hill Hospital, New York City.

Statement, Boehringer Ingelheim US, Ridgefield, Connecticut.

New England Journal of Medicine

A new blood thinner touted for its convenience and low maintenance may have hidden problems that could threaten the lives of certain patients, a report suggests.

A letter to the editor of *The New England Journal of Medicine* reports severe bleeding complications among trauma patients on the anti-clotting medicine *dabigatran etexilate* (Pradaxa).

In one case, a patient died, the letter said.

"We have noted on multiple occasions patients who have 'bleeding out' from Pradaxa and our hands are tied," said Bryan Cotton, MD, lead letter author and a trauma surgeon with the University of Texas Health Science Center at Memorial Hermann Hospital in Houston.

REVERSIBILITY A PROBLEM FOR PRADAXA

The main problem, Dr. Cotton said, is that there's no real way to reverse the anti-clotting effect of the drug, unlike older agents such as *warfarin*.

The only way to reverse Pradaxa is with emergency dialysis but, said Dr. Cotton, "in a patient bleeding to death, that's not really a practical or pragmatic option."

BACKGROUND

Warfarin (Coumadin, Jantoven) has been the mainstay of blood-thinning medications to manage heart and stroke patients for decades.

But the drug is notoriously difficult to manage, requiring frequent lab tests and having interactions with multiple foods and other medications. Its one big advantage, however, is that its blood-thinning properties are easily reversible when needed.

Enter the new, easier-to-use blood thinner, Pradaxa, first approved by the US Food and Drug Administration in late 2010 for use in patients with atrial fibrillation, a common and dangerous form of irregular heartbeat.

"There is an advantage over warfarin in many ways because of the simplicity and ease of management," said Jack Ansell, MD, chairman of the department of medicine at Lenox Hill Hospital in New York City. "There are very few interactions with other drugs or foods." On the other hand, he says, "warfarin is relatively easy to reverse."

OTHER ISSUES

Pradaxa also has other problems in addition to the irreversibility, the letter said, namely that there are no readily available tests to assess how well it's working or not working.

"You can't really check the labs. There's no easy, cheap, readily available lab test," Dr. Cotton noted.

The information provided in the letter, said Lisandro Irizarry, MD, chair of emergency medi-

cine at the Brooklyn Hospital Center in New York City, is "incredibly useful and incredibly timely."

"Although this medication provides enhanced quality of life, it does have a significant impact on how we manage patients because there's no way to reverse it and no way to measure how thin the blood is," he said.

Dr. Cotton and his coauthors urged the US Food and Drug Administration (FDA) to support more trials to assess the potentially wide-ranging effects of the drug.

"We absolutely understand that it's a lot better for patients from a convenience standpoint…but when something goes wrong, it can go wrong very badly," Dr. Cotton said.

SAFETY A PRIORITY, SAYS MANUFACTURER

In a statement, Pradaxa's maker, Boehringer Ingelheim, confirmed that, "At this time, there is no reversal agent available" for the blood thinner. The company says that dialysis can lead to "the removal of about 60% of the drug over two to three hours; however, data supporting this approach are limited."

In the meantime, "Patient safety is our top priority and we frequently communicate with the FDA and regulatory agencies around the world to ensure they have the most up-to-date information regarding the safety profile of Pradaxa," the company said. "All treatment decisions should be made on an individual basis between patients and their health care providers and should take into consideration the overall benefits and risks associated with various treatment options."

Pradaxa is not the only new-generation blood thinner to be approved recently—the anti-clotting drug *ticagrelor* (Brilinta) gained FDA approval for use in heart patients this past summer. However, according to Dr. Ansell, there is no "reversibility" problem with Brilinta.

info The Web site of the National Library of Medicine has more on blood thinners. Visit *www.nlm.nih.gov/medlineplus/bloodthin ners.html*.

New Drug Helps Some Patients Avoid Heart Attack and Stroke

Eugene Braunwald, MD, professor, medicine, Harvard Medical School, and cardiologist, Brigham and Women's Hospital, Boston.

C. Michael Gibson, MD, chief of clinical research, Division of Cardiology, Beth Israel Deaconess Medical Center, Boston.

Gordon F. Tomaselli, MD, chief of cardiology, Johns Hopkins University School of Medicine, Baltimore, and past president, American Heart Association.

New England Journal of Medicine

When added to standard treatment, a new blood-thinning drug called *rivaroxaban* (Xarelto) may help people with "acute coronary syndrome" lower their risk of death, subsequent heart attack or stroke, a recent study finds.

Acute coronary syndrome is an umbrella term that includes people with angina (chest pain) or prior history of heart attack.

The finding "opens up a new area for treating this very common condition," said study coauthor Eugene Braunwald, MD, professor of medicine at Harvard Medical School and a cardiologist at Brigham and Women's Hospital in Boston.

The study could help Xarelto expand the ranks of common blood thinners, which for decades were dominated by old standbys such as *warfarin* (Coumadin) or, more recently, *clopidogrel* (Plavix).

Xarelto has been approved by the US Food and Drug Administration to treat an abnormal heart rhythm called atrial fibrillation and to prevent the formation of blood clots after hip and knee replacement surgery.

STUDY DETAILS

The recent trial included more than 15,500 people who had been hospitalized for acute coronary syndrome. Participants received either a low dose (5 milligrams [mg]) or a very low dose (2.5 mg) of the new blood thinner or a placebo, in addition to standard care. The medications were given twice daily for an average of 13 months.

People who received either dosage of Xarelto had a lower risk of heart attack, stroke or death when compared with their counterparts given a placebo. Specifically, there was a 16% decrease among patients in the 2.5-mg group and a 15% decrease in the 5-mg group, the researchers reported.

Among the participants taking the 2.5-mg dose, there was a 34% reduced risk of cardiovascular death and a 32% lower risk for death from any cause. Similar reductions were not seen among people taking the 5-mg dose, however.

Xarelto also reduced the risk of blood clots forming within arteries that were held open by stents—small mesh tubes used to widen narrowed arteries.

However, addition of the new drug did boost the odds of a common blood-thinner side effect: bleeding, including bleeds within the brain. However, this increase in risk was confined to nonfatal bleeds, the research team reported, and the incidence of bleeding fell when patients took the smaller versus the larger dose of Xarelto.

Dr. Braunwald said risks for bleeding must always be balanced against the benefits of any anti-clotting medication. "I'd rather have a patient walk out of a hospital with a bleed than [leave through] the morgue," he said.

The study, funded by the drug's makers, Johnson & Johnson and Bayer Healthcare, was published in the *New England Journal of Medicine* and presented at the annual meeting of the American Heart Association in Orlando, Florida.

IMPLICATIONS

Another study author, C. Michael Gibson, MD, was encouraged by the findings.

"We have not seen a mortality reduction like this in cardiology for a few decades," said Dr. Gibson, who is chief of clinical research in the Division of Cardiology at Beth Israel Deaconess Medical Center in Boston. "This is secondary prevention for people who have weathered the storm and survived."

Secondary prevention refers to staving off a future coronary event among people who have already had a first one. By contrast, primary prevention is aimed at keeping that first event from occurring.

The benefit from Xarelto was consistent across all subgroups, Dr. Gibson said. "There is more bleeding," he said, "but no excess fatal bleeding or bleeding that leads to disability. I think it will be a game-changer."

According to Dr. Gibson, one big issue with the old standby drug Coumadin is that doses must often be adjusted. However, using Xarelto to manage atrial fibrillation has typically been more of a "one-size-fits-all" situation, he noted.

When it comes to managing acute coronary syndrome, this trial has shown a "smallest-size-fits-all" result for Xarelto, Dr. Gibson said, with the 2.5 mg dosage performing better. "Less is more," he added.

EXPERT REACTION

Before moving forward, Xarelto needs further study among people who are at high risk for bleeding, Matthew T. Roe, MD, and E. Magnus Ohman, MD, of Duke University Medical Center in Durham, North Carolina, wrote in an accompanying editorial in the journal.

They point out that better ways of predicting which patients are at risk for drug-related bleeds is also needed. Still, they wrote, "the results of this study indicate that rivaroxaban (Xarelto) will play an important role in the future of optimized secondary prevention."

For his part, American Heart Association past president Gordon F. Tomaselli, MD, said that Xarelto and other, newer drugs may offer options to patients beyond warfarin. Other members of this relatively new class of drugs now include *dabigatran* (Pradaxa) and *ticagrelor* (Brilinta).

"Xarelto and the others are important new medications that are easier for patients to take and do not interact as much with other medications or foods," said Dr. Tomaselli, who is chief of cardiology at Johns Hopkins University School of Medicine in Baltimore. They do cost more, but they don't require as much monitoring, including frequent blood draws, he explained.

"For many people who hate taking warfarin, because it interferes with what they eat or take, these drugs are good alternatives," he said.

SIMILAR DRUGS NOT AS EFFECTIVE

Other anti-clotting medications in development did not perform as well, according to two other studies also presented at the heart association meeting, and also published in the *New England Journal of Medicine*.

One study, led by Pierlugi Tricoci, MD, PhD, of Duke University, looked at a blood thinner called *vorapaxar*. In a study involving nearly 13,000 patients with acute coronary syndromes, adding vorapaxar to standard treatment did not significantly reduce patients' risk of dying from heart disease, risk of heart attack, stroke or rehospitalization. The drug did boost patients' odds for major bleeding, however.

And in another trial, the drug *apixaban* (Eliquis) was pitted against another mainstay blood thinner, *enoxaparin* (Lovenox), in more than 6,500 patients with congestive heart failure at high risk for dangerous clots. Researchers led by Samuel Goldhaber, MD, of Brigham and Women's Hospital and Harvard Medical School found that Eliquis did not outperform Lovenox and was also linked to more bleeding.

The vorapaxar study was funded by drug maker Merck, while Bristol-Myers Squibb and Pfizer supported the Eliquis/Lovenox trial.

■ ■ ■ ■

New Drugs for Hepatitis C Boost Cure Rate

Either *boceprevir* (Victrelis) or *telaprevir* (Incivek) is taken with two other drugs—*pegylated interferon alpha* and *ribavirin*.

Recent finding: The three-drug combination effectively cured more than 70% of patients in clinical trials, compared with 20% to 40% cured by the two-drug treatment. The treatments are expensive, and insurance coverage varies.

Robert G. Gish, MD, clinical professor of medicine, University of California, San Diego.

■ ■ ■ ■

Seniors—Beware These ER Drugs

Some drugs prescribed in ERs, such as *propoxyphene* for pain, may be dangerous for older adults who already are taking a variety of drugs. The medications prescribed may have a larger and longer-lasting sedating effect on older adults and may increase the risk for falls at home and other complications.

Self-defense: Carry a list of all medicines and supplements that you use with you at all times, including dosage information. If someone is bringing you to the hospital, be sure that person has a copy of the list to give to hospital personnel. Consider asking the physician if there are safer alternatives to the drugs prescribed, especially pain medications.

William J. Meurer, MD, assistant professor, department of emergency medicine, University of Michigan, Ann Arbor, and coauthor of a study of 1.5 billion emergency room visits, published in *Academic Emergency Medicine*.

Painful News About Common Painkillers

Harlan Krumholz, MD, professor of cardiology at Yale School of Medicine, New Haven, Connecticut, and author of *The Expert Guide to Beating Heart Disease: What You Absolutely Must Know* (HarperCollins).

Several years ago, people in pain were horrified to learn that certain prescription medications—Vioxx and Bextra, in particular—were dangerous and put them at significant risk for cardiovascular problems. Not only were these people rightfully outraged at having been misled about the safety of these drugs, they were outraged as well at the prospect of having to endure more of the pain they were trying to escape. Many switched to other, more well-known, over-the-counter brands of nonsteroidal anti-inflammatory drugs (NSAIDs), such as Advil, Motrin, Aleve. Now a recent study delivers yet more painful news—it seems that these drugs also carry stroke risks.

STUDY DETAILS

A group of researchers at the University of Bern recently conducted a meta-analysis of more than 30 randomized trials with a combined total of 116,429 patients taking placebo or NSAIDs. The researchers found abundant evidence of a heightened risk for cardiovascular events and found that taking drugs containing *ibuprofen*, including brand names such as Motrin, Advil and Nuprin, and those containing *naproxen* (such as the brand Aleve and a few others) raises the likelihood of suffering a stroke.

These are everyday drugs that sit in most of America's medicine cabinets right now. So, even though this finding is based on a "study of studies" rather than a customized clinical trial that is the gold standard, it's an important one—as many people take these drugs often and without giving it much thought.

CAUTION FROM AN EXPERT

According to Harlan Krumholz, MD, professor of cardiology at Yale School of Medicine and author of the book *The Expert Guide to Beating Heart Disease: What You Absolutely Must Know*, the reason NSAIDs carry cardiovascular risk is that these drugs "disturb the balance of the blood's clotting system, and some of them tend to cause clot formation." He cautions that everyone who takes NSAIDs is at some risk for heart problems. "In particular, people with heart disease should avoid using these medications," Dr. Krumholz said.

Since there is also some risk (albeit small) associated with products containing *acetaminophen* (such as Tylenol), Dr. Krumholz said that for people with heart issues, aspirin is probably the safest pain reliever. It is, after all, recommended for this group as protection against future heart attacks.

■ ■ ■ ■

Narcotic Painkillers May Harm Your Heart

Older patients taking opioids such as hydrocodone or codeine face a higher risk for heart attack, bone fracture and death, compared with similar patients taking non-narcotic drugs, such as *ibuprofen*. If an opioid is necessary to control pain, it is best to take the medicine for as short a time as possible in the lowest effective dose.

Daniel H. Solomon, MD, MPH, associate physician, division of pharmaco-epidemiology, Brigham & Women's Hospital, Boston. He led an analysis of painkillers published in *Archives of Internal Medicine*.

■ ■ ■ ■

Zocor Dosage Danger

Zocor should not be taken in an 80-milligram dose. The FDA says that the 80-mg dose of the statin drug Zocor (*simvastatin*) can cause *myopathy*, a potentially severe muscle disorder. A patient taking the 40-mg dose who still has not reached his/her cholesterol goal should be switched to another statin, such as Lipitor (*atorvastatin*) or Crestor (*rosuvastatin*).

Caution: Never change your medication or dose without your doctor's OK.

Steven E. Nissen, MD, chairman of cardiovascular medicine, Cleveland Clinic, Ohio.

The Deadly Dangers of Off-Label Drugs

Randall S. Stafford, MD, PhD, director of the Program on Prevention Outcomes and Practices at the Stanford Prevention Research Center and associate professor of medicine at Stanford University.

At least 21% of prescriptions written by American doctors are written for medical conditions that the drugs have not been proven to treat. The prescriptions are "off-label," which means that the drugs are being used in ways that have not been formally tested or approved by the Food and Drug Administration (FDA) as safe and effective.

A drug also is considered off-label if it's used…

•**For a type of person that the drug has not been tested on** (such as children or the elderly).

•**At a dosage not approved by the FDA.**

•**By itself,** when labeling specifies it should be used with other drugs.

•**With other drugs,** when labeling specifies it should be used alone.

Key finding: A study in *Archives of Internal Medicine* showed that 73% of off-label prescriptions do not have good scientific evidence justifying their use.

OFF-LABEL, ON TRIAL

It is illegal for pharmaceutical companies to promote their drugs for off-label use, but billions of dollars in possible profits are a strong incentive to circumvent the law. In a study published in *PLoS Medicine*, researchers from Harvard Medical School analyzed 18 cases where drug companies were prosecuted for off-label marketing that resulted in $7.9 billion in judgments against the companies.

The researchers found that the drug companies tried to expand the use of the drugs to unapproved diseases…to unapproved disease subtypes (such as prescribing an antidepressant for mild depression when it has been approved only for severe depression)…and to unapproved drug doses.

They also found that the drug companies used marketing schemes to influence doctors, including "direct financial incentives" (85% of the time)…"self-serving presentations" of the scientific literature about the drug (76%)…sponsorships of teaching (54%) and research (20%)…and free drug samples (20%).

In other words, doctors were essentially being bribed and duped by drug companies to prescribe drugs off-label.

Randall S. Stafford, MD, PhD, from the Stanford Prevention Research Center, and his colleagues conducted research to identify the most problematic off-label drugs, publishing the results in *Pharmacotherapy. Each of the riskiest drugs had one or more of the following problems…*

1. It lacked scientific evidence for off-label use.

2. It raised safety concerns.

3. It was newer to the marketplace, meaning that rare or long-term adverse effects were less likely to be known.

4. It cost more than FDA-approved drugs for the same problem.

5. It was marketed heavily by drug companies.

Most of these drugs fall into three classes of medications…

ATYPICAL ANTIPSYCHOTICS

This new generation of medicines is now the top-selling class of drugs in the US, replacing cholesterol-lowering agents as number one. They're called "atypical" to distinguish them from older antipsychotics. The drugs are approved to treat the psychosis of schizophrenia and bipolar disorder.

Main off-label uses: In 2008, there were 9 million off-label prescriptions written for antipsychotic drugs in the US, more than double the amount in 1995. They are used for a wide range of psychiatric conditions, including the behavioral problems of dementia, such as severe agitation (the most common use)…depression…long-term maintenance in bipolar disorder (the drugs are approved only for short-term use)…obsessive-compulsive disorder…and post-traumatic stress disorder (PTSD).

Biggest risks: With long-term use, the drugs tend to cause weight gain and the subsequent development of type 2 diabetes. And in the elderly with dementia, they are linked to an increased incidence of heart problems and a higher death rate.

The drugs: *Quetiapine* (Seroquel), *risperidone* (Risperdal), *olanzapine* (Zyprexa), *aripiprazole* (Abilify) and *ziprasidone* (Geodon).

Shocking finding: Researchers in the department of psychiatry at the University of Pennsylvania studied 2,597 people with Parkinson's disease and psychosis (hallucinations and delusional thinking), a common symptom of the disease. Fifty percent of the patients were prescribed antipsychotic drugs. Of those, most received off-label atypical antipsychotics—in spite of the fact that there are no scientific studies showing that the prescribed drugs work for psychosis in Parkinson's…that two of the drugs (Zyprexa and Risperdal) have been shown to worsen Parkinson's symptoms…and that there is a "black box" warning on these antipsychotics alerting doctors that they increase the risk for death in those patients who have been studied. Less than 2% of the patients received *clozapine* (Clozaril)—an older atypical antipsychotic that scientific studies show does improve psychosis in Parkinson's. The study was reported in the *Archives of Neurology*.

ANTIDEPRESSANTS

This is another top-selling class of drugs, approved for major depression and a few other conditions.

Main off-label uses: In a study of Medicaid patients, 75% of prescriptions for antidepressants were off-label. Off-label uses include treating mild depression (dysthymia)…bipolar disorder…insomnia…hot flashes…urinary incontinence and bladder infections…diabetic neuropathy…and chronic pain.

Biggest risks: Antidepressants don't pose the same level of health risk as antipsychotics. But while they may have a low risk of harming you, there is little scientific evidence showing that their off-label use helps the conditions for which they are being prescribed. Why spend money on a drug with potential side effects and no proven benefit?

The drugs: *Escitalopram* (Lexapro), *bupropion* (Wellbutrin), *sertraline* (Zoloft), *venlafaxine* (Effexor) and *duloxetine* (Cymbalta).

ANTISEIZURE DRUGS

These drugs are approved to treat epilepsy.

Main off-label uses: They're commonly prescribed for chronic pain—in fact, they're often used without making certain that other approaches have been tried.

Biggest risks: When an off-label drug replaces approved therapies for chronic pain and when there's evidence that the pharmaceutical industry is promoting that particular use, then there's a serious question as to whether that drug is the best treatment for chronic pain.

The drugs: *Gabapentin* (Neurontin) and *pregabalin* (Lyrica).

QUESTIONS TO ASK YOUR DOCTOR

If you or a family member is prescribed an antipsychotic, antidepressant or antiseizure drug, ask your doctor the following question…

•**Could you give me more background on the evidence that this drug will work for the condition I have and be beneficial for me?**

Best answer: The drug is FDA-approved for the condition and has been recommended by an expert group based on a review of the available scientific literature.

If that's not the answer, consider other treatment options.

Also, many doctors tend to prescribe new, expensive, brand-name drugs over tried-and-true drugs.

Example: The newer diabetes drug *sitagliptin* (Januvia) is often prescribed over the generic drug *metformin*—even though Januvia has not been proven to work better than metformin.

This practice is widespread for both off-label and FDA-approved drugs, so ask your doctor…

•**What's the rationale for putting me on this expensive new drug?**

Best answer: The newer drug was proven in clinical studies to work better than the older drug. (This is rarely the case.) If that's not the answer, consider the older, safer, proven drug.

■ **More from Dr. Randall S. Stafford…**

When Off-Label Drugs Are OK

There are several situations where off-label drugs may be helpful…

Your doctor has tried FDA-approved drugs for your condition and they haven't worked… or there are no approved drugs for your condition. Using an off-label drug allows the doctor to explore other options that might work. The drug is moving through the process of FDA approval for your condition. An off-label prescription for that drug gives you early access to a valuable medication.

■ ■ ■ ■

Antibiotics vs. Laser Surgery

Low-dose antibiotics for gum disease may contribute to antibiotic resistance. Dentists often use the antibiotic *doxycycline hyclate* (Periostat) to prevent infection during traditional oral surgery for gum disease—but this means that the patient may not respond when he/she later needs an antibiotic for an illness.

Self-defense: Laser surgery for gum disease. The laser kills bacteria, reducing risk for infection.

Victor Zeines, DDS, dentist in private practice in New York City and author, most recently, of *Your Tongue Never Lies* (Perio-Ventures LLC).

Bacteria Behind 75% of Urinary Tract Infections Is Resistant to Drugs

Guillermo Sanchez, researcher, physician assistant program, George Washington University in Washington, DC.

Jose Bordon, MD, PhD, infectious disease specialist at Providence Hospital in Washington, DC.

George Washington University Medical Center, news release

Escherichia coli (E. coli) bacteria's resistance to *ciprofloxacin* (Cipro), the most widely prescribed antimicrobial for urinary tract infections in the United States, increased fivefold between 2000 and 2010, according to a recent study.

E. coli accounts for 75% to 95% of urinary tract infections, which are among the most common infections in humans. Half of all women experience at least one urinary tract infection in their lifetime.

E. coli antimicrobial resistance reduces the likelihood of clinical cure, increases the risk of infection recurrence and increases treatment costs and hospitalization rates.

The surveillance study of more than 12 million bacteria also found that nearly one-fourth of E. coli in 2010 were resistant to *trimethoprim-sulfamethoxazole* (brand name Bactrim), the second most commonly prescribed drug for urinary tract infections.

The study was published in the journal *Antimicrobial Agents and Chemotherapy*.

"Our study is important because it shows that E. coli resistance to two common drugs to treat [urinary tract infections] rose substantially over the last decade," said lead study author and researcher Guillermo Sanchez, physician assistant program, George Washington University in Washington, DC.

WHAT THIS MEANS FOR PATIENTS

"For patients, this will ultimately translate into more expensive and sometimes more complex antimicrobial treatments," Sanchez said. "What is more concerning, however, is the lack of new antimicrobial drug development, which has been declining for decades."

There are other antimicrobial drugs available to treat urinary tract infections, but they are more likely to cause side effects such as gastrointestinal problems, nausea and vomiting.

"Our study reveals that *ciprofloxacin* and [*trimethoprim-sulfamethoxazole*] are no longer safe for outpatient urinary tract infection," said Jose Bordon, MD, PhD, an infectious disease specialist at Providence Hospital in Washington, DC. "Our study indicates that safer antimicrobials for outpatient [urinary tract infection] are *nitrofurantoin* in patients without kidney insufficiency and *amoxicillin/clavulanate* and third-generation *cephalosporins* for all others."

info For more information on urinary tract infections visit the Web site of the American Academy of Family Physicians, *www.family doctor.org* (Click "Diseases & Conditions").

■ ■ ■ ■

Is It Safe to Take a "Drug Break"?

Drug holidays—going off medications for a period of time for various reasons, such as assessing side effects—should not be done without the consent of your physician. The dosage of some drugs, including selective serotonin reuptake inhibitor antidepressants, such as *paroxetine* (Paxil) and *fluoxetine* (Prozac), needs to be gradually decreased, since withdrawal symptoms can occur if you abruptly stop taking them. Also, drugs that treat chronic conditions, such as asthma or high blood pressure, need to be continuously taken to be effective. A pharmacist can also advise you on how best to discontinue or taper off some prescription and OTC medications. If you feel that you are taking too many drugs, you need to discuss how best to reduce or eliminate them with your physician.

Jack E. Fincham, PhD, RPh, professor of pharmacy practice and administration, University of Missouri–Kansas City School of Pharmacy.

Emotional Well-Being

Surprising Secrets From the World's Happiest People

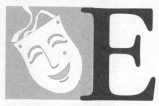

Everyone's heard the phrase "wealth does not buy happiness." Neither, it turns out, does social status, youth or beauty.

Social scientists have collected tens of millions of data points that help identify what truly makes people happy. Genetics and life circumstances can influence happiness, but personal choices account for about 55% of it. That means we all have more control over our happiness than we may realize.

National Geographic author and explorer Dan Buettner spent five years talking to people in areas identified by researchers as the world leaders in happiness—Denmark's Jutland Peninsula…Singapore…Nuevo León, Mexico…and the town of San Luis Obispo in California.

In his book, *Thrive*, he identified the main characteristics of what he calls thrivers, people who consistently report the highest levels of well-being. *Here, secrets from the world's happiest people…*

•**Own one TV, no more.** Americans spend more than four hours a day, on average, in front of the television. This is time that they're not spending with other people, including their families. (Family time in front of the television is not the same as real interaction.)

In the places where happiness is highest, people spend the least time watching television. It's not that they never watch—they just watch less than most people.

I advise people to own no more than one television—and to keep it in an out-of-the-way place, such as the basement. You still can watch your favorite programs, but watching will become a

Dan Buettner, founder of Blue Zones, an organization that studies the regions of the world where people commonly live active lives past the age of 100. Based in Minneapolis, he is a writer for *National Geographic* and author of *Thrive: Finding Happiness the Blue Zones Way* (National Geographic). *www.bluezones.com*

deliberate activity, not something you just do automatically.

•Create a "flow room." In Danish society, most families have an area in the house where everyone naturally congregates. I call these rooms "flow rooms" because they're places where time seems to flow away when people are engaged and enjoying one another's company. Flow rooms have no screens (TVs or computers) and no clocks. They are quiet environments where it's easy to engage in meaningful activities with family.

In our house, I chose a room with good lighting and the best views—it's comfortable, and everyone in the family wants to be there. I keep it stocked with good books, musical instruments and the best family games.

There's nothing formal about our gatherings. People wander in and out. Because it's so pleasant, we spend a lot more time there than in front of the TV or separated in different parts of the house.

•Experience the "sun bonus." By most standard measures, people in Mexico should be less happy than those in other countries. About 60% of the population is poor. Education and health care are less than optimal. Yet on the happiness scale, Mexico ranks high.

This is partly due to the "sun bonus." People in sunnier climates are consistently happier than those who live in northern countries.

Those of us who live in colder, less sunny climates still can take advantage of the sunny days we do have by getting out and enjoying the sun. The vitamin D that is produced in the body from sun exposure is sometimes called the "happiness vitamin" because it increases brain levels of serotonin, the same neurotransmitter that is increased by some antidepressant medications.

•Stop shopping. The satisfaction that we get from buying things—an expensive watch, a new suit, a fancy car—wears off within 14 months. Yet in the US, we're pressured by the media and social expectations to always want more. In order to get it, we have to work longer hours and take fewer vacations, which generally reduces happiness.

In Denmark, regulations limit the number of hours that shops can be open. In Mexico, most of the inhabitants are not running a status race with their neighbors.

For more happiness, take the money that you could spend on nonessential items and spend it on something that lasts. For example, take a vacation with your family or sign up for a painting class. The experiences and good memories will continue to give satisfaction for the rest of your life.

•Employ yourself. Self-employed workers and business owners report some of the highest levels of well-being. It may be because they are more likely to pursue work that they love or simply because they feel more in control.

The happiness zone of San Luis Obispo, California, has far more self-employed people per capita than the average community in the US. These self-employed workers are shop owners, graphic designers, artists, wine-makers and the like. The more autonomy and control you have over your job, the more likely you will be satisfied with your work.

•Make new friends. People around the world report higher levels of satisfaction when they spend time with family and friends. Every additional friend that you make (assuming that these friends are upbeat) increases your chances of being happy by 9%.

People who get together with others for at least seven hours a day have the highest levels of happiness. That sounds like a lot, but the time quickly adds up.

For example, everyone eats lunch. Ask a coworker to join you, or sit with a group in a cafeteria. Talk with friends during coffee breaks. After work, encourage the family to eat and socialize together, rather than dispersing to separate rooms. Take classes or join a club.

The Danes don't identify themselves as being particularly outgoing, yet 19 out of 20 Danish adults belong to clubs dedicated to arts, exercise and hobbies.

•Get addicted to serving others. The happiest people almost always volunteer in some fashion—at their church, with environmental groups, for social-service organizations and the like. Volunteering means spending time with others, and it also takes your mind off your own problems and increases self-worth and pride in your community.

Studies have shown that altruism has an effect on the brain that is similar to that of sugar and cocaine. It creates feelings of well-being, along with an addictive feedback loop that encourages people to keep doing it.

Also, volunteers are healthier. They tend to weigh less than those who don't volunteer, and they're even less likely to suffer a heart attack.

Commit to volunteering for a set period of time—say, once a week for four weeks. People are more likely to keep doing it when they make this initial commitment—and then get "hooked" on the rewards.

•**Keep the faith.** Religious people tend to be happier than those without faith. It's not clear whether religion makes people happy or if happy people tend to be drawn to religious practices. Either way, those who are religious have less disease, live longer and are less likely to engage in dangerous behavior (such as smoking and heavy drinking).

In Mexico, for example, more than 80% of people who were asked, "How important is God in your life?" responded with a 10 on a scale of one to 10, compared with only 58% in the US. This helps explain why people in some parts of Mexico, despite the hardships of daily life, tend to thrive emotionally.

Even if you're not religious, you can achieve similar benefits by cultivating a sense of spirituality—and a belief in giving back to your community and making the world a better place.

■ ■ ■ ■

Smiling Is Youthful

Study participants who looked at photos of happy people underestimated their age by two years, says a *Psychology and Aging* study. They accurately guessed age when the same people looked angry or expressionless.

Best aging remedy: Smiling.

Mark A. Stengler, NMD, naturopathic medical doctor in private practice, Encinitas, California…adjunct associate clinical professor at the National College of Natural Medicine, Portland, Oregon…author of *The Natural Physician's Healing Therapies* and coauthor of *Prescription for Natural Cures* (both from Bottom Line Books).

Bipolar Disorder— It's More Common Than You Might Think

David J. Miklowitz, PhD, a professor of psychiatry at University of California, Los Angeles, School of Medicine. He is author of *The Bipolar Disorder Survival Guide: What You and Your Family Need to Know* (Guilford).

Bipolar disorder has gotten lots of press lately. Several celebrities have received treatment for this disorder—some of whom have been quite open about it. But many people who have it don't realize that they do. *Here's what you need to know…*

WHAT IS IT?

Bipolar disorder is a psychiatric illness that also is known as manic-depressive disorder because many patients alternate between manic highs and severe lows. These episodes of mania and/or depression can last for days, weeks or months. A UCLA study found that someone who has had one manic or depressive episode has a 60% chance of having another within two years and a 73% chance of a repeat over four to five years.

An imbalance in naturally occurring brain chemicals called neurotransmitters seems to play a role in bipolar disorder, but stress plays a role, too. It's estimated that between one in 25 and one in 50 Americans suffers from bipolar disorder, and it is more common in people who have a blood relative (such as a sibling or parent) with the condition.

People with the disorder have a high risk for alcoholism and substance abuse, and serious difficulties with work and/or family. About 15% commit suicide, and about 33% will attempt suicide at least once in their lives.

A DIAGNOSTIC CHALLENGE

There are no clinical tests for bipolar disorder. The diagnosis largely depends on the patient's description (or descriptions from family members) of symptoms. These include extreme euphoria and manic energy during the "up" phase and severe depression when they're "down."

On average, there's a 10-year lag between the onset of symptoms and diagnosis. That's because symptoms vary widely from patient to patient and often go unrecognized by the mental health profession.

For example: Mania occurs initially in less than 50% of cases. Bipolar patients are more likely to see a doctor for, and be diagnosed with, depression. Mania might not appear for months or even years after a first episode of depression, which can confuse the diagnosis.

Alcoholism or other forms of substance abuse can "mask" the underlying disorder. It's also common for those with bipolar disorder to insist that their emotions and behavior are normal or even desirable. During a manic phase, for example, they might thrive on their creativity and high energy, even though observers might describe them as grandiose, boisterous or hostile.

Bottom line: Patients typically are diagnosed with bipolar disorder when they experience at least one week of manic symptoms, accompanied by work and/or family difficulties, and they've also had severe depression lasting two weeks or more. Some people have only mild high periods, called "hypomanias," which alternate with episodes of depression.

GAINING CONTROL

Drug therapy is essential for virtually all bipolar patients, but it's also important to identify triggers that can bring on episodes of mania or depression and to make behavioral adjustments to prevent and/or manage these episodes. *Important…*

•**Keep a mood chart.** Use it to track your daily moods and mood changes and to identify factors that you think might be triggering mood cycles.

By keeping and reviewing the chart, you will learn to identify minor mood fluctuations that may predict a full-fledged manic or depressive episode—and to make the necessary adjustments to prevent it.

Example: After a period of relative mood stability, one of my patients started having mood swings. After reviewing the chart, she realized that the changes were due in part to changes in her sleep cycle and conflicts with her father and boyfriend.

You can download a blank mood chart, and instructions for filling it out, at *www.manic depressive.org/images/moodchart.pdf.*

•**Maintain regular sleep.** Changes in sleep patterns are one of the most common triggers for mood cycling. Sleep changes also are a symptom that can occur with both mania and depression.

Try to go to bed and get up at the same times every day. If you're having trouble sleeping, don't make up for it with sleep bingeing. Sleeping more than usual can increase depression and anxiety and make it harder to sleep well on subsequent nights.

•**Abstain from alcohol.** Bipolar patients tend to be more strongly affected by alcohol than those without the disorder. I know very few people with bipolar disorder who can consume any alcohol and still maintain good control.

Also, alcohol—along with marijuana or other recreational drugs—can disrupt sleep-wake cycles. And even small amounts of alcohol can interfere with your medications.

•**Anticipate stress.** No one can avoid stressful events altogether, but you can minimize the negative effects. It's important to manage stress in healthy ways because bipolar patients are particularly vulnerable to "escapes," such as alcohol or drug use.

Keep your schedule and activities as close to normal as possible. Also, be sure to get help when you need it. If you have a sick child, for example, ask a friend or relative to help out. If you're anticipating a difficult period in your life, ask your doctor if you should change medications or doses during that time.

•**See a therapist.** Patients who get regular therapy do better at monitoring their moods, anticipating manic/depressive episodes, identifying triggers and maintaining a regular medication schedule. We've found that patients who engage in cognitive-behavioral therapy (aimed at identifying and evaluating patterns of negative thinking), family-focused therapy (which deals with communication/problem-solving within families) or interpersonal therapy (which focuses on how moods affect or are affected by relationships) have success rates that are about three times higher than patients who depend on medications alone.

Also, consider a self-help group. One study found that 95% of those who attended support groups had significant improvements.

MEDICATIONS

Most patients will take medications for the rest of their lives, particularly if they've had more than one major episode of mania and depression or if they have a family history of the disorder.

Warning: More than 50% of bipolar patients stop taking their medications at some point. In some cases, they stop because they don't believe that they need medication or because they miss the euphoria that is part of the illness or they don't like the side effects such as weight gain and/or shaky hands.

Many people want to go on "drug holidays," thinking that if they get worse, they can always go back on the drug and return to normal. Because the consequences of discontinuing medications are not always immediate (that is, you can temporarily feel better after stopping your medications), you may feel that you can go on living your life without them.

I advise patients to make a list of the pros and cons of going off medications and a list of things they can do to make medications feel more acceptable to them. Family members may be able to help. You can take the lists to your doctor to discuss issues of concern to you.

Homeopathy Can Make You Happier

Mark A. Stengler, NMD, naturopathic medical doctor in private practice, Encinitas, California…adjunct associate clinical professor at the National College of Natural Medicine, Portland, Oregon…author of *The Natural Physician's Healing Therapies* and coauthor of *Prescription for Natural Cures* (both from Bottom Line Books).

More than one out of every 20 Americans experiences depression at any given time, yet fewer than one-third seek help from a mental health professional for this condition, according to the Centers for Disease Control and Prevention.

One of the reasons for this reluctance is that patients expect to be prescribed antidepressants, and many have concerns about taking these drugs, which is understandable. Antidepressant drugs are supposed to help patients with severe depression, but studies show that they have a low success rate—and have many serious side effects, including suicidal thoughts.

Depression should be diagnosed and treated by carefully evaluating and addressing each person's nutritional, hormonal and emotional profile. One underrated therapy for depression is homeopathy, which can help on its own or in conjunction with nutritional and/or hormone therapy.

Homeopathy, by its very nature, requires holistic practitioners to take into account the whole person. After an extensive interview with a patient, a practitioner will consult a *repertory*, a catalog of symptoms and the homeopathic remedies associated with relieving those symptoms. The correct remedy is believed to stimulate the body's natural healing response.

FOR HELP WITH DEPRESSION

There are dozens of homeopathic remedies to choose from based on an individual's personality, symptoms and disposition.

The challenge: To find the remedy that works best for your profile. Four of the most common remedies used to treat depression are described on the next page. You can begin with the one that best matches your symptoms. As you will see, some of the symptoms overlap.

Homeopathic remedies can be dispensed in different dosing amounts. One dose with a high potency, such as 200C or higher, usually is prescribed by a holistic practitioner (this high dose should not be taken by a patient on his own). The patient then waits a month or two to see if it has helped. Sometimes patients feel much better after taking just one high dose.

Lower doses (such as 6C or 30C) can be taken by a patient on his own. Lower doses usually are taken once or twice daily for about two to four weeks. If one homeopathic remedy doesn't start to relieve symptoms within that time, stop taking it and try another remedy. These remedies have no known side effects.

•**For acute depression following a recent grief,** such as the loss of a loved one or a job, the breakup of a relationship or a recent experience of abuse…

Symptoms: Sighing, a lump in the throat, frequently alternating moods.

Remedy: Ignatia amara, derived from the seeds of the St. Ignatius bean tree.

•**For depression that arises following a humiliating experience,** insult or loss of pride…

Symptoms: Bouts of anger aimed at yourself or someone else.

Remedy: Staphysagria, derived from the herb stavesacre.

•**For depression related to loss or grief,** particularly if you tend to dwell in the past, suppress your grief or have haunting memories…

Symptoms: You are easily aggravated by consolation, and you do not like to express your emotions. You prefer to be alone.

Remedy: Natrum muriaticum, derived from sodium chloride (table salt).

•**For chronic depression,** including depression marked by feelings of despair and lack of meaning in life…

Symptoms: You engage in self-condemnation, self-reproach and self-criticism. You imagine that obstacles are in your way and impede the reaching of goals. You expect bad news and things to go wrong.

Remedy: Aurum metallicum, derived from gold.

If none of the treatments above helps you, there are many more homeopathic remedies to try. A trained practitioner can pick up the nuances of your symptoms and match you to the most helpful remedy.

To find a licensed homeopathic practitioner in your area, contact the American Institute of Homeopathy (888-445-9988, *http://homeopathyUSA.org*). A practitioner can work with you and your doctor to help you make the transition from antidepressant drugs to homeopathic remedies.

Caution: Do not stop taking an antidepressant drug on your own—this can be dangerous. If you have severe depression or suicidal thoughts, you should be under the care of a psychiatrist.

■ ■ ■ ■

Painkillers Lower Antidepressant Effectiveness by 25%

Painkillers may make antidepressants less effective. Selective serotonin reuptake inhibitor (SSRI) antidepressants, such as *fluoxetine* (Prozac) and *citalopram* (Celexa), are 25% less effective when the patient also is taking a painkiller, such as *acetaminophen* (Tylenol), *ibuprofen* (Advil) or aspirin. Talk to your doctor about switching to another type of antidepressant, such as *amitriptyline* (Elavil) or *buproprion* (Wellbutrin) if you take painkillers regularly, for example, for arthritis.

Jennifer Warner-Schmidt, PhD, research associate in Dr. Paul Greengard's Laboratory of Molecular and Cellular Neuroscience, The Rockefeller University, New York City, and leader of a study published in *Proceedings of the National Academy of Sciences*.

■ ■ ■ ■

Shot Blunts Trauma

In a double-blind study, victims of trauma who were given a shot of cortisone up to six hours after the trauma were more than 60% less likely to develop post-traumatic stress disorder than those who didn't get the shot.

European Neuropsychopharmacology

Study Explains How Shock Therapy Works

Christian Schwarzbauer, PhD, chair, neuroimaging, University of Aberdeen, Aberdeen, Scotland.

Jennifer Perrin, PhD, research fellow, University of Aberdeen, Scotland.

Tony Tang, PhD, adjunct professor, psychology, Weinberg College of Arts & Sciences, Northwestern University, Chicago.

A small recent study gives insight into how electroshock therapy, an effective yet poorly understood treatment for severe depression, affects the brains of depressed people.

Researchers used functional MRI scans to look at brain activity in nine adults with severe depression before and after electroshock therapy. The investigators found that electroshock, or electroconvulsive therapy (ECT), dampens the connections between different areas of the brain in depressed people.

"With our study we were able to confirm that there is hyperconnectivity [in depression], and in addition we could show that treatment removes it," said study coauthor Christian Schwarzbauer, PhD, a professor of neuroimaging at the University of Aberdeen in Scotland.

Although it may seem counterintuitive that people with severe depression, who are often also lethargic, would have brains on overdrive, one explanation could be that they have too much internal brain activity and cannot deal as well with external stimulation, Dr. Schwarzbauer said.

This study could point to ways to improve electroshock therapy's effectiveness and safety, he added. In its 76-year history, the treatment has met with opposition from doctors because of concerns of its side effects, such as memory loss.

Electroshock therapy is typically only used for patients who have not responded to antidepressants or other types of treatment and are at risk of hurting themselves or others.

"I think the fact that now there's more of an explanation, I think that's reassuring to the clinician as well as the patient," said Jennifer Perrin, PhD, who is a research fellow at the University of Aberdeen and lead author of the study published in the *Proceedings of the National Academy of Sciences.*

STUDY DETAILS

For the study, nine severely depressed participants underwent functional MRI scans of their whole brain before and after a series of electroshock therapy. They received the treatment twice a week until their symptoms, including sadness and fatigue, subsided.

The participants had not responded to antidepressant drugs before the study or received electroshock therapy in the previous six months, although four of the patients were taking antipsychotic medications.

The researchers zeroed in on an area in the front of the brain called the dorsolateral prefrontal cortex. It had fewer and less intense connections with a number of other areas of the brain following electroshock therapy, the scans showed.

This particular part of the brain is involved in cognition [thought processes] and social behavior and has been implicated in depression, so this finding is not surprising, said Tony Tang, PhD, an adjunct professor of psychology at Northwestern University. What is surprising, he said, is that none of the many other brain areas that have been associated with depression were found to have cut-off lines of communication following electroshock therapy.

"ECT is a rather invasive, drastic procedure and you see a lot of changes in patients, so we would probably speculate that there would be some sort of widespread brain connectivity changes," Dr. Tang said. This study "found it to be localized, and I found that to be rather amazing."

During electroshock treatment, clinicians place electrodes on the scalp and, while the patient is under anesthesia, deliver enough electric current to induce a seizure. The therapy is more effective when electrodes are on both sides of the head, as opposed to just one, but unfortunately this also carries greater risk of side effects.

Having electrodes on both sides of the head may be more effective because it triggers a more widespread seizure, but the current findings suggest another possibility, Dr. Tang said.

When clinicians put electrodes just on one side of the scalp, they usually put them over the right half of the brain because it is less dominant (for right-handed people). However, according to this study, the dorsolateral prefrontal cortex, in the left side of the brain, could be the crucial area to target.

"Most localized forms of stimulation we've tried so far don't work as well [as having electrodes on both sides], but this type of study could potentially point to the right direction," Dr. Tang said.

IMPLICATIONS

Looking at brain connections in people with severe depression could help clinicians predict who will benefit from electroshock therapy as well as who will relapse after treatment, Dr. Schwarzbauer suggested. Between about 60% and 80% of people become depressed again, usually within six months of the treatment.

Beyond depression, functional MRI of the entire brain could offer insights into other conditions that could be related to changes in brain networks, including autism, schizophrenia and dementia, Dr. Schwarzbauer said.

info For more information on electroshock therapy and other brain stimulation therapies, visit the Web site of the US National Institute of Mental Health, *www.nimh.nih.gov*, and search "brain stimulation therapies."

Working Too Much Can Give You the Blues

PLoS ONE, news release

People who work overtime are at much greater risk for depression, according to a recent study.

Researchers followed roughly 2,000 middle-aged British government workers and after taking other risk factors for depression into account, found that workers on the job for 11 hours or more each day are twice as likely to suffer from depression as those who work just seven to eight hours daily.

The study was published online in the journal *PLoS ONE*.

"Although occasionally working overtime may have benefits for the individual and society, it is important to recognize that working excessive hours is also associated with an increased risk of major depression," said study author Marianna Virtanen, PhD, of the Finnish Institute of Occupational Health and University College London.

info For more information on depression, visit the Web site of the US National Institute of Mental Health, *www.nimh.nih.gov*, and search "depression."

Think Positive To Land a New Job

Ruth Kanfer, PhD, professor, psychology, Georgia Institute of Technology, Atlanta.
Eva J. Parsons, executive coach, Eva Parsons Executive Development.
Academy of Management Journal

A study that followed recently unemployed people for five months—or until they landed a new job—found that staying positive and being persistent helped people find work sooner.

In early 2008, the US unemployment rate ranged from 4.9% to 5.6%, according to the US Bureau of Labor Statistics. In March 2012, the unemployment rate was 8.2%.

"It's very, very tough," said study coauthor Ruth Kanfer, PhD, professor of psychology at the Georgia Institute of Technology. "It's not like learning a skill, where maintaining a positive attitude can be easier as you see improvement with your effort. You submit resumes, but get almost no feedback on how you're doing or what you could do to improve your chances of finding a job."

STUDY DETAILS

The study took place between January and July 2008. During that time, 128 of the 177 people (72%) found new jobs.

Study participants had not been fired or quit, but were laid off, downsized or otherwise let go. All received Minnesota unemployment benefits, were between the ages of 25 and 50, and had at least a bachelor's degree. Most were caucasian. Sixty percent had recently lost professional, technical or managerial jobs—the rest were in clerical, sales or other fields.

On average, participants put in 17 hours searching for a job each week, but that dipped to 14 hours toward the study's end. Mental health gradually rose, and then declined slightly with a final uptick.

Weekly online assessments of participants uncovered either an "approach" attitude—striving for personal growth, developing skills and energetically pursuing goals—or one of "avoidance."

"Avoiders" had a more defensive posture and were most concerned with avoiding failure and emotional disruption. They were also more sensitive to criticism.

Dr. Kanfer said self-defeating thinking includes: "I can't do this," "I'm not likely to find a job," "I keep getting no's," "No leads." Job seekers should not allow those thoughts to dominate, she said.

Not surprisingly, those with a positive, go-getter outlook did better than those who were more fearful and anxious. But personality traits were secondary to self-management in terms of success. From week to week, those who did the most to develop routines, seek support and keep self-defeating thoughts in check were those who put in the most hours on their search.

The findings are published in the *Academy of Management Journal*.

JOB SEEKERS NEED TO KEEP WORKING

Eva Parsons is an executive coach. "Over the years, especially in the last few years, I have talked to quite a few executives who have been laid-off or downsized in an organization," she said.

Parsons recalled one client: "He was a senior executive in a global company and he was laid off. He went right to work and said, 'I'm approaching this as if this is my job now.' He was at his desk every day and he had a list of things he wanted to accomplish. Mostly networking initially, but also revisiting his resume or his CV and making sure that everything was current."

Parsons said job seekers "have to do the usual things that people do to stay healthy and to keep their spirits up: eat properly, get enough sleep, exercise, all the things you normally do to manage stress."

She added, "When they feel like they've been hit in the gut and they've gotten this sort of bad news—a lot of people's initial reaction is to want to curl up and go hide in the corner.

"People need to do the opposite—Reach out to friends. Keep making that part of the discipline."

If a job search drags on, Parsons recommended finding or starting a support group, "so that you can have other people to share your strategy with and touch base with on a weekly or biweekly basis, and compare notes and keep each other motivated. If it's too solitary a process, it can be really hard for people."

info The American Psychological Association has more about recovering from job loss. Visit its Web site at *www.apa.org* (search "job loss").

Do Men Think About Sex All the Time? Maybe Not

Ohio State University, news release

A recent study is challenging the widely held notion that men's minds are preoccupied with one topic—sex.

The research in college-age participants suggests that while men do think about sex more often than women, the subject crosses their mind an average of only about 19 times per day, compared with 10 times per day for women.

The results seem to disprove the popular notion that men think about sex every seven seconds, which would total more than 8,000 thoughts about sex in 16 waking hours, the Ohio State University researchers said.

"It's amazing the way people will spout off these fake statistics that men think about sex nearly constantly and so much more often than women do," said lead author Terri Fisher, PhD, a professor of psychology. "When a man hears a statement like that, he might think there's something wrong with him because he's not spending that much time thinking about sexuality, and when women hear about this, if they spend significant time thinking about sex they might think there's something wrong with them."

The study, published in the *Journal of Sex Research*, also found that men spend more time than women thinking about other biological needs, such as food and sleep.

STUDY DETAILS

The study included 163 female and 120 male college students, ages 18 to 25, who recorded their thoughts about sex, sleeping and eating every day for a week.

The frequency of thoughts about sex ranged widely between individual men and individual women—between one and 388 thoughts per day among the men, and between one and 140 times a day among the women.

"For women, that's a broader range than many people would have expected. And there were no women who reported zero thoughts per day. So women are also thinking about sexuality," Dr. Fisher said.

The researchers also found that a person's comfort with sexuality was the best predictor of which people would have sex on the brain most often.

"If you had to know one thing about a person to best predict how often they would be thinking about sex, you'd be better off knowing their emotional orientation toward sexuality, as opposed to knowing whether they were male or female," Dr. Fisher said.

"Frequency of thinking about sex is related to variables beyond one's biological sex," she added.

THOUGHTS ABOUT FOOD AND SLEEP

Dr. Fisher and her colleagues also found that men thought about food an average of nearly 18 times per day and sleep almost 11 times per day. Women thought about food an average of nearly 15 times per day and about sleep 8.5 times per day.

"Since we looked at those other types of need-related thoughts, we found that it appears that there's not just a sex difference with regard to thoughts about sex, but also with regard to thoughts about sleep and food," Dr. Fisher said.

"That's very significant. This suggests males might be having more of these thoughts than women are or they have an easier time identifying the thoughts. It's difficult to know, but what is clear is it's not uniquely sex that they're spending more time thinking about, but other issues related to their biological needs, as well."

info For more information on sexual health, visit the Web site of the US Centers for Disease Control and Prevention, *www.cdc.gov/sexualhealth/*.

■ ■ ■ ■

Sex Fantasies Raise Analytical-Thinking Skills

People who thought about casual sex with someone they did not love did better on a test filled with analytical questions and worse on a creativity test. People who thought about taking a long, loving walk with their partner were more creative and less analytical.

Possible reason: Love is a broad, long-term emotion that may help people make big-picture associations and connect differing ideas. Sex is more intensely connected to a focus on details.

Jens Förster, PhD, social psychologist, University of Amsterdam, the Netherlands, and senior author of a study published in *Personality and Social Psychology Bulletin*.

Can a Stranger Make You Feel Left Out?

Psychological Science, news release

The need for a connection to other people is so powerful that being ignored by a stranger can make someone feel left out, according to a recent study.

People need to feel they are part of a group or connected to others in order to be happy, the researchers explained. This sense of belonging can come from joining a club, a friendly neighbor or—as this study reveals—even eye contact from a stranger.

STUDY DETAILS

In conducting the study, researchers randomly chose people walking on the Purdue University campus in West Lafayette, Indiana. A research assistant looked them in the eye, looked them in the eye and smiled or looked in their general direction but not directly at them. Once they passed the research assistant, the study subjects were asked how connected they felt to others.

The study, published in *Psychological Science*, found those who had gotten eye contact from the research assistant felt less disconnected than those who were ignored—even when they didn't get a smile.

IMPLICATIONS

"These are people that you don't know, just walking by you, but them looking at you or giving you the air gaze—looking through you— seemed to have at least momentary effect," said study coauthor Eric Wesselmann, MD, of Purdue University. "What we find so interesting about this is that now we can further speak to the power of human social connection. It seems to be a very strong phenomenon."

The researchers noted previous studies have shown that being excluded by a group—even one that they condemn—can make people feel left out.

info For more on friendship research, visit the Stanford University Encyclopedia of Philosophy Web site at *http://plato.stanford. edu/entries/friendship.*

Lost Love Can Mean A Lifetime of Regret

Kellogg School of Management, Northwestern University, Evanston, Illinois, news release

A recent study suggests lost love causes the greatest regret of all in life. Researchers report that people have stronger feelings of regret about decisions involving romance and family than those involving work.

The findings underscore the importance of social relationships, according to Neal Roese, PhD, professor of marketing at the Kellogg School of Management at Northwestern University, and his colleagues.

"Social relationships, we suggest, are the most pivotal component of life regrets. Failed marriages, turbulent romances and lost time with family may elicit regrets that last a lifetime," according to the study researchers.

The study was published in *Social Psychological and Personality Science.*

Regrets about social relationships are intense because they threaten a person's need to belong. "Belonging, as a core human motive, powerfully connects to well-being and mental health," said the researchers.

STUDY DETAILS

Northwestern University researchers conducted a series of five experiments, with participants ranging from 108 to 549 men and women. Some focused on college students and others on a representative sample of adult Americans. Studies involved rating intensity of life regrets and connecting that with the social impact of decisions.

Results suggested that love or other social decisions, such as ending a relationship or being unfaithful, are more intense than those involving work or nonsocial decisions, such as quitting a job or dropping out of college.

CONCLUSION

"What our research makes clear is that, while regrets are multifaceted with diverse consequences, their social impact looms especially large," the researchers concluded. "Regrets can stem from love or work, but those stemming from the former seem to be the toughest to overcome. The need to belong is not just a fundamental human motive but a fundamental component of regret."

info For research about the value of regret, visit the Web site of *Harvard Medical School's Harvard Health Newsletter* at *http:// harvardhealth.staywell.com/viewnewsletter. aspx?NLID=85&INC=yes.*

Do Worry! It Helps You Live Longer

Howard S. Friedman, PhD, distinguished professor of psychology at University of California, Riverside. He is author, with Leslie R. Martin, PhD, of *The Longevity Project: Surprising Discoveries for Health and Long Life from the Landmark Eight-Decade Study* (Plume). *www. howardsfriedman.com/longevityproject*

Much of the common advice about living a long life—chill out and don't work too much—is wrong. These surprising findings emerged from a groundbreaking eight-decade study that followed 1,528 Americans from early childhood until their deaths. The study, which began in 1921, gathered information from interviews conducted every five to 10 years. It looked at nearly 10 million pieces of data, including work habits, exercise routines, social relations and personality traits.

The study revealed that people who plan and worry tend to stay healthier and live longer than those who don't—and that hard work and the accompanying stress actually are good for you.

Here's what really does extend life...

CONSCIENTIOUSNESS

People who are detail-oriented, responsible and organized live longer than those who aren't. By about the year 2000, 70% of the men and 51% of the women in the study had died. The majority of deaths occurred among those with low conscientiousness scores.

Conscientious people are more prudent in their personal habits. They're less likely to smoke or consume excessive amounts of alcohol. They have healthier, more stable relationships and better work lives.

Scientists speculate that conscientious people have higher levels of serotonin and/or other neurotransmitters that curb impulsive, risk-taking behavior—and so they have a biological tendency toward being prudent and staying healthy.

The good news is that you can become more conscientious. A number of the study participants originally tested in the bottom 25% for conscientiousness. A decade or more later, as they became less impulsive, more mature and more motivated, they scored in the upper 25% and lived long, healthy lives.

WORRY IS GOOD

It's a myth that people who are really cheerful tend to be healthier and live longer than those who view the world through a darker lens. In the study, children who were described by their parents as being unusually cheerful and worry-free tended to die sooner than their less optimistic counterparts.

Those with an excess of optimism may feel so invincible that they don't take reasonable precautions. They might ignore medical advice, for example.

Better: A personality trait known as "realistic optimism." People with this trait are optimistic at the right times...and they worry when they should.

Example: Someone with troublesome health symptoms doesn't just ignore them but makes an appointment to see his/her doctor.

A separate study of Medicare patients found that those who were somewhat neurotic—and worried too much at times—tended to be healthier than those who worried less.

BUT DON'T BE A CHICKEN LITTLE

Too much optimism isn't good, but neither is too much pessimism. People who think that the sky is falling tend to die sooner than those who are more optimistic. They're especially more likely to die from accidents and violence (including suicide), as well as from diseases such as cancer.

You don't have to suffer from persistent negative thinking. The first step is to understand that thoughts, including negative thoughts, are only thoughts—and thoughts can be changed.

Cognitive therapy teaches patients how to recognize negative, harmful thoughts and then replace them with more sensible ones.

Example: Someone who tells himself that *all my friends hate me* can learn to recognize how distorted that is. He will be taught to replace the negative thought with one that is more realistic, such as *I had dinner with John last night, and we had a wonderful time, even though we disagree about politics.*

STAY BUSY

Starting in the 1980s, we followed study participants who were by then over the age of 70. Over the next 20 years, those who stayed productive in some fashion lived much longer than those who took it easy.

That's partly because people who are busy and productive tend to have healthier habits. They have things to look forward to and to get them out of their chairs. They also tend to have stable relationships—good partners and/or friends.

Older people often are told to "take it easy" and "avoid stress." Our study shows that this is rotten advice. Productivity and pressure are signs of healthy engagement. Productive people strive to achieve goals and then set new goals when the old ones are reached.

MORE FRIENDS

It's true that steadily married men tend to live longer than single or remarried men, and much longer than divorced men. However, women who are divorced or those who never married live just about as long as women who were steadily married. The difference is due to relationships—women usually find it easier than men to have fulfilling social relationships outside of marriage.

The best social networks are those that involve helping others. Being loved makes people happy, but it doesn't prolong their lives. Those who help others are the ones who live longest.

Study Shows Fear Makes Spiders Seem Extra Large

Ohio State University, news release

People with an intense fear of spiders perceive the creatures to be larger than they actually are, a recent study has found.

While a warped perception of spiders likely won't interfere with daily living, other types of phobias could prove debilitating or even harmful, according to the Ohio State University researchers.

For example, people who are afraid of needles and perceive them to be larger than they actually are may avoid shots and put their health at risk.

STUDY DETAILS

In this study, 57 people with a fear of spiders were asked to undergo five encounters with tarantulas and then estimate the size of the spiders. The more afraid participants were of spiders, the larger they estimated the spiders' sizes to be, according to the study published in the *Journal of Anxiety Disorders*.

IMPLICATIONS

"If one is afraid of spiders, and by virtue of being afraid of spiders one tends to perceive spiders as bigger than they really are, that may feed the fear, foster that fear and make it difficult

to overcome," said lead author and professor of psychology Michael Vasey, PhD.

"When it comes to phobias, it's all about avoidance as a primary means of keeping oneself safe. As long as you avoid, you can't discover that you're wrong. And you're stuck. So to the extent that perceiving spiders as bigger than they really are fosters fear and avoidance, it then potentially is part of this cycle that feeds the phobia that leads to its persistence," he explained.

Learning more about how a phobia affects a person's perception of a feared object may help lead to more effective treatments for people who want to overcome their fears, the researchers said.

info For more information about phobias, visit the Web site of the American Psychiatric Association, *http://healthyminds.org*, and search "phobia."

Could Trans Fats Make You Cranky?

University of California, San Diego Health Sciences, news release

Eating a diet high in trans fatty acids, an ingredient found in fried foods, baked goods and other prepared meals and snacks, might be associated with negative—and even aggressive—behavior, recent research suggests.

Trans fat is made through a process called *hydrogenation*, which makes oil less likely to spoil and helps foods stay fresher longer. Previous research has found that these trans fatty acids raise LDL "bad" cholesterol and lower HDL "good" cholesterol, raise triglyceride (fat) levels, which can increase risk for stroke, heart disease and diabetes and promote inflammation.

STUDY DETAILS

In conducting the study, researchers from the University of California, San Diego School of Medicine analyzed the diet and behavior of 945 men and women. They also considered other possible contributing factors, such as the participants' history of aggression as well as alcohol and tobacco use.

The study, published online in PLoS ONE, found that people who consumed more trans fats were more likely to demonstrate negative behaviors, such as impatience, irritability and aggression.

Study leader Beatrice Golomb, MD, PhD, an associate professor in the UC San Diego department of medicine, explained that higher levels of trans fatty acids in the diet were "significantly associated with greater aggression."

However, while the study uncovered an association between dietary trans fatty acids and negative behavior, it did not prove a cause-and-effect relationship.

IMPLICATIONS

"If the association between trans fats and aggressive behavior proves to be causal, this adds further rationale to recommendations to avoid eating trans fats, or including them in foods provided at institutions like schools and prisons, since the detrimental effects of trans fats may extend beyond the person who consumes them to affect others," Dr. Golomb concluded.

info For more about trans fatty acids, visit the American Heart Association Web site, *www.heart.org*, and search "trans fats."

■ ■ ■ ■

Fats That Increase Depression Risk 48%

Trans fats increase depression risk. *Recent finding:* People who consumed more than 1.5 grams of trans fats per day increased their risk for clinical depression by 48%. The more trans fats, the higher the risk. (None of the study volunteers suffered from depression at the start of the study.) Trans fats increase inflammation, which may interfere with brain transmitters and disrupts mood.

Almudena Sánchez-Villegas, BPharm, PhD, associate professor of preventive medicine, University of Las Palmas de Gran Canaria, Las Palmas, Spain, and lead author of a study of 12,059 people, published in *PLoS One*.

How to Spot a "Mean Drunk" Before They Take a Sip

Ohio State University, news release

People who lack the ability to consider the future consequences of their current actions are more likely to be aggressive when they're drunk, a recent study indicates.

"People who focus on the here and now, without thinking about the impact on the future, are more aggressive than others when they are sober, but the effect is magnified greatly when they're drunk," said study author Brad Bushman, PhD, professor of communication and psychology at Ohio State University.

"If you carefully consider the consequences of your actions, it is unlikely getting drunk is going to make you any more aggressive than you usually are," he added.

STUDY DETAILS

The study included 495 adults with an average age of 23 who were social drinkers. They were given a test to determine their ability to think about the future impact of their current actions.

The participants then received either mixed drinks with a 1:5 ratio of alcohol/orange juice (alcohol group) or drinks that had orange juice with a tiny amount of alcohol (placebo group).

Aggression in both groups was assessed using computer-based speed reaction tests in which the participants believed they were competing against other people. The winner gave a harmless, but somewhat painful electric shock, to the loser. The winner determined the length and intensity of the shock.

There were no actual opponents. The researchers controlled the outcomes and increased the intensity and length of the electric shocks given to the participants to assess their level of retaliation.

SHOCKING RESULTS

"The less people thought about the future, the more likely they were to retaliate, but especially when they were drunk. People who were present-focused and drunk shocked their opponents longer and harder than anyone else in the study," Dr. Bushman said.

"Alcohol didn't have much effect on the aggressiveness of people who were future-focused," he added.

Men were more aggressive than women overall, but members of both genders who were "here and now" focused grew progressively more retaliatory when intoxicated.

The study appears in the *Journal of Experimental Social Psychology*.

info The US National Institute on Alcohol Abuse and Alcoholism offers an overview of alcohol and your health at its Web site, *http://rethinkingdrinking.niaaa.nih.gov/*.

How Former Heavy Drinkers Can Protect Their Health

John Newport, PhD, author of *The Wellness–Recovery Connection: Charting Your Pathway to Optimal Health While Recovering from Alcoholism and Drug Addiction* (Health Communications). He has worked in the fields of addiction and health services for more than 30 years and is based in Tucson, Arizona.

Recovery from alcoholism can be really, really hard—so if you've been sober for some time, congratulations! It's prudent, though, to recognize that those years of drinking may have taken a long-lasting toll on your body.

"Alcohol abuse can do cumulative damage to the brain, heart, liver, digestive tract and other parts of the body. Unfortunately, millions of people in recovery unwittingly shortchange themselves of years, if not decades, of joyful living by succumbing to illnesses associated with self-destructive lifestyle patterns," said John Newport, PhD, author of *The Wellness–Recovery Connection: Charting Your Pathway to Optimal Health While Recovering from Alcoholism and Drug Addiction*. What can you do now to protect your future health from the excesses of the past? *Steps to take…*

●**Make a healthful diet a cornerstone of your sobriety.** Many active alcoholics (those still drinking) are malnourished because alcohol, which has virtually none of the nutrients of healthful food, provides a large proportion of their calories. Thus, you probably entered recovery with nutritional deficiencies that can exacerbate alcohol-induced health problems.

Also: Alcohol causes blood sugar spikes and plunges that, over time, may increase the risk for chronic inflammation, insulin resistance, cardiovascular disease, certain cancers, belly fat accumulation, slowed metabolism and impaired cognitive function.

Many recovering alcoholics continue to eat in ways that keep them on the blood sugar roller coaster, including overindulging in sweets. This can create a chronic feeling of being "out of sorts" that can tip the scales in the direction of relapse, Dr. Newport cautioned.

Self-defense: To replenish nutrients your body needs for self-repair, stabilize blood sugar and reduce cravings for sweets, adopt a "Mediterranean diet" high in whole grains, fruits, vegetables and plant-based protein sources (such as legumes)…and low in processed foods and saturated fats.

Important: Some Mediterranean diet descriptions include a moderate amount of red wine, but no amount of wine is appropriate for a person in recovery.

●**Supplement with the nutrients recovering alcoholics need most.** While not a substitute for a healthful diet, supplementation can provide a nutritional insurance policy. Consider taking a daily multivitamin or consult a physician with expertise in nutrition and recovery for individualized guidance on supplements and dosages, Dr. Newport suggested. *Recovery supporters include…*

●L-glutamine. This amino acid may help curb cravings for sugar, alcohol and other drugs.

●Milk thistle. Some evidence suggests that this herb can assist a damaged liver in rebuilding itself.

But: "If you have been diagnosed with liver damage, be sure to also follow through with appropriate medical treatment. I wouldn't want anyone to think that milk thistle will fix cirrhosis, for instance," Dr. Newport emphasized.

• Omega-3 fatty acids. These have anti-inflammatory effects that may help repair your heart, digestive system and other alcohol-damaged tissues. Omega-3s also are highly concentrated in the brain and thus may help combat depression and aid cognitive function and memory (which can be impaired by years of heavy drinking). Supplement sources include fish oil, evening primrose oil, black currant oil and borage seed oil.

• Vitamin A. This antioxidant helps repair damaged cells of the bones, teeth and soft tissues. It also may reduce the risk for cancer, many types of which are seen in higher levels among heavy drinkers.

• Vitamin B complex. The B vitamins improve nervous system function. They also help the body and brain cope with stress, which is important since stress is a risk factor for relapse.

• Vitamin C. This stimulates the immune system, promotes blood vessel health and helps detoxify the liver—all of which may have been compromised by excessive alcohol.

• Vitamin E. This improves the function of heart and muscle cells and reduces cardiovascular risk.

• **Curb caffeine consumption.** It's fine to have a cup or two of joe in the morning. But unfortunately, said Dr. Newport, many recovering alcoholics radically increase their caffeine intake, overstimulating the adrenal glands and elevating blood sugar. Symptoms of caffeine overload include anxiety, irritability and insomnia (which won't help your sobriety), plus frequent urination that can deplete water-soluble vitamins. If you consume more than five servings of caffeine daily from coffee, black tea, soft drinks and/or chocolate, cut back gradually to avoid triggering withdrawal headaches…and substitute herbal tea, decaffeinated green tea, spring water or fruit juice mixed with sparkling water.

• **If you smoke, make quitting part of your recovery.** Smoking rates are significantly higher among active alcoholics than nonalcoholics—and many people in recovery from alcoholism continue to smoke. You can see that at

Alcoholics Anonymous meetings, Dr. Newport said, because there is almost always a group of people smoking outside the door.

Smoking is harmful for everyone, but particularly for alcoholics because it exacerbates chronic alcohol-induced nerve cell injury and cell membrane damage in the brain. It also impedes cerebral blood flow and thus slows the process of healing the damage caused to the brain by excessive alcohol consumption—so the longer you continue to smoke, the more you interfere with that process.

Recovering alcoholics may hesitate to give up cigarettes for fear that doing so would jeopardize their sobriety—but recent research contradicts this notion. Because smoking and drinking behavior often go together, continued smoking actually can trigger cravings for alcohol and thus reduce your chances of staying sober.

The same sorts of tools that helped you quit drinking also can help you give up cigarettes. Ask your doctor about smoking cessation aids, including nicotine replacement products, medication, psychotherapy, group support and 12-step programs (such as Nicotine Anonymous, *www.nicotine-anonymous.org*).

Also helpful: Call 800-QUIT-NOW (800-784-8669) to reach the smoking quit line sponsored by your state health department. "This gives you access to trained counselors who can help you over the hump," Dr. Newport said. Beating your nicotine addiction not only will do wonders for your physical health, it also will support your recovery from alcoholism.

■ ■ ■ ■

Fish Oil May Lower Suicide Risk

Recent research showed that military service members with low levels of the omega-3 fatty acid DHA were 62% more likely to commit suicide. Some earlier research has shown that omega-3s in fish oil may relieve symptoms of certain forms of depression, but larger, more rigorous studies are needed.

Captain Joseph Hibbeln, MD, acting chief, section of nutritional neuroscience, National Institutes of Health, Bethesda, Maryland, and coauthor of a study published in *The Journal of Clinical Psychiatry*.

■ ■ ■ ■

Love Helps Your Heart

When researchers surveyed 5,654 adults, those who were secure in their romantic relationships (that is, able to get close to others and willing to let others depend on them) had lower rates of high blood pressure, heart attack and stroke than those who were anxious in their relationships (for example, needy and worried about rejection).

Theory: Anxiety in relationships can negatively affect your cardiovascular system.

Self-defense: If you are having problems in your relationships, consider seeking advice from a therapist, who may help you learn more about your relationship style.

Lachlan McWilliams, PhD, associate professor of psychology, Acadia University, Nova Scotia, Canada.

■ ■ ■ ■

Boost Your Self-Esteem at 60+

Researchers who surveyed 3,617 adults four times over 16 years found that self-esteem generally began to decline around age 60—a time when factors such as retirement, poor health, disability and reduced income may come into play. Self-esteem was determined by how participants responded to statements such as "I take a positive attitude toward myself." People who are less confident and less satisfied with life are more susceptible to depression.

To maintain your self-esteem: Exercise regularly, eat healthfully and stay socially connected—volunteer in your community, join groups and/or regularly contact family and friends.

Richard W. Robins, PhD, professor of psychology, University of California, Davis.

■ ■ ■ ■

If You Don't Like Your Body...

People who hate their bodies have different activity patterns in areas of the brain devoted to visual processing than people with normal views of their bodies. Body dysmorphic disorder (BDD), a syndrome in which people become overly focused on a perceived body defect, is estimated to affect about 1% to 2% of Americans. Treatment includes a combination of drug treatments and cognitive behavior therapy.

Jamie D. Feusner, MD, director, BDD Research Program, David Geffen School of Medicine, University of California at Los Angeles.

You Don't Have to Be Young (or a Woman) to Have an Eating Disorder

Cynthia M. Bulik, PhD, director of The University of North Carolina (UNC) at Chapel Hill Eating Disorders Program. She is author of *Crave: Why You Binge Eat and How to Stop* and *The Woman in the Mirror: How to Stop Confusing What You Look Like with Who You Are* (both published by Walker & Company).

Until recently, eating disorders have been primarily associated with adolescent girls who don't eat enough—or eat far too much.

Now: The landscape of these disorders has changed. More and more women (and men) in their 40s, 50s, 60s and beyond are struggling with these sometimes life-threatening conditions.

Most of the 11 million Americans—10 million women and one million men—who struggle with an eating disorder, such as anorexia nervosa, bulimia nervosa or binge-eating disorder (a condition that's only recently been recognized by health professionals), are under age 30.

However, in the last 10 years, there has been a substantial increase in the number of women over age 30 who seek treatment for an eating disorder. There are no up-to-date data to tell us whether eating disorders are increasing in men, but clinical experience suggests that they are.

WHAT IS AN EATING DISORDER?

Scientists aren't sure exactly what causes an eating disorder, but research shows that genetics play a role. People who have a first-degree relative, such as a parent or sibling, with an eating disorder are generally at greater risk themselves. When this genetic predisposition is combined with certain psychological and emotional triggers, an eating disorder may result.

Older adults battling an eating disorder fall into three categories—those who have struggled their entire lives…those who struggled as adolescents, recovered to some degree, then relapsed…and those who have recently developed the problem for the first time. *Eating disorders can be divided into the following categories…*

•**Anorexia nervosa is characterized by low weight** (typically less than 85% of normal weight for one's age and height), fear of weight gain, denial of illness and distorted body image—typically, thinking you are overweight when you are not. Anorexia nervosa can lead to a number of complications, such as hair loss, osteoporosis, electrolyte imbalances, cardiac problems and organ failure.

•**Bulimia nervosa occurs in people at all weights and is marked by binge eating—** uncontrolled consumption of unusually large amounts of food—accompanied by purging that seeks to "undo" the binge in the form of vomiting, unnecessary use of laxatives or excessive exercise. Bulimia causes many of the same health consequences as anorexia.

•**Binge-eating disorder (BED) is similar to bulimia but without the purging.** BED differs from simple overeating in that sufferers feel a loss of control over what they eat. The condition can lead not only to obesity but also to problems such as insomnia and body aches.

AREN'T I TOO OLD FOR THIS?

Older women (and men) face a number of situations that can trigger an eating disorder…

•**Hormonal changes.** At menopause, most women are unprepared for the physical changes, including a hormonally driven redistribution of fat from other parts of the body to the abdomen. This can result in extreme weight-loss strategies to try to retain a youthful body. Hormonal changes also can lead to mood swings and sleep disturbances that often trigger cravings and increase appetite, setting the stage for binge eating. In men, decreases in testosterone and age-related changes in their bodies can trigger eating disorders.

•**Divorce.** Following a breakup, women may seek a new mate and want to appear as physically attractive as possible. This can prompt some women to take extreme measures to lose weight. If a man's wife initiates the divorce, he can feel lost and abandoned and turn to food for comfort.

•**Empty-nest syndrome.** A mother who has spent many years attending to her children can experience a sense of loneliness, uselessness and boredom when they leave home. This is a classic set-up for binge eating—often seen as a desperate attempt to find a sense of "fullness" in the pantry.

•**Depression.** Older women and men must contend with the deaths of friends and other life events that can trigger depression. Reduced appetite is a common symptom of depression and can lead to anorexia in some cases.

•**Overdoing fitness regimens.** Anorexia can develop in people who are overly zealous in diet and fitness regimens. Their good intentions can quickly cross the line from healthful to obsessive.

HOW TO GET HELP

One of the challenges of treating older adults is that, unlike a teenager, a 60-year-old woman or man cannot be compelled to enter treatment. It's crucial that women or men who experience thoughts and behaviors that characterize eating disorders (such as distorted body image, irrational fears of being overweight and an inability to control bingeing) realize that it may not be just a passing phase, and the earlier they seek help, the better.

In the case of anorexia, inpatient treatment is often necessary. With anorexia, the brain is unable to function properly because of malnutrition (decision-making can be impaired and brain shrinkage may occur). About 10% of patients with anorexia die from medical complications of starvation, such as heart failure, or suicide.

Insurance companies often cover inpatient treatment for anorexia but tend to deny coverage for inpatient treatment of bulimia and BED.

For anyone struggling with bulimia or BED…

•**Find the right professional.** The most effective treatment includes a therapist (a psychiatrist, psychologist, social worker or other experienced health professional) with a background in treating eating disorders. To find a practitioner in your area, consult the National Eating Disorders Association, *www.national eatingdisorders.org*…or the Binge Eating Disorder Association, *www.bedaonline.com*. A registered dietitian should be consulted to offer advice on proper nutrition and healthful eating habits.

Also, be sure that the symptoms—mental and physical—are discussed with the patient's primary care physician. This is important to ensure that the doctor takes the patient's eating disorder into account when offering medical advice.

Caution: Some doctors are not educated about the growing prevalence of eating disorders among older patients. If you believe that you or a loved one has symptoms of one of these conditions but your doctor doesn't agree, get help from a therapist on your own and seek a second medical opinion.

•**Start therapy.** Cognitive behavioral therapy, a form of psychotherapy that teaches patients how to understand their own patterns of thinking and behavior, is the most effective treatment for eating disorders. With the help of a therapist, you will explore why you starve yourself and when you're more likely to binge so you can work to change these habits.

•**Consider medication.** The only FDA-approved medication for eating disorders is the antidepressant *fluoxetine* (Prozac), which is approved for the treatment of bulimia. This drug can decrease the frequency of binge eating and purging but does not offer a permanent solution.

If you suspect that a loved one may have an eating disorder: Have a conversation that begins with a loving message such as "I care about you, and I care about your health. And I worry about how much you seem to be struggling with your eating."

Try to persuade your loved one to at least undergo a professional evaluation (with a dietitian or psychologist or psychiatrist) and to then think through the options. Point out that it's always better to have information and an expert's opinions than to make decisions in a vacuum.

A Diagnosis of ADD Can Change Your Life For the Better

Edward M. Hallowell, MD, instructor at Harvard Medical School and director of the Hallowell Centers for Cognitive and Emotional Health, with locations in Sudbury, Massachusetts, and New York City. Dr. Hallowell, who has ADD, is coauthor of *Delivered from Distraction: Getting the Most Out of Life with Attention Deficit Disorder* (Ballantine). *www.drhallowell.com*

Attention deficit disorder (ADD), characterized by distractibility, impulsivity and restlessness, affects millions of children. About 60% of those children will continue to have symptoms as adults. In fact, ADD affects 10 million American adults.

The main symptom of childhood ADD—the inability to give sustained or close attention to tasks—often persists into adulthood. However, because most people think of ADD as a childhood condition, nearly nine out of 10 adults with ADD remain undiagnosed and untreated.

That means the biggest downside of adult ADD—unexplained underachievement, when you don't perform as well as you know you could or should—can become a lifelong problem, leading to chronic frustration and depression.

How to figure out if you have adult ADD—and steps to take if you do…

DO YOU HAVE IT?

Because there is no clear cause or biological marker for ADD, there is no definitive test to diagnose it. Combining several tests is the best approach. *The two most important…*

•**Your history.** This is the most powerful "test"—your story, which tells your doctor how your attention has varied in different settings throughout your life at school, at work and at home. A lifetime of inconsistent focus is the hallmark of adult ADD. If the diagnosis is obvious from the history, the diagnostic process can end there.

•**Neuropsychological testing.** This is the second-most important diagnostic tool. A psychologist performs a variety of tests that attempt to quantify levels of distractibility as well as impulsivity.

For an accurate diagnosis, see a health professional who has extensive experience diagnosing and treating ADD—perhaps a child psychiatrist or psychologist who specializes in ADD (most child psychiatrists and psychologists also treat adults).

BUILD CONFIDENCE

To foster self-esteem…

•**Educate yourself.** By learning what ADD is and is not—and also by helping your spouse and family understand it—you put an entirely new "frame" on your life and your experience. When you're diagnosed with ADD, all the bad that may have happened to you because of the disorder—the inability to focus that caused opportunities to disappear and/or the impulsivity that led to huge mistakes—shift out of the darkness of moral condemnation into the light of science. You're not lazy, weak and undisciplined. You have a particular type of brain that generates a particular set of behaviors.

In fact, certain positive traits are associated with adult ADD, including original thinking, a zany sense of humor, remarkable persistence and resilience, warmhearted and generous behavior, and a highly intuitive learning style.

•**Identify and implement talents and strengths.** Instead of focusing on what's wrong, focus on what's right—your hidden strengths and potential talents—and developing those. Think about what you love to do. It could be related to the arts or nature or science or helping others—any activity in which your brain "lights up" and you forget who you are and where you are. Practice that activity. Mastery is the key to self-esteem and confidence.

SIMPLE LIFESTYLE CHANGES

Many lifestyle changes can improve brain functioning. *These include…*

•**More sleep.** Most people with ADD don't get enough sleep for optimal functioning, usually staying up too late on their computers or watching TV. The amount of sleep you need is the amount that it takes for you to wake up without an alarm clock.

•**Better diet.** Poor nutrition can harm the brain, causing distractibility, impulsivity and restlessness. *Sensible dietary recommendations for people with ADD include…*

•Eat citrus fruits and other foods that contain vitamin C. They help control the action of dopamine, a neurotransmitter needed in treating ADD. Opt for eating the fruit as opposed to drinking juice—juice is higher in sugar.

•Avoid refined carbohydrates, such as sugar and white flour.

•**Supplements.** *You can try the following…*

•Vitamin-mineral supplement that contains recommended daily levels of B-12 and folic acid (which improve cognition)…vitamin D and selenium (which improve brain function)…and zinc (research links low levels to ADD symptoms).

•Fish oil, which provides omega-3 fatty acids, increases dopamine levels. An adult can safely take up to three grams daily.

•**Alcohol avoidance.** People with ADD are more likely to develop alcohol dependence.

•**Regular exercise.** Regular physical exercise is one of the best treatments for ADD. Thirty minutes a day of aerobic exercise is plenty, and brisk walking is an excellent choice.

When you are starting to daydream or get spacey, a quick burst of exercise—25 jumping jacks or running up and down a flight of stairs—is like pushing the restart button on your brain, leaving you refreshed and focused.

•**Prayer or meditation.** Both help focus and calm the mind.

•**Structure.** This is any habit or external device—such as a list or a filing cabinet—that you set up outside your brain to help you make up for what may be missing inside it.

•**Help from a counselor.** Various kinds of counseling can help with adult ADD. For example, a "life coach" can help you get organized and make plans to achieve goals. Group therapy for adults with ADD also is a very helpful intervention—talk to your doctor about finding a group.

•**Medication.** Medication is a mainstay of the treatment of adult ADD and works in 80% of people who use it. The most commonly used drugs are stimulants, including *methylphenidate* (Ritalin) and the combination of *dextroamphetamine* and *amphetamine* (Adderall).

Talk to your doctor about whether medication is right for you. The goal is to have symptom improvement with no side effects (other than the common symptom of appetite suppression).

That's an achievable goal with the right medication, at the right dose, prescribed by a doctor with extensive experience in treating adult ADD.

Recent finding: A study in *The Journal of the American Medical Association* showed that people with adult ADD who took medication and underwent cognitive behavioral therapy (in which they learned such skills as how to organize and plan) had a 30% greater improvement in symptoms than people taking medication only. This study shows that medication is one valuable element but that it should not be the only element.

ADD TEST

The World Health Organization and a team of experts led by doctors from Harvard and New York University developed the *Adult Self-Report Scale* (ASRS), a brief self-screening test for adults who suspect that they might have ADD. It's not a definitive diagnosis—but 80% of adults who score positive turn out to have ADD. Answer each of the following questions with one of the following responses…"N" for never… "R" for rarely…"S" for sometimes…"O" for often …or "V" for very often.

1. How often do you have trouble wrapping up the final details of a project, once the challenging parts have been done?

2. How often do you have difficulty getting things done in order when you have to do a task that requires organization?

3. How often do you have problems remembering appointments or obligations?

4. When you have a task that requires a lot of thought, how often do you avoid or delay getting started?

5. How often do you fidget or squirm with your hands and feet when you have to sit down for a long time?

6. How often do you feel overly active and compelled to do things, as if you were driven by a motor?

Scoring: If you answered "S," "O" or "V" for questions 1, 2 or 3, give yourself one point for each. If you answered "O," or "V" for questions 4, 5 or 6, give yourself one point for each. Now add up your points. A score of 4 or higher means that you may have ADD. The next step is to find a health-care provider experienced with ADD.

■ ■ ■ ■

Happiness Is Overrated

Don't try too hard to be happy. Making happiness a personal goal actually makes it harder to achieve.

Recent finding: Women who actively strive for happiness tend to set higher goals for themselves and fall short more often…and thus are likely to be more depressed.

Iris Mauss, PhD, assistant professor of psychology, University of Denver, and leader of two studies published online in *Emotion*.

Family Matters

Autism: Closer to Finding a Cause

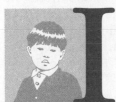

It wasn't so long ago that psychologists theorized that autism was caused by mothers who were unable to show affection toward their children. It's hard to believe, but these moms were actually referred to as "refrigerator mothers." Huge strides have been made in terms of understanding that autism is not a result of something a parent does to a child. The condition remains heartbreaking, however.

These days the term "autism" is applied to a range of brain disorders characterized by poor communication and interaction with others. According to the most current statistics from the Centers for Disease Control and Prevention, autism now affects one out of every 110 American children between ages three and eight. (That is when the condition is typically diagnosed.) And while experts still don't know for sure what the cause is, researchers are making some impressive strides toward solving the mystery.

Irva Hertz-Picciotto, PhD, MPH, a professor at the School of Medicine at the University of California in Davis (UC Davis), is one of the authors of two recent studies on autism, both reported in *Epidemiology*. One study shows that children conceived during winter months (December through March) have an increased chance of being autistic. The other shows that women who take prenatal vitamin supplements in the three months prior to conception and the first month after conception are less likely to bear autistic children.

"The studies present us with more evidence that autism isn't caused by a single factor," Dr. Hertz-Picciotto said. In fact, she said there's mounting evidence that autism is caused by

---

Irva Hertz-Picciotto, PhD, MPH, chief, division of environmental and occupational medicine, professor, School of Medicine, University of California, Davis. She is also affiliated with the UC Davis MIND (Medical Investigation of Neurodevelopmental Disorders) Institute in Sacramento, an interdisciplinary research center for the study and treatment of autism and other neurodevelopmental disorders.

a combination of genetic and environmental factors…which aren't necessarily the same in each case.

In one of the studies, researchers at UC Davis looked at approximately 6.6 million birth records in California filed from 1990 through 2002, correlating the rates of autism for children conceived in December through March with those conceived in July.

The results were surprising: Children conceived in December had an 8% greater chance of being autistic than those conceived in July… and the percentage of increase over the July rate kept rising for subsequent winter months, reaching a high of 16% in March.

"We don't believe the calendar month itself is a cause of autism, but it's a marker for other potential causes that may vary with the season," said Dr. Hertz-Picciotto, who is also affiliated with the UC Davis MIND Institute, a research center for the study of autism and other neurodevelopmental disorders. She said these other seasonal factors may include viruses that are more common in winter months or the change in the amount of daylight, which affects, among other things, the body's production of vitamin D.

VITAMINS MAY HAVE A CRITICAL ROLE

In the second study, researchers collected data from some 700 California families who had children with autism. Results of the study, Dr. Hertz-Picciotto said, showed a reduction of about 40% in autism rates in cases in which the mother had taken prenatal vitamin supplements during the three months before conception through the first month after conception. In other words, a buildup of vitamins before the crucial first month of embryonic development seems to be key to healthy neural growth. Prenatal supplements typically contain vitamin A, niacin (vitamin B-3), folic acid (vitamin B-9), vitamin B-12, vitamin C, vitamin D, vitamin E, calcium, iron, pyridoxine, riboflavin, thiamine and zinc.

Folic acid may be the critical component, said Dr. Hertz-Picciotto, because the vitamin is known to protect against defects in the embryo's neural tube, which develops into the brain and spinal cord. With so many factors still unknown, Dr. Hertz-Picciotto said, more studies are expected to be conducted in the near future, especially research into B and D vitamins as well as fevers, infections and exposure to pesticides during pregnancy.

In the meantime, given the vitamin study's finding of a 40% reduction in autism rates, it's certainly wise to take prenatal vitamin supplements three months before potential conception through the first month after conception.

Swaddling Infants Too Tightly May Cause Hip Problems

Pediatric Orthopaedic Society of North America, news release

When swaddling an infant, make sure to leave the blankets loose enough to allow leg and hip movement, experts say.

Wrapping infants too tightly may cause their hip joints to develop abnormally, causing the ball of the thighbone to dislocate from the socket. The condition, called developmental dysplasia of the hip, can lead to limping, differences in limb length, pain and arthritis, according to the Pediatric Orthopaedic Society of North America.

"Many cultures, and a growing number of Americans, practice traditional swaddling—the tight wrapping of infants with their legs together and fully extended," said orthopedic surgeon Peter Waters, MD, president of the society.

"Unfortunately, this practice places infants at a high risk for dysplasia," he said. "Instead, the infant's arms and torso should be snugly wrapped, while the legs are wrapped loosely, ensuring the legs are bent up and out. The legs should be free to move, and, most importantly, the legs should never be wrapped in a straight-down position."

Animal studies confirm that forcing the hip and knee to extend right after birth increases tension in the hamstring and hip muscles, increasing the risk of loose ligaments, instability and dislocation of the thigh bone from the hip socket.

The society joined the American Academy of Pediatrics and the International Hip Dysplasia Institute in recommending an updated method of swaddling that allows more wiggle room for infants.

info The International Hip Dysplasia Institute provides more information on infant hip dysplasia at its Web site, *www.hipdysplasia.org.*

Babies May Be Smarter Than You Think

University of Pennsylvania, news release

Babies can understand many words sooner than they can actually say them, a recent study indicates.

Researchers from the University of Pennsylvania say six- to nine-month old babies learn the meaning of the words for certain foods and body parts through their daily exposure to language. The general view among most psychologists is that this type of word comprehension is not possible until a child is closer to one year.

"I think it's surprising in the sense that the kids at this age aren't saying anything, they're not pointing, they're not walking," said the study's coauthor, Elika Bergelson, a doctoral student, University of Pennsylvania department of psychology. "But actually, under the surface, they're trying to put together the things in the world with the words that go with them."

HOW THE STUDY WORKED

In conducting the study, researchers had 33 babies between six and nine months old view a screen with a picture of a food item and a body part while sitting with their parents. The parents were given phrases to say to the child, asking them to find the apple, for instance. An eye-tracking device revealed the babies' responses to the phrases.

In a second test, the children went through the same process but saw pictures of typical food scenes and a whole person, not just body parts.

After taking into account possible reasons for errors or distraction among the babies, the researchers compared the responses of the six- to nine-month-old infants with those of 50 other babies ranging from 10 to 20 months of age.

In both tests, the researchers found the six- to nine-month-olds looked more often at the picture that was named than any other images. The researchers argued this was a sign that they knew what the word meant.

"There had been a few demonstrations of understanding before, involving words like 'mommy' and 'daddy,'" said study coauthor Daniel Swingley, PhD, an associate professor in the psychology department at University of Pennsylvania. "Our study is different in looking at more generic words, words that refer to categories."

Bergelson added, "We're testing things that look different every time you see them. There's some variety in apples and noses, and 'nose' doesn't just mean your nose; it could mean anybody's nose. This is one of the things that makes word learning complicated: Words often refer to categories, not just individuals."

The study's authors said babies at eight and nine months performed no better than six- and seven-month-old infants. They said no significant improvement was seen until the children reached about 14 months of age. They could not explain exactly why performance did not improve for so long.

Their study was published online in the *Proceedings of the National Academy of Sciences.*

IMPLICATIONS

"I think this study presents a great message to parents: You can talk to your babies and they're going to understand a bit of what you're saying," Dr. Swingley concluded. "They're not going to give us back witty repartee, but they understand some of it. And the more they know, the more they can build on what they know."

info The US National Institutes of Health provides more information on infant development at its Web site, *http://www.nlm. nih.gov/medlineplus/infantandnewborndevel opment.html.*

Common Household Chemicals Might Harm Kids' Immunity

Philippe Grandjean, MD, DMSc, adjunct professor, environmental health, Harvard School of Public Health, Boston.

Jerome Paulson, MD, medical director, Child Health Advocacy Institute, Children's National Medical Center, Washington, DC.
Journal of the American Medical Association

Exposure to high levels of a group of common household chemicals may impair children's immunity, a recent study suggests.

The team of researchers, from the United States and Denmark, showed that elevated exposures to perfluorinated compounds (PFCs) in early childhood was associated with a reduced immune response to two routine immunizations.

"We found that PFC pollution is apparently making the immune system more sluggish, so that it doesn't react as vigorously to vaccines as it should," said study author Philippe Grandjean, MD, DMSc, an adjunct professor of environmental health at the Harvard School of Public Health in Boston.

The findings were published in the *Journal of the American Medical Association*.

ABOUT PERFLUORINATED COMPOUNDS

PFCs are commonly used in a wide range of household products including nonstick cookware, carpets, upholstery and food packaging such as microwave popcorn bags. Previous research has found that the chemicals are present in most people's bloodstreams.

Other recent studies have linked increased exposure to the chemicals with early menopause and elevated cholesterol levels.

THE STUDY

Dr. Grandjean and his colleagues followed 587 children born in the Faroe Islands between 1999 and 2001. In the Faroes, located in the North Atlantic Sea between Iceland and Norway, frequent intake of seafood is associated with increased exposure to PFCs.

To examine the chemicals' effects on immunity, the research looked at antibody levels to the tetanus and diphtheria vaccines, which children in the Faroes are given at three, five and 12 months of age, with a booster shot at five years of age.

The children's prenatal exposures to five kinds of PFCs were measured by conducting blood tests on their mothers in the last weeks of their pregnancies. Postnatal exposure was assessed through blood tests at age five. The researchers then measured serum antibody concentrations against tetanus and diphtheria vaccines at ages five and seven.

Dr. Grandjean's team found that all of the five PFCs measured showed negative associations with antibody levels. In children who had twice the average levels of PFCs in their blood at age five, their immune response to the tetanus and diphtheria vaccines at age seven was only half of what it should have been, Dr. Grandjean said.

IMPLICATIONS

Dr. Grandjean said this is the first study in humans to find an association between high levels of PFCs in the blood and an impaired immune response.

"What we don't know is whether this association represents a general immune system dysfunction, and if it has implications in regards to infections, allergies or even cancer," Dr. Grandjean said. "We are looking at something that appears to be just the tip of the iceberg, and we'd very much like to know what the rest of the iceberg looks like."

The researchers noted that most levels of PFCs measured in the children studied at age five were lower than the levels found in a group of three-year-olds to five-year-olds in the United States studied in 2001 and 2002.

EXPERT REACTION

Another children's environmental health expert said the findings were concerning. "It's one more thing, along with a number of other findings about perfluorinated chemicals, that suggests we should all be concerned about them in general and try to decrease everybody's exposure to them," said Jerome Paulson, MD, medical director of the Child Health Advocacy Institute at Children's National Medical Center in Washington, DC.

HOW TO AVOID PFCS

Dr. Grandjean said that in addition to avoiding products made with PFCs such as microwave popcorn and nonstick cookware, parents who want to reduce their young children's exposure to PFCs should vacuum their rugs and upholstery more frequently "to control the levels of house dust."

info For more information on PFCs and other potentially harmful environmental chemicals, visit the Web site of the Environmental Working Group, *www.ewg.org/node/19261.*

Homeopathic Help for Kids with Colds and Flu

Edward Shalts, MD, DHt (diplomate in homeotherapeutics), private practitioner in New York City and author of *The American Institute of Homeopathy Handbook for Parents* (Jossey-Bass) and *Easy Homeopathy* (McGraw-Hill). *www.homeopathynewyork.com*

Children and colds go hand in hand every winter. Homeopathic remedies are safe, mild and effective alternatives to over-the-counter children's medicines.

Often effective is Children's Oscillococcinum, a proprietary remedy from the company Boiron (available at many health-food stores and online). Give it at the first sign of a cold or flu, following instructions on the label.

If Oscillococcinum fails to help within four hours, individualize the treatment by using the remedy below that most closely matches the child's symptoms. *Try…*

•**Aconitum napellus** when symptoms come on suddenly (as frequently happens after exposure to cold wind)…significant chills precede a fever that rises in the evening or at night…pupils of the eyes are small…the child is scared, restless and thirsty.

•**Arsenicum album** when the child is anxious and restless…complains of burning pains (for example, in the throat) that improve when warm compresses or pads are applied…and has signs of stomach flu (nausea, vomiting, diarrhea).

•**Belladonna** when there is very rapid onset of symptoms and high fever…eyes are glassy and pupils large…there is perhaps slight twitching of the face and body…the child seems confused…and the child is not thirsty (or he or she may specifically crave lemonade!).

•**Bryonia alba** when fever develops slowly …chills (if any) begin around 9 am or 9 pm and start in the fingers, toes or lips…the child craves lots of cold water, complains of pain (including a painful cough) and wants to be absolutely still, quiet and left alone.

•**Gelsemium sempervirens** when fever is accompanied by tremendous weakness and sleepiness (for instance, he won't even open his eyes)…chills run up and down the back…the head feels heavy and perhaps achy…limbs feel heavy…the child is not thirsty.

•**Ferrum phosphoricum** when the child has a fever but his symptoms do not match any of the other descriptions above.

The remedies above are safe and appropriate for children age two years and up. Give five pellets of a 30C concentration, then wait 30 minutes. If there is no change, try a different remedy. If the child improves somewhat, repeat the dosage once or twice at hourly intervals, for a maximum of three doses per day. If the child is not significantly better in 24 hours or if symptoms are severe, consult your pediatrician.

■ ■ ■ ■

Antibiotics Unnecessary for 80% of Ear Infections

Antibiotics may not be necessary for most kids' ear infections. Eighty percent of children with ear infections get better on their own in about three days, according to a recent study. Antibiotics may cause side effects such as rash or diarrhea. And overuse of antibiotics may be responsible for the increase in stronger, drug-resistant bacteria.

Helpful: Ask your pediatrician to write a prescription for antibiotics to be filled only if your child gets worse or if the infection has not cleared up within two to three days. Give your child *ibuprofen* or *acetaminophen* to help relieve pain.

Tumaini Coker, MD, pediatrician, Mattel Children's Hospital, University of California, Los Angeles, and leader of a systematic review of 135 studies on acute ear infections, published in *The Journal of the American Medical Association*.

Get Rid of Bumpers, Stuffed Animals in Baby's Crib

Loyola University Health System, news release

Acomfortable and safe sleep environment is crucial for infants and could mean the difference between life and death, pediatricians say.

Sudden infant death syndrome (SIDS) remains the leading cause of death for children younger than one year, according to the US Centers for Disease Control and Prevention. There's been a significant decline in the number of SIDS-related deaths since the American Academy of Pediatrics (AAP) recommended that all babies be placed on their backs.

DEATHS DUE TO CRIB DANGERS INCREASED

But sleep-related deaths caused by entrapment, suffocation and asphyxia have increased, leading the AAP to expand its sleep safety guidelines.

"These new guidelines will help enlighten parents about what items and behaviors can lead to infant sleep-related deaths," said Lisa Martin, MD, a pediatrician at Loyola University Health System and an associate professor of pediatrics at Loyola University Chicago Stritch School of Medicine.

"Infants, especially young infants, are completely dependent on their caregivers to provide a safe sleep environment, since they don't have the ability to roll away from objects that are restricting their breathing," she noted.

IMPORTANT NEW INFANT GUIDELINES

As well as always placing infants on their backs to sleep, the AAP says babies should be placed on a firm sleep surface and the crib should be free of objects such as loose bedding, bumper pads, pillows and stuffed animals.

"There are numerous products out there that are not necessary and could even become death traps for a baby. Items like bumper pads and sleep positioners have not been shown to prevent injuries, and the concern is that an infant can get trapped and suffocate," Dr. Martin said.

"Babies don't care if they have a boring crib. They do care if it's safe. The more objects in a sleeping space, the more dangerous it is for a baby," she added.

RECOMMENDATIONS FOR COMFORT

A good rule of thumb for keeping babies warm is to dress them in one additional layer of clothing above what a parent is wearing, Dr. Martin advised. For example, if a parent is wearing two layers, a baby will need three.

Another AAP recommendation is to offer infants a pacifier at nap and bedtime.

"Pacifiers have been shown to protect against SIDS, but if a mother is planning on breast-feeding, wait to offer it until the baby is three or four weeks old and make sure breast-feeding habits have been established," Dr. Martin said.

info To read the complete list of AAP recommendations for reducing the risk for SIDS, go to *www.healthychildren.org* and search "reduce the risk of SIDS."

Missed Naps Could Put Toddlers at Risk for Mood Disorders

University of Colorado Boulder, news release

Toddlers who miss daytime naps may be at increased risk for mood disorders later in life, a recent study indicates.

Researchers found that depriving toddlers of a single daily nap resulted in more anxiety, lower levels of joy and interest, and reduced problem-solving abilities.

The study was published in the *Journal of Sleep Research.*

THE STUDY

The researchers videotaped the emotional expressions of toddlers, ages 30 months to 36 months, while they worked on solvable and unsolvable picture puzzles on two different days. One day, the test was conducted an hour after the toddlers had their normal 90-minute daytime nap. On another day, the toddlers were deprived of their naps and tested an hour after their normal naptime.

When they were nap-deprived, the toddlers had a 34% decrease in positive emotional responses after completing the solvable puzzles, a 31% increase in negative emotional responses when they were unable to complete the unsolvable puzzles, and a 39% decrease in the expression of confusion when they tried to complete the unsolvable puzzles.

"Confusion is not bad—it's a complex emotion showing a child knows something does not add up," noted study leader Monique LeBourgeois, PhD, an assistant professor in the integrative physiology department at the University of Colorado, Boulder. "When well-slept toddlers experience confusion, they are more likely to elicit help from others, which is a positive, adaptive response indicating they are cognitively engaged with their world."

IMPLICATIONS

"Many young children today are not getting enough sleep, and for toddlers, daytime naps are one way of making sure their 'sleep tanks' are set to full each day," said Dr. LeBourgeois.

"This study shows insufficient sleep in the form of missing a nap taxes the way toddlers express different feelings, and, over time, may shape their developing emotional brains and put them at risk for lifelong, mood-related problems," she explained.

Missing a daytime nap may make it more difficult for toddlers to take full advantage of exciting and interesting experiences and to adapt to new frustrations.

"Just like good nutrition, adequate sleep is a basic need that gives children the best chance of getting what is most important from the people and things they experience each day," Dr. LeBourgeois said.

info For more information about the importance of naps for children, visit the Web site of The Nemours Foundation, *http://kidshealth.org/parent* and search "naps."

■ ■ ■ ■

Prenatal Operation Works Best

Children with spina bifida, a debilitating spinal abnormality, were more likely to walk and had fewer neurological problems if they were operated on before birth rather than after. Researchers hope that this will open the door for more fetal procedures to address such problems as heart defects and bladder blockages.

Diane Farmer, MD, professor, department of surgery, UC Davis School of Medicine, Sacramento, California, and coauthor of a study of 158 women, published in *The New England Journal of Medicine*.

Kids' Diarrhea Vaccine Seems Safe After All

Irene M. Shui, ScD, postdoctoral fellow, Harvard Medical School and Harvard Pilgrim Health Care Institute, Boston.
Jeffrey P. Brosco, MD, PhD, professor, clinical pediatrics, University of Miami Miller School of Medicine.
Journal of the American Medical Association

Despite earlier research that suggested the rotavirus vaccine increased the risk of intussusception—when a portion of the intestine slides forward into itself—a large recent study finds this is not the case.

"The findings of our study are reassuring and add to the evidence that the benefits of rotavirus vaccine, in terms of reducing doctor's visits, hospitalizations and deaths from rotavirus disease, is far greater than any low-level risk for intussusception that may exist," said lead researcher Irene Shui, postdoctoral fellow at Harvard Medical School and Harvard Pilgrim Health Care Institute in Boston.

Intussusception is a serious condition in which one part of the large or small intestine slides into another part, which can block food or fluid from passing through. Intussusception also cuts off the blood supply to the part of the intestine that's affected. However, with prompt detection and treatment, almost all patients recover, Dr. Shui said.

BACKGROUND

In 1999, the first rotavirus vaccine was taken off the US market due to increased risk of intussusception. The US Food and Drug Administration has since approved two new vaccines to prevent the infection—Rota Teq in 2006, and Rotarix in 2008.

Before the introduction of the rotavirus vaccine, rotavirus disease occurred in the majority of young children, causing a substantial public health burden from severe cases of diarrhea, Dr. Shui said.

"Since its introduction, health care utilization for diarrhea has decreased dramatically and more than 50,000 hospitalizations a year in the United States due to rotavirus have been prevented," she said.

STUDY DETAILS

For the study, Dr. Shui's team looked at the risk of intussusception from the vaccine, focusing on the first week after the first dose of the vaccine was given.

Included in the study were infants aged four weeks to 34 weeks who were given the vaccine between May 2006 and February 2010. In all, this included almost 800,000 doses of the vaccine.

The researchers found no statistically significant increased risks for intussusception in either the month or week after the vaccine was given.

In the month following vaccination, there were 21 cases of intussusception compared with 20.9 expected cases. For the week following vaccination, there were four cases compared with 4.3 expected cases, the researchers found.

That works out to a risk of one case of intussusception for every 65,287 vaccine doses. The risk might even be lower, the researchers added.

The study appeared in the *Journal of the American Medical Association*.

BENEFITS OUTWEIGH RISK

Recent reports from international studies in Mexico and Australia found some evidence for a low-level risk, especially in the week following the first dose of vaccine, Dr. Shui said.

That's because intussusception is rare and cases may be due to chance and not the vaccine, or due to genetic variations in populations where the vaccine was tested, the researchers noted.

"Given the rarity of intussusception, we cannot rule out that a small excess risk may exist following vaccination; however, this potential low-level risk is far smaller than the overall benefits from the vaccine," Dr. Shui said.

EXPERT COMMENTARY AND GUIDANCE

Commenting on the study, Jeffrey Brosco, MD, PhD, professor of clinical pediatrics at the University of Miami Miller School of Medicine, said that "it confirms what we already know. The benefits of the rotavirus vaccine far outweigh the risks."

The vaccine drastically reduces rotavirus infections that cause vomiting and diarrhea, he said. "It prevented about 55,000 hospitalizations in the United States in 2008 alone."

Outside the United States, it's even more important, Dr. Brosco said. "Here kids get hospitalized and get better, but across the world it's one of the leading causes of death for infants," he noted.

Children should get three doses of this oral vaccine at two, four and six months of age, Dr. Brosco said. "It's very safe and effective, and parents needn't worry," he added.

The study was supported in part by the Vaccine Safety Datalink contract with American Health Insurance Plans, funded by the US Centers for Disease Control and Prevention.

info For more information on rotavirus, visit the US Centers for Disease Control and Prevention at its Web site, *http://www.cdc.gov/rotavirus/index.html*.

Students Report Playing Deadly "Choking Game"

Sam Houston State University, news release

The "choking game" has been played by nearly one in seven students who were surveyed at a Texas university, a recent study finds.

This so-called "game" is played individually or in groups and involves deliberately cutting off blood flow to the brain in order to achieve a high. This is done by choking oneself or others, applying a ligature around the neck, placing a plastic bag over the head, placing heavy objects on the chest, or hyperventilating.

The dangerous behavior—also called the "fainting game," "pass out" or "space monkey" —has led to several suffocation deaths in Texas and around the country, according to researchers at the Crime Victims' Institute at Sam Houston State University.

"This study was undertaken to determine who is playing the game, in what context and how they learned about it," said Glen Kercher, director of the Crime Victims' Institute. "It is our hope that these findings will inform efforts by parents, schools and community agencies to warn young people about the dangers of participating in the choking game."

SURVEY CONDUCTED

The investigators conducted a survey of 837 university students and found that 16% reported having played the choking game and 72% of those students said they had done so more than once. The average age when students first played the choking game was 14, and 90% of those who had played the game first heard about it from peers.

Curiosity was the primary motivation for playing the choking game and most of those who had participated said others were present. Males were more likely to have participated than females, the findings showed.

Learning about the potential dangers of the choking game acted as a deterrent for most the students who had never engaged in this behavior.

"This 'game,' as it is often called, does not require obtaining any drugs or alcohol, is free, and can go undetected by many parents, teachers, physicians and other authority figures. Most importantly, many of those who engage in this activity do not understand that the practice can be just as deadly as the illegal substances youth have been warned against," the study authors pointed out.

info The US Centers for Disease Control and Prevention has more information about the choking game. Visit its Web site at *http://www.cdc.gov/homeandrecreationalsafety/Choking/choking_game.html*.

Teens' IQ May Change Over Time

Cathy Price, PhD, professor, Wellcome Trust Centre for Neuroimaging, University College London, UK.

Paul Sanberg, PhD, DSc, distinguished professor of neurosurgery and director, University of South Florida Center for Aging and Brain Repair, Tampa.

Michael P. Carey, PhD, assistant professor of psychiatry and behavioral science, Texas A&M Health Science Center College of Medicine and psychologist, Scott & White Hospital, Temple, Texas.
Nature

Parents, you may be onto something: A small recent study suggests that teens' intelligence, as measured by the IQ test, may fluctuate throughout adolescence.

The changes—in both verbal and nonverbal IQ—ranged as much as 20 points and were correlated with specific brain areas.

IQ has long been thought to remain stable over a person's lifetime.

IMPLICATIONS

The findings might have implications for kids' educations, the researchers said. Children, especially those with lower IQs, should not be pigeonholed into specific educational and career trajectories based on their IQ alone.

"Approximately one-fifth of our sample had very substantial changes such that they moved from above average to below average or vice versa," said Cathy Price, PhD, senior study author and professor at the Wellcome Trust Centre for Neuroimaging, University College London, UK.

Dr. Price hasn't yet measured whether or not IQ changes in adults, "but my guess would be yes, because intensive skill training in adults causes brain changes."

STUDY DETAILS

In their research, Dr. Price and her colleagues measured the IQs of 33 individuals aged 12 to 16 in 2004. They performed MRI brain imaging of the adolescents' brains at the same time.

Four years later, the same group of individuals, now between 15 and 20 years old, were tested and underwent additional MRI scans.

The team reported that changes in IQ did seem to occur, with some participants improving their scores by as much as 20 points over time, relative to people of similar age, while other kids saw declines in IQ levels.

"A change in 20 points is a huge difference," Dr. Price said. "If an individual moved from an IQ of 110 to an IQ of 130 they move from being 'average' to 'gifted.' And if they moved from 104 to 84 they move from being high average to below average."

The fluctuations seemed correlated to changes in certain brain areas, with verbal IQ (such as might be used in language and math) corresponding to a different part of the brain than nonverbal changes (involving visual questions).

Dr. Price explained that "the degree to which verbal IQ changed correlated with the degree to which brain structure changed in an area of the brain that we are referring to as a 'motor speech area.'" She added that this region, the brain's left motor cortex, "is very active when we (including the participants in our study) articulate speech."

Nonverbal performance correlated to changes in the anterior cerebellum, which is also activated when making hand movements, Dr. Price noted.

The authors don't know yet what is driving these variations in IQ over time.

"It could either be an active environmental effect (such as education/learning) or it could relate to developmental differences (late developers/early developers) or it could be both," Dr.

Price said. "This is the classic nature/nurture debate. I am pretty sure that there is a strong environmental effect because we know that the adult brain changes with learning. In this case, intensive training causes brain changes."

According to the study authors, prior studies have shown changes in IQ in individuals over time, but those studies hadn't been able to rule out the possibility of chance.

The findings were published in the journal *Nature*.

EXPERT COMMENTARY

The take-home message, according to one expert, is that intelligence may not be as "fixed" in adolescence as once thought.

"The brain is clearly, at least in the teenage years, more plastic and amenable to change," said Paul Sanberg, PhD, DSc, distinguished professor of neurosurgery and director of the University of South Florida Center for Aging and Brain Repair in Tampa. "The real question is, does this continue into adulthood? Is this reflective of changes we now see in plasticity in the brain in adulthood? The data is suggesting that things can get better."

However, another expert cautioned that the study did have some limitations. Michael Carey, PhD, assistant professor of psychiatry and behavioral science at Texas A&M Health Science Center College of Medicine, believes that some of the IQ tests used in the study were outdated, nor did they take into account other factors, such as age, gender or whether a person is right-handed or left-handed when identifying brain structures related to the change.

"It's a relatively small sample and pretty selective. The average IQs are above average, even though there's a lot of variation," said Dr. Carey, who is also a psychologist with Scott & White Hospital, in Temple, Texas. "The question is, how representative is this of natural day-to-day adolescence?"

info Find out more on the developing brain at the US National Institute of Mental Health Web site, *http://www.nimh.nih.gov/media/video/giedd.shtml.*

Nearly One in Four Teenage Girls Has a Sexually Transmitted Infection (STI)

Within one year of starting to have sex, 19.2% of girls ages 14 to 19 are infected with at least one of the five most common STIs—human papillomavirus (HPV), herpes simplex virus type 2, chlamydia, gonorrhea or trichomoniasis. The most common sexually transmitted infection is HPV, found in 18.3% of girls.

Sara E. Forhan, MD, MPH, researcher, National Center for HIV/AIDS Viral Hepatitis, STD and TB Prevention, Centers for Disease Control and Prevention, Atlanta, and leader of the analysis of STIs from National Health and Nutrition Survey (NHANES) 2003–2004 data from 838 teenage girls, published in *Pediatrics*.

Suicide Attempts More Likely Among Girls

Drug-related suicide attempts are almost three times as likely among girls as boys. A study that analyzed emergency room visits from 2004 to 2008 found that the number of drug-related suicide attempts during this period for adolescent girls ages 12 to 17 was 15,552, and for boys it was 5,283. The study did not look at the reasons for the suicide attempts and only included incidents that ended in an ER visit.

Substance Abuse and Mental Health Services Administration, Rockville, Maryland. *www.samhsa.gov*

Better ADHD Solutions

There's a better way to treat children with ADHD than the medications most doctors prescribe.

My experience is that most children with attention-deficit/hyperactivity disorder (ADHD) do not require pharmaceutical medications. Brain biochemistry can be balanced naturally, beginning with diet.

There is some evidence that food sensitivities in children can lead to ADHD. Common culprits can include dairy, gluten, sugar and artificial sweeteners and dyes. Try to notice if any of these foods triggers a reaction in your child—and have him/her avoid these foods. Make sure that your child eats a high-protein, low-sugar breakfast and gets plenty of protein in every meal throughout the day to maintain blood sugar levels.

There are several supplements that have been found to ease ADHD in children, including high-dose fish oil, which helps brain function…*phosphatidylserine* (also called PS), a type of fat that normalizes brain chemistry…and Pycnogenol, an extract from the bark of the French maritime pine, which can help regulate brain chemistry. Lastly, biofeedback with a practitioner can help a child focus and improve restlessness.

Mark A. Stengler, NMD, naturopathic medical doctor in private practice, Encinitas, California…adjunct associate clinical professor at the National College of Natural Medicine, Portland, Oregon…author of *The Natural Physicians Healing Therapies* and coauthor of *Prescription for Natural Cures* (both from Bottom Line Books).

Youngest Students More Likely to Be Labeled ADHD

Richard Morrow, PhD, health research analyst, University of British Columbia, Vancouver, Canada.
Richard Milich, PhD, professor, psychology, University of Kentucky, Louisville.
CMAJ (Canadian Medical Association Journal)

A recent Canadian study provides more evidence that too many young kids may be diagnosed with attention-deficit/hyperactivity disorder, or ADHD, simply because they're younger than their peers in the same classrooms.

Researchers found that nearly 7% of boys ages six to 12 were diagnosed with ADHD overall, but the percentage ranged from 5.7% for those who were the oldest in their grade levels to 7.4% for the youngest. There was a similar gap for girls, although they're much less likely to be diagnosed.

The findings, which are similar to those from US studies, don't prove definitively that any kids are being wrongly diagnosed with ADHD or being diagnosed purely because they're younger than their peers.

Still, "it's good for parents to know about this," said study author Richard Morrow, PhD, a health research analyst at the University of British Columbia. "In general, the younger you are within your grade, the more likely you are to receive this diagnosis and get treatment."

BACKGROUND

ADHD is a controversial developmental disorder, and there's been debate about whether it is overdiagnosed. The researchers launched the study to determine whether a student's age in relation to his or her peers may have something to do with the likelihood of diagnosis.

STUDY FINDINGS

The study authors examined the records of more than 930,000 kids in British Columbia who were between the ages of six and 12, during the time period from 1997 to 2008. They focused on differences between kids born in January (who'd typically be the oldest in their classes) and December (who'd typically be the youngest due to cut-off dates for school enrollment).

The level of ADHD diagnosis was lowest for kids born early in the year—the oldest ones in their classes—and highest for those born later in the year.

Kids born in January and December had the lowest and highest rates, respectively: 5.7% of boys and 1.6% of girls for those born in January, and 7.4% of boys and 2.7% of girls among those born in December.

Boys born in December were 30% more likely to be diagnosed and 41% more likely to be treated with ADHD medications than boys born in January were, while the youngest girls were 70% more likely to be diagnosed and 77% more likely to be treated with medications than the oldest girls were, the study found.

The study was published in the *CMAJ* (*Canadian Medical Association Journal*).

IMPLICATIONS

"There is no reason for them to have this kind of difference in their diagnosis," Dr. Morrow said. "The way we would interpret that is that there are differences in maturity that are coming into play."

In other words, physicians and teachers may think kids have ADHD when they're actually just younger and less mature than their peers.

EXPERT REACTION

Richard Milich, PhD, a professor of psychology at the University of Kentucky who studies ADHD, said the findings make sense considering that the disorder is difficult to diagnose, especially at younger ages.

When ADHD becomes an issue, Dr. Milich said, parents should be aware of this kind of research and bring it up with their pediatrician or whomever else is appropriate. However, "I hope it doesn't get to the point that people say it's not a valid disorder," he said.

Kids with ADHD "do poorer in school, they're more likely to be left behind and more likely to drop out of school early. Across the board, they are impaired," Dr. Milich said.

The Truth About Stuttering

Jane Fraser, president of The Stuttering Foundation of America, based in Memphis. She is coauthor, with Stanley Ainsworth, PhD, of If Your Child Stutters: A Guide for Parents (The Stuttering Foundation of America). *www. StutteringHelp.org*

The Academy Award–winning movie *The King's Speech* is a reminder that stuttering can be a devastating disability. But we know much more now about the causes of stuttering and how to treat it than we did back when King George VI struggled to overcome his stammer. *Here, the latest findings…*

Who stutters and why: Stuttering almost always begins in early childhood. About 80% of children who stutter outgrow it within six months to a year—of those who don't, only about 1% have problems as adults.

Contrary to popular opinion, stuttering is not caused by psychological problems, emotional trauma or stress. Stress can make it worse, but the underlying causes are thought to involve genetics, as well as factors such as neurophysiology. About 60% of those who stutter have a family member with the same problem.

Nearly everyone who stutters can benefit from the latest treatments, which typically are used in combination and include…

•**Fluency-shaping therapy.** Patients work with a speech therapist to correct some of the "errors" that can lead to stuttering. *Example:* Speaking too quickly or trying to say too much. It's easier to speak fluently when you slow down and use shorter sentences.

King George VI broke down his speeches into groups of three or four words and allowed time for pauses—a technique known as pausing and phrasing.

•**Stuttering modification therapy.** This technique, combined with fluency shaping, isn't meant to eliminate stuttering. It helps patients overcome a stutter as it occurs. *Example:* When a stutter is imminent, the speaker stops speaking for a moment…releases tension from the lips… breathes normally…and then resumes speaking.

•**Cognitive behavior therapy.** With cognitive behavior therapy, a person might predict the worst thing that could happen in a feared situation, such as being ridiculed for ordering a h-h-h-amburger. Then the stutterer and therapist work together to test the prediction in some way, such as going together to order a hamburger and really paying attention to others' reactions. Once people experience that the "worst" they imagine usually does not come true, it makes it easier to face other feared situations.

•**Electronic therapy.** Antistuttering devices change how the stutterer hears his/her own voice. Units vary in size from small enough to be worn in the ear to the size of a deck of cards. There are different types. One type produces "white" noise that distracts stutterers so that they're less focused on their own voices when speaking.

Drawbacks: The units are expensive. Some cost as much as $5,000. They're also awkward to use in real-life situations, in part because the listener can overhear the sounds from the headset. But they can be effective when people are reading or giving a presentation in a classroom or business setting.

•**Medications.** There are no medications for stuttering, although some patients report that they do better when they take antianxiety drugs, such as *paroxetine* (Paxil).

To find a speech therapist who specializes in stuttering in your area, go to *www.stuttering help.org* and click on "Resources" and then "Therapy Referral Lists."

Children Suffer in Overcrowded ERs

University of Colorado School of Medicine, Denver, news release

Overcrowding in emergency rooms appears to keep children with broken arms and legs from getting pain relief in a timely manner, according to a recent study.

Researchers from the University of Colorado School of Medicine said their findings are significant since these injuries, known as long bone fractures, are common among children and very painful.

"Pain associated with long bone fractures can be pretty severe," said study author Marion Sills, MD, associate professor of pediatrics at the University of Colorado School of Medicine. "But crowded emergency departments are impacting the delivery of care on many levels, including the delivery of pain medication."

STUDY DETAILS

In conducting the study, published in the journal *Academic Emergency Medicine*, researchers examined 1,229 children treated in an ER over the course of one year. They found the children were 4% to 47% less likely to receive treatment in a timely fashion when the ER was very crowded (at the 90th percentile) than when it was less crowded (at the 10th percentile). The researchers also found the children were 3% to 17% less likely to receive effective care in these crowded conditions.

"The relationship between emergency department crowding and pain treatment is not unexpected," noted Dr. Sills. "When the emergency department gets busier, staff may be less responsive to the needs of individual patients and, as a result, patients have a higher likelihood of non-treatment and delays in treatment."

POSSIBLE SOLUTIONS

The authors said delays happen in some cases when only doctors are permitted to provide certain pain medications to patients.

"The expensive way to mitigate crowding is to hire more staff. Another way is to leverage the staff you have," Dr. Sills said. "Institutions can use techniques like protocols for pain management with standing orders for nurses, and computer- or phone-based alerts to call attention to under-treated pain."

Crowding is a serious issue, said Dr. Sills. "It is caused by a variety of things, from patients who too readily use emergency departments to federal policies that exacerbate the problem," she noted. "We as a nation need to get serious about this. Crowding needs to be a policy priority at every level."

info For more information on pain relievers, visit the Web site of the US National Institutes of Health, *www.nlm.nih.gov/medline plus/painrelievers.html.*

■■■■

Children and Radiation

Did you know the average American child is exposed to medical radiation more than seven times by age 18? X-rays and other medical tests that use radiation increase risk for cancer. Of particular concern are CT scans, which use more radiation than X-rays.

Adam L. Dorfman, MD, assistant professor, departments of pediatrics and radiology, University of Michigan Medical School, Ann Arbor, and leader of a study of 355,088 children, published in *Archives of Pediatrics and Adolescent Medicine.*

■■■■

Sleeping Alongside Pets Can Make You Sick

A recent review of medical journals found that pets can carry pathogens for such bacterial infections as *pasteurellosis* and cat-scratch disease. The risk is rare, but it's still wise not to have your pet in bed with you. The pet can sleep next to the bed, not on it.

Bruno Chomel, DVM, PhD, professor, School of Veterinary Medicine, University of California-Davis, published in *Emerging Infectious Diseases*.

■■■■

Keep Your Medications Out of Reach of Pets

Many medicines that are safe for people are not safe for pets. *Examples…*

•**Nonsteroidal anti-inflammatory drugs (NSAIDs),** such as Advil and Aleve, can cause kidney failure and serious ulcers in dogs, cats, birds and other pets.

•*Acetaminophen,* such as Tylenol, can severely damage cats' red blood cells and may cause liver failure in dogs.

•**Antidepressants** are sometimes used in pets in small doses, but human-strength pills can cause tremors, seizures, elevated heart rate and other dangerous conditions.

•**ADD/ADHD medicines** can cause life-threatening tremors, seizures and heart problems.

•**Medical marijuana** can affect a dog's heart and cause a comalike stupor, loss of bladder control and more.

Other human medicines that are dangerous to pets: Sleep aids, birth-control pills, heart medicines, thyroid hormones and more. Ask your veterinarian for details. If you think your pet has swallowed any human medicine, immediately call your vet or the Pet Poison Helpline, 800-213-6680.

Jon Geller, DVM, Diplomate, American Board of Veterinary Practitioners, Fort Collins, Colorado.

Teenage All-Nighters Raise Risk for MS!

Anna Karin Hedström, MD, staff physician, department of environmental medicine, Karolinska Institute, Stockholm, Sweden.

Lots of teens earn extra cash by working overnight, when most of us are sleeping. But a recent study has just shown that clocking in between 9 pm and 7 am may do more than make them tired—it actually may ruin their health by raising their risk for multiple sclerosis (MS)!

Anna Hedström, MD, the study's lead researcher, who works as a staff physician in the department of environmental medicine at the Karolinska Institute in Sweden, said that the potential association between night-shift work and risk for MS, an autoimmune disease, had never before been studied. She was inspired to investigate after learning that previous research showed links between working nights and developing autoimmune thyroid disorders, cardiovascular disease and even some cancers. Her study was published in *Annals of Neurology*.

THE RISK OF WORKING ALL-NIGHTERS

Dr. Hedström's research evaluated data from two separate Swedish studies, which included a total of more than 6,000 patients, ages 16 to 70, with MS and more than 7,000 "control" patients in the same age range who did not have MS. Participants gave detailed information about their health and lifestyle—including their workplace history, with details such as what kind of work they had done over the years and what the hours had been.

Dr. Hedström and her team compared the number of MS cases among those who had worked between 9 pm and 7 am at some point in their lifetimes with those who had never worked during those hours.

Results: People who had worked either regular or alternating graveyard shifts as teens were between 30% and 60% more likely to develop MS at some point in their lives compared with people who had never worked graveyard shifts. The average age of onset of MS in these people was 33, said Dr. Hedström.

The type of overnight work that had been done in the teen years—whether it was unloading trucks or dishing out fast food—didn't matter. The risk did rise the most, however, in those who worked these shifts for a long time (three years or more) and/or more frequently (10 night shifts or more per month). Dr. Hedström and her team factored out the influence of many other previously known MS risk factors, such as smoking, family history and body mass index

(BMI), in reaching their conclusion. But it is important to note, said Dr. Hedström, that genetics and environmental factors may also affect MS risk—and those factors were not studied.

LATE-NIGHT LINK TO DISEASE

It's never a good idea to constantly disrupt natural sleep patterns and the body's circadian rhythm—aka the body's "biological clock"—said Dr. Hedström. She said that it disrupts the release of the hormone melatonin, which affects the immune system and may trigger a system-wide inflammatory response, and that is what causes MS and other autoimmune diseases to develop. Since MS can bring on symptoms that range from uncomfortable to debilitating—from balance problems to vision loss to paralysis—it's definitely a disease that you want to avoid at all costs.

So pay attention to any teen you know who pulls "all-nighters" while studying for high school or college exams. Encourage students to keep all-nighters to a minimum instead of treating them as just another way to study.

How Secondhand Smoke Saps Hearing

Anil Lalwani, MD, surgeon and researcher, professor of otolaryngology, physiology and neuroscience, and pediatrics, New York University School of Medicine, NYU Langone Medical Center, New York City.

Most of us barely pay attention to background noises like engines, fans or groups of people talking loudly. That's because most of us have the ability to block out those annoying distractions when we want to. But sadly, that's not the case for a large group of youngsters whose ability to separate those sounds from what they do want to hear—for instance, a conversation in a noisy room—has already been compromised, even at their young ages, because of their exposure to secondhand smoke.

In a recent study by Anil Lalwani, MD, professor of otolaryngology, pediatrics and physiology and neuroscience at New York University Langone Medical Center in New York City, 12- to 19-year-olds who had been exposed to secondhand smoke were found to be nearly twice as likely as other teenagers to suffer irreversible *sensorineural hearing loss* (SNHL) in their teen years—even though that kind of hearing loss typically tends to occur among older adults.

About 80% of the teenagers with SNHL had no idea that their hearing had been affected. But even if damage is mild, it can impair one's ability to function. While smoke-exposed adolescents performed worse across every sound frequency tested, their scores showed the most impairment in the mid- to high-frequency levels, which are crucial for understanding speech and for pulling any relevant sounds out of the din. Because kids who can't always understand what's being said in the classroom are easily distracted, they may be misdiagnosed with attention deficit hyperactivity disorder or at the very least labeled as troublemakers. And of course, their schoolwork may suffer.

ADD HEARING LOSS TO THE LIST

Dr. Lalwani pointed out that secondhand smoke has already been impacting those he calls "innocent bystanders," since it has been linked to a wide range of other health issues—including low birth weight, sudden infant death syndrome (SIDS), childhood asthma, inner ear infections and behavioral and cognitive problems. "In the last one to two decades," said Dr. Lalwani, "we've seen a huge amount of evidence mounting about the health consequences of secondhand smoke"—and now we have to add hearing loss to that list.

How did he discover this particular effect of secondhand smoke? Dr. Lalwani and his colleagues studied data on more than 1,500 12- to 19-year-olds selected from the 2005–2006 National Health and Nutrition Examination Survey, which gathered health information from adults and kids around the US. First, the youngsters were evaluated by National Center for Health Statistics personnel in 2005–2006, including at-home visits to determine family medical history, whether or not smokers lived in the home and other demographic information. Then the teens were given extensive hearing tests. They were also given blood tests measuring the level of a nicotine-related substance called *cotinine* that can objectively tell how much secondhand smoke one has been exposed to.

Dr. Lalwani's results were compelling—the higher the teens' levels of cotinine, the higher their chances of having SNHL. The cotinine acted as a remarkably accurate biomarker—or barometer, if you will—of the hearing damage. His findings were published in a recent issue of *Archives of Otolaryngology-Head & Neck Surgery*. The study authors did note that among the drawbacks of the study was that data on noise levels in the homes was not available.

Perhaps the biggest question to be answered now is, how is it that smoke can affect people's ability to hear—especially young people with robust constitutions? Dr. Lalwani's study didn't look for the cause, but he has many theories. "We know smoking leads to reduced oxygen in the blood, so that may be an issue," he said. "The ear is a high-energy-requirement organ. We also know that smoking causes vascular issues (blood vessel problems), so a variety of factors could be contributing."

SOUND ADVICE

There is an obvious and surefire answer to this health problem among teens—parents who smoke should stop! Beyond that, Dr. Lalwani hopes that standard newborn hearing screenings can be expanded to include older kids, since only newborns and young children are routinely given hearing tests in the US. "I think it will happen eventually," he said optimistically, "and I think this is part of the evidence that will drive it." Until then, if you're a concerned parent, discuss with your child's pediatrician whether your child should have the test.

Teens May Need a Second Meningitis Shot

A vaccine for meningococcal meningitis is recommended for children ages 11 or 12—the disease is common in adolescents and spreads readily in crowded places, such as camps and dorm rooms. The shot was originally thought to last for at least 10 years.

But: New research shows that the vaccine may last for less than five years—so a federal advisory panel now recommends a booster shot at age 16. The recommendation has recently been adopted by the Centers for Disease Control and Prevention. Ask your doctor for details.

James Turner, MD, executive director, department of student health, University of Virginia, Charlottesville.

Lack of Sun Hurts Kids' Eyes

Studies in the US, Singapore and China have found a consistent link between the time spent outdoors and myopia (nearsightedness). Children who spent the most time outdoors—10 to 14 hours a week—were half as likely to have myopia as children who were outdoors only three to six hours a week. Avoiding the outdoors causes a lack of retinal *dopamine*, which can lead to myopia.

Kathryn Rose, PhD, associate professor, Faculty of Health Sciences, University of Sydney, Australia, and coauthor of a study of 4,132 children, published in *Ophthalmology*.

Tanning Beds Raise Melanoma Risk 75%

Did you know that risk for skin melanoma in later life rises by 75% when tanning beds are used before age 30? The International Agency for Research on Cancer places UV tanning beds in its highest cancer-risk category, labeling these "carcinogenic to humans."

Review of more than 20 studies of skin cancer by Cancer Monograph Working Group, International Agency for Research on Cancer, published in *The Lancet Oncology*.

Pitching Limits Protect Kids from Injury

Glenn S. Fleisig, PhD, research director, American Sports Medicine Institute, adjunct professor, department of biomedical engineering, University of Alabama at Birmingham, and pitching safety consultant for Little League Baseball & Softball.

In past generations, overuse injuries from tennis, basketball, baseball and other sports were pretty much the province of professional athletes and aging men and women. Now, because of kids' aggressive sports schedules, pediatricians and orthopedic physicians report that they are seeing "wear and tear" injuries in children of younger and younger ages, which is of great concern for those young bodies.

In fact, new research from the American Sports Medicine Institute (ASMI) in Birmingham, Alabama, has found a direct correlation between the number of innings played by the pitchers in youth baseball and the likelihood of injury in years to come. Based on the findings, researchers hope that youth leagues will establish and enforce a 100-inning-per-year limit.

THE REAL BOYS OF SUMMER PLAY ALL YEAR

"Years ago, most youngsters played organized baseball only in Little League and school teams," says Glenn Fleisig, PhD, lead author of the pitching study and research director for ASMI. "But a sharp rise in travel teams is giving kids the opportunity to play organized baseball more months of the year." Today, a young pitcher might pitch 30 or 40 games a year (at six innings per game, that's as many as 240 innings)—compared with 10 games a year in previous generations—which has led to an increased number of elbow and shoulder injuries. And these are kids in primary and secondary school!

The study participants included 481 boys between the ages of nine and 14 who were followed for a decade. They were asked, yearly, whether they had pitched...if so, how many innings...whether they had had an elbow or shoulder injury that resulted in surgery or retirement from baseball. Researchers found that boys who pitched more than 100 innings in a year were 3.5 times more likely to be injured. Playing pitcher and catcher in the same game also appeared to increase the risk for injury.

LITTLE PITCHERS

Pitching brings stress to the bones, tendons and ligaments of the elbows and shoulder at any age—and there's a reason why childhood and adolescence are called "the tender years." "Kids' bones are still growing, with soft areas at the ends of their bones—the so-called growth plates," said Dr. Fleisig. "Young pitchers are especially susceptible to injuries at the growth plates of the elbow and shoulder."

Most elbow injuries involve the ulnar collateral ligament of the elbow, known as the Tommy John injury after the professional pitcher who tore this ligament in the 1970s and then made a very unlikely comeback after innovative surgery to replace it. Shoulder injuries usually involve the rotator cuff tendons or the shoulder capsule (the ligaments that wrap around the upper arm bone connecting it to the shoulder socket).

SAFE PITCHING

If you know and care about young pitchers (male or female), you'll want to encourage them along with their coaches to consider these guidelines offered by Dr. Fleisig…

•**Stop when tired.** Pitchers who end up needing surgery as a result of overuse tend to be the ones who kept pitching when they were fatigued.

•**Take rejuvenating breaks.** Pitchers should avoid overhead throwing completely for at least two to three months a year—although a four-month break from competitive baseball pitching every year is preferred.

•**Keep track of innings pitched.** Learn and adhere to the recommended limits for pitch counts and days of rest (one to four days, depending on the number of pitches). You can find details on the ASMI Web site, *http://www.asmi.org/asmiweb/position_statement.htm.*

•**Do not pitch on multiple teams with overlapping seasons** unless you can keep to the guidelines above.

•**Learn and use good throwing mechanics (just as pro pitchers do).** There are many young pitchers who are effective on the mound—for now—but whose pitching form is almost guaranteed to overstress their arms and shoulders. Working with a fitness coach and pitching coach/instructor is a good idea.

•**Avoid using radar guns to frequently measure the speed of young pitchers' throws.** This may lead them to focus too heavily on speed at the expense of protecting their arms.

•**Do not pitch and catch in the same game.**

•**Don't "push through" pain.** If a pitcher complains of pain in his elbow or shoulder, get an evaluation from a sports medicine physician.

Encourage young pitchers to have fun playing a variety of sports so that they strengthen different combinations of muscle groups and avoid overuse.

"The issue of overuse comes largely from playing the same sport year-round," said Dr. Fleisig. "For children to be as healthy as possible, they need athletic activity, but they develop best if they engage in multiple activities using a variety of muscles rather than specializing in one sport or position."

■ ■ ■ ■

Close Scores Increase Fatal Accidents

Sports events with a very close score increased the risk for fatal traffic accidents among the winning team's supporters by 133%. The excitement of the game increases testosterone among fans, increasing aggression. That, combined with alcohol consumption, results in more accidents after the game.

Melayne McInnes, PhD, associate professor, economics department, The Darla Moore School of Business, University of South Carolina, Columbia, and an author of a study published in *Journal of Consumer Research.*

Heart & Stroke

Standard Heart Tests Fail to Show True Risks

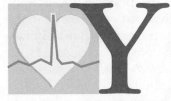

You may think that you are at low risk for a heart attack because the heart tests that your doctor has ordered had "negative" results. The standard blood test that you received may show that your cholesterol and triglyceride levels are fine. And you may have even received a clean bill of health after taking a cardiac stress test (exercising on a treadmill while heart rhythms are electronically monitored).

Surprising fact: Those two standard heart tests miss many high-risk individuals with early heart disease. For example, a study published in the *Journal of the American College of Cardiology* found that 95% of women who had heart attacks at age 65 or younger were considered low risk.

For the greatest protection: In addition to the standard heart tests, all adults should consider receiving the highly accurate heart tests described in this article, which are not regularly ordered by most physicians but serve as stronger predictors of cardiovascular disease.

Why don't more doctors have conversations with their patients about these important tests? Many physicians closely adhere to the guidelines of the government's Preventive Services Task Force, whose evidence-based recommendations tend to include tests that are less sophisticated and less expensive.

But if your primary care physician or cardiologist does not mention these tests, ask him/her which ones might be right for you. The results will provide the best possible information for your doctor to create a customized medical and lifestyle regimen that can help prevent heart attacks and strokes.

James Ehrlich, MD, a clinical associate professor of endocrinology at the University of Colorado, Denver. The chief medical officer of United Cardio Systems, based in Castle Rock, Colorado, Dr. Ehrlich is a coauthor of *The Physician's Guide to Coronary Imaging*, a multimedia CD (available to physicians only).

CORONARY CALCIUM CT SCAN

This radiological imaging test—also called a CT heart scan—detects and quantifies calcified plaque, a marker for atherosclerosis (fatty buildup in the arteries). This test is up to 10 times more predictive of future heart problems than a cholesterol test and can detect early heart disease that often goes undetected by a stress test.

My advice: Men over age 35 and women over age 40 with one to two risk factors for cardiovascular disease are good candidates for screening with a heart scan. Risk factors include being overweight…having hypertension, diabetes (or prediabetes), high LDL "bad" cholesterol, low HDL "good" cholesterol, elevated triglycerides, a family history of heart disease…and/or smoking.

Risks: Cardiac CT tests expose patients to ionizing radiation (the same type used in X-rays), which has been linked to an increased risk for cancer. Heart scans, such as electron-beam CT scans and late-generation spiral CT scans, now are performed at lower radiation doses—the equivalent of 10 to 25 chest X-rays is typical. These CT scans use faster speeds than standard CT scans to produce the image, are accurate and expose you to less radiation.

Cost and coverage: $150 to $500 and may be covered by insurance.

CAROTID TEST

An ultrasound test of the carotid (neck) arteries leading to the brain does not involve radiation and measures two important conditions that help predict cardiovascular disease—the dangerous presence of plaque and the thickness of the two inner layers of each artery (the intima and media).

The carotid test is a stronger predictor of a future stroke than coronary calcium and a moderate predictor of heart attack risk.

My advice: I recommend this test for men over age 35 and women over age 40 with one to two risk factors such as hypertension and/or a family history of heart disease or stroke. People with such risk factors as high cholesterol and type 2 diabetes also may benefit from the test.

Results: If there is any noticeable plaque or the thickness of the intima/media is in the top 25% for people of your age, sex and ethnicity, you are at a higher than desirable cardiovascular risk and should pay close attention to all risk factors—especially hypertension.

Cost and coverage: $100 to $500 and often is covered by insurance.

ADVANCED LIPOPROTEIN ANALYSIS

Advanced lipoprotein analysis includes blood tests that measure hidden risk factors such as…

•**Lp(a),** a dangerous particle that often is elevated in families with a history of premature heart attacks.

•**ApoB/ApoAI,** a ratio of dangerous particles to protective particles.

My advice: This analysis is especially useful for people with heart disease that occurs in the absence of risk factors or who have a family history of premature heart disease (heart attack before age 55 in a father or brother and before age 65 in a mother or sister, for example). Those with type 2 diabetes (or prediabetes) or "metabolic syndrome"—often with a bulging waistline, hypertension, low HDL, elevated triglycerides and/or elevated blood sugar—also are good candidates.

Cost and coverage: Varies widely from as little as $40 to as much as $400—often covered by insurance.

However, not all labs perform these tests. Labs that perform advanced lipoprotein analysis: Atherotech (*www.atherotech.com*)…Berkeley Heart Lab (*www.bhlinc.com*)…Boston Heart Diagnostics (*www.bostonheartdiagnostics.com*)…Health Diagnostic Laboratory (*www.hdlabinc.com*)…LipoScience(*www.liposcience.com*)…and SpectraCell (*www.spectracell.com*).

OTHER BIOMARKERS

•**Lp-PLA2 (PLAC test).** This blood test, which measures inflammation in blood vessels themselves, is a powerful predictor of the most common type of stroke (ischemic stroke). The test is more specific for vascular disease than the commonly ordered test for C-reactive protein (which is elevated with any type of inflammation in the body).

Cost and coverage: About $50 to $200 and may be covered by insurance.

• **BNP or NT-proBNP (B-type natriuretic peptide).** This is an early indicator of a weakening heart muscle (even before overt heart failure) and an excellent test for managing patients with heart failure. The test can also be used to help predict risk for heart attack.

Cost and coverage: About $50 to $250 and may be covered by insurance.

ASPIRIN RESISTANCE TESTING

Aspirin helps stop blood components called platelets from sticking together, which reduces the risk for an artery-plugging blood clot. A daily "baby" aspirin (81 mg) or higher doses usually are prescribed for anyone who has had a heart attack or stroke…or for someone who is at risk for either condition.

However, 25% of people are aspirin resistant—the drug doesn't effectively prevent platelet "stickiness."

Aspirin resistance testing measures a urinary metabolite (11-dehydrothromboxane B2), which is high if you are aspirin resistant.

Who should be tested: Anyone taking aspirin to treat or prevent cardiovascular disease.

Cost and coverage: $30 to $150 and often covered by insurance.

Good news: Recent research published in the Journal of the American College of Cardiology shows that supplementing the diet with omega-3 fatty acids can overcome aspirin resistance.

SOBERING STATISTICS

About 81 million American adults have cardiovascular disease. This may include narrowed, blocked arteries (coronary artery disease)…irregular heartbeats (arrhythmia)…and/or a weakened heart muscle (heart failure).

Every year, 1.5 million of those Americans have heart attacks and 500,000 of them die. Another 800,000 have strokes, 140,000 of whom die.

■ ■ ■ ■

Urgent Test for Heart Disease

In a study in *Circulation,* researchers at Harvard Medical School tracked levels of Lp-PLA2 in more than 3,000 patients who had survived a heart attack or a serious episode of unstable angina, a type of heart pain caused by a lack of oxygen. After two years, people with the highest Lp-PLA2 levels were 33% more likely to suffer another heart attack, stroke or cardiovascular-related death.

My advice: Ask your doctor to measure your blood levels of Lp-PLA2 if you are at risk for cardiovascular disease…if your low-density lipoprotein (LDL) cholesterol or CRP levels are high…or if you have survived a heart attack or stroke. The FDA-approved Lp-PLA2 test is called the PLAC test. The lower your Lp-PLA2, the better. If your Lp-PLA2 is 235 ng/mL or higher, you have an above-average risk for a heart attack or stroke.

Mark A. Stengler, NMD, naturopathic medical doctor in private practice, Encinitas, California…adjunct associate clinical professor at the National College of Natural Medicine, Portland, Oregon…author of *The Natural Physicians Healing Therapies* and coauthor of *Prescription for Natural Cures* (both from Bottom Line Books).

FDA OKs Valve That Does Not Require Open-Heart Surgery

Gregory Crooke, MD, assistant director, cardiothoracic surgery, Maimonides Medical Center, New York City.
James Slater, MD, director, Cardiac Catheterization Lab, NYU Langone Medical Center, New York City.
US Food and Drug Administration.

The first artificial heart valve that can be implanted without open-heart surgery has been approved by the US Food and Drug Administration.

The Sapien Transcatheter Heart Valve is designed to replace an aortic heart valve damaged by senile aortic valve stenosis, a progressive and age-related illness caused by calcium deposits that cause the valve to narrow.

One expert called the advent of the device "a revolutionary breakthrough" in terms of expanding access for sick or frail patients.

"This new approach to valve replacement is designed for the elderly and the highest risk patients who are inoperable—or nearly inoperable—by conventional criteria," said Gregory

Crooke, MD, assistant director of cardiothoracic surgery at Maimonides Medical Center in New York City, which is already offering the device to select patients. "As has been shown in trials, it should greatly improve the survival and quality of life for this cohort of patients," he said.

ABOUT AORTIC STENOSIS

In aortic stenosis, the heart has to work harder to pump sufficient amounts of blood through the narrowed valve opening. This eventually causes the heart to weaken, leading to problems such as fainting, chest pain, heart failure, irregular heart rhythms or cardiac arrest.

More than half of patients with symptoms of senile aortic valve stenosis die within two years. Open-heart surgery to replace the diseased valve can restore blood flow, but the procedure is too dangerous for some patients, the FDA noted in a news release.

HOW THE ARTIFICIAL HEART VALVE WORKS

The new artificial valve—made of cow tissue and polyester supported with a stainless steel mesh—provides an option for these patients. The valve is compressed into the end of a catheter that's inserted into a femoral artery (large artery in the thigh) and threaded to the site of the diseased valve. The artificial valve is then released from the catheter and expanded with a balloon. The valve is immediately functional, according to information in the FDA news release.

STUDY FINDINGS

The FDA's approval of the valve is based on a study of 365 patients with the condition who weren't eligible for open-heart surgery. Half of the patients received the artificial valve while the other patients received alternative treatments, such as one that enlarges the aortic valve opening by stretching it with a balloon.

Patients who received the new valve did have eight times as many vascular and bleeding complications and 2.5 times more strokes than those who did not receive the valve. However, patients who received the valve were also more likely to be living one year after surgery than those who received an alternative treatment—69% versus 50%, respectively, the investigators found.

SIDE EFFECTS

The most common serious side effects associated with the artificial valve and its implantation include death, stroke, perforation of blood vessels or ventricular or valvular structures in the heart, significant bleeding, leaks around the new valve, and damage to the heart's conduction system, which is responsible for a consistent and healthy heart beat.

EXPERT COMMENTARY

"Often these patients are elderly with numerous other medical ailments that make standard aortic valve surgery too risky to perform," said James Slater, MD, director of the Cardiac Catheterization Lab at NYU Langone Medical Center in New York City. "Medical [drug] therapy is generally not effective and the availability of a therapy that is less invasive and traumatic than standard surgery is an important advance," he added.

Dr. Slater also hopes that "further improvements in these devices will decrease the rate of complications and that further investigations will allow this therapy to be available to a wider range of patients with this disease."

California-based Edwards Lifescience, which makes the new valve, says it will continue to evaluate patient outcomes through a national registry.

PATIENT ELIGIBILITY

The FDA approved the Sapien Transcatheter Heart Valve for patients who are not eligible for open-heart surgery, but it is not approved for those who can be treated by open-heart surgery. The agency also said that patients with congenital heart valve abnormalities, masses or an infection in their hearts, or those who cannot tolerate anticoagulation/antiplatelet therapy should not receive the new valve.

The valve's product label says a heart surgeon should be involved in determining if a patient is a suitable candidate for the artificial valve.

info For more on heart valve disease, visit the Web site of the US National Heart, Lung, and Blood Institute, *www.nhlbi.nih.gov/health/health-topics/topics/hvd/*.

Drug-Coated Balloons Open Arteries Blocked By Narrowed Stents

Mariusz Zadura, MD, senior cardiologist, Heart and Diabetes Center of Mecklenburg-Vorpommern, Karlsburg, Germany.

Gregg Fonarow, MD, professor, cardiology, University of California, Los Angeles, and spokesman, American Heart Association presentation, American Heart Association annual meeting, Orlando, Florida.

Balloons coated with a drug used to open blocked stents in heart arteries restore blood flow and also reduce bleeding in some high-risk patients, recent research shows.

BACKGROUND

Bare-metal stents, implanted to keep a blood vessel in the heart open during angioplasty, can narrow over time as scar tissue develops, which restricts blood flow and requires another procedure to widen the vessel, the researchers say.

In the new balloon procedure, a catheter with a drug-coated balloon is passed through the narrowed stent to restore blood flow. The procedure leaves behind the drug, which acts to prevent the stent from renarrowing.

Gregg Fonarow, MD, a professor of cardiology at the University of California, Los Angeles, and a spokesman for the American Heart Association, said, "drug-eluting stents significantly attenuate scar formation and the need for repeat procedures." However, dependency on prolonged therapy with two anti-clotting drugs and late-stent thrombosis have led to investigations of alternative treatments, he added.

In recent years, drug-eluting balloons have emerged as an alternative to drug-eluting stents to address blocking of arteries and avoid the need for prolonged dual anti-clotting therapy. The drug *paclitaxel* (Taxol) is used to coat the balloons and minimize cell growth, he said.

STUDY #1

Mariusz Zadura, MD, a senior cardiologist at the Heart and Diabetes Center of Mecklenburg-Vorpommern in Karlsburg, Germany, and his team studied the responses of 84 patients who had narrowed bare metal stents reopened. The balloons used in the procedure were coated with paclitaxel, a cancer drug also used to prevent blocking of arteries.

In all, 91 stented arteries were treated. After six to nine months, the procedure kept 85 of the arteries open.

New blockages occurred in six stented arteries, but only three patients needed an additional procedure, the researchers noted.

STUDY #2

The research team followed 63 patients who were at high risk of bleeding. These patients were being treated with anti-clotting drugs for other medical problems, such as mechanical heart valves, atrial fibrillation and pulmonary embolism.

These patients also had narrowed stented arteries. Over six to nine months, drug-coated balloon procedures were effective in keeping 69 of 73 narrowed arteries open.

Although narrowing occurred in four stents, only two patients needed another procedure, the researchers reported.

The study findings were presented at the American Heart Association's annual meeting in Orlando, Florida.

CONCLUSION

Using the drug-eluting balloon is better than using drug-eluting stents, according to the researchers.

"Drug-eluting [emitting] balloons are, in my opinion, the therapy of choice in case of bare-metal stent restenosis," said Dr. Zadura, the lead researcher of both studies

Also, patients treated with drug-eluting metal stents need daily aspirin and other anti-clotting drugs for at least one year, which can increase the risk of bleeding, the researchers said.

However, they said, patients treated with a drug-coated balloon only need to take dual anti-clotting therapy for one month.

EXPERT COMMENTARY

"Drug-eluting balloon technology has been demonstrated to be safe and potentially efficacious in small studies," Dr. Fonarow said.

Both of these studies on patients showed very good efficacy and safety. These promising findings should be further evaluated in prospective randomized clinical trials, he said.

info For more information on angioplasty, visit the US National Heart, Lung, and Blood Institute Web site, *www.nhlbi.nih.gov,* and search "coronary angioplasty."

Aspirin Works As Well As Warfarin for Heart Failure Patients

Kenneth Ong, MD, cardiologist, The Brooklyn Hospital Center, New York City.

Shunichi Homma, MD, professor of medicine, Columbia University, New York City.

American Stroke Association, news release

A major head-to-head trial finds that aspirin is equally as good as *warfarin* (Coumadin) in preventing stroke and death in heart failure patients. Heart failure patients are at increased risk for blood clots, stroke and death.

The researchers said that, all things being equal, the findings raise questions about the wisdom of routinely using warfarin, which can cause dangerous bleeding.

The findings were presented at the annual meeting of the American Stroke Association in New Orleans.

STUDY DETAILS

The study is the largest and longest of its kind to date and included more than 2,300 patients averaging 61 years of age. All patients had heart failure and a normal heart rhythm, and were followed for up to six years (average 3.5 years).

The patients were randomly assigned to receive either 325 milligrams a day of aspirin, or warfarin doses meant to achieve a pre-specified degree of blood thinning.

Death, ischemic stroke (caused by blockage of an artery carrying blood to the brain) or bleeding inside the brain (intracerebral hemorrhage) occurred in about 8% of the patients taking aspirin and about 7.5% of those taking warfarin. This difference was not found to be statistically significant, the research team said.

Among patients who were followed for more than three years, strokes occurred in 0.72% of those taking warfarin and in 1.36% of those taking aspirin, according to the study. While warfarin users had half the stroke risk of those on aspirin, the overall risk for stroke for patients in either group was considered low.

On the other hand, the researchers found that major bleeding (other than intracerebral hemorrhage) occurred in 0.9% of the patients on aspirin each year, compared with 1.8% of those on warfarin. That was a statistically significant difference, the team said.

"Although there was a warfarin benefit for patients treated for four or more years, overall, warfarin and aspirin were similar," said lead author Shunichi Homma, MD, a professor of medicine at Columbia University in New York City.

CONCLUSION

Given that there is no overall difference between the two treatments, there is no compelling reason to use warfarin, especially considering the bleeding risk, Dr. Homma noted.

EXPERT COMMENTARY

"There has always been a question about whether warfarin or aspirin is better when treating heart failure in patients with normal heart rhythms, so this is a very important study," noted Kenneth Ong, MD, a cardiologist at The Brooklyn Hospital Center in New York City.

"Until now, we considered warfarin a more potent anti-clotting drug than aspirin, though each affects a different mechanism of clotting," he explained. "In the past, the only reason to put heart failure patients on warfarin was in the case of patients with a history of strokes, transient ischemic strokes (TIA or 'mini-stroke') or an irregular heart rhythm. This study confirms current standards of treatment. Aspirin is just as effective as warfarin in the treatment of heart failure, but warfarin is indicated for high-risk patients."

The US Agency for Healthcare Research and Quality has more about blood thinners on its Web site, *www.ahrq.gov/consumer/btpills.htm.*

Fried Foods That Won't Harm Your Heart

Pilar Guallar-Castillon, MD, PhD, MPH, associate professor of preventive medicine at Universidad Autonoma de Madrid.

Michael Leitzmann, MD, chair of the department of epidemiology, University of Regensburg, Germany.

BMJ (*British Medical Journal*) online

Researchers in Spain have some good news for people who enjoy eating fried food—cooking in olive or sunflower oil is not linked to heart disease or premature death.

Because heart disease risk factors—such as high blood pressure, high cholesterol and obesity—have been linked to eating fried foods, the study authors decided to investigate the association.

STUDY DETAILS

For the study, the researchers examined the cooking habits and health of nearly 41,000 adults, aged 29 to 69, who did not have heart disease at the start of the 11-year study. The participants were split into four groups depending on how much fried food they consumed.

There were 606 heart disease-related events and 1,134 deaths during the study follow-up period, according to a report published in the online edition of the *BMJ*.

"In a Mediterranean country where olive and sunflower oils are the most commonly used fats for frying, and where large amounts of fried foods are consumed both at and away from home, no association was observed between fried food consumption and the risk of coronary heart disease or death," according to the research team, led by Pilar Guallar-Castillon, MD, PhD, MPH, associate professor of preventive medicine at Universidad Autonoma de Madrid.

FRIED FOOD CAVEAT

The study authors pointed out that because their research was conducted in Spain, where olive and sunflower oil are used for cooking, the findings might not apply in other countries where other types of oil are more commonly used. For example, when food is fried in solid and re-used oils (as in the Western diet), it absorbs the fat of the oils, which increases the calories of the food.

EXPERT COMMENTARY

In an accompanying editorial on the study, Michael Leitzmann, MD, chair of the department of epidemiology, University of Regensburg, Germany, wrote that the findings challenge the prevalent belief that "frying food is generally bad for the heart."

However, he added that this "does not mean that frequent meals of fish and chips will have no health consequences."

info Learn more about how to eat for a healthy heart at the US Food and Drug Administration Web site, *http://www.fda.gov* (search "eat for a healthy heart").

Four Heart-Healing Supplements You Need Now

Mark A. Stengler, NMD, naturopathic medical doctor in private practice, Encinitas, California...adjunct associate clinical professor at the National College of Natural Medicine, Portland, Oregon...author of *The Natural Physicians Healing Therapies* and coauthor of *Prescription for Natural Cures* (both from Bottom Line Books).

Several nutrients help patients immediately after a heart attack. The four nutrients below can help anyone who has had a heart attack or is at risk for one. People who are not at risk but who want to prevent a heart attack can take the first two supplements. Except as noted, most of these nutrients are safe to take with other medications and there are no side effects. They all are available at health-food stores.

•**Coenzyme Q10 (CoQ10).** Heart cells cannot produce energy without CoQ10. This nutrient has been found to reduce the risk for subsequent cardiac events, which usually are increased in people who have had a heart attack. I recommend that patients take 100 milligrams (mg)—and optimally 300 mg—daily of CoQ10 with food.

Caution: CoQ10 may interfere with some blood-thinning and blood pressure medications (and heart attack patients often are on both), so take CoQ10 only while supervised by a physician.

●**Magnesium.** This mineral enables the heart to manufacture enough energy to beat properly. It also contributes to blood-clot prevention. I usually suggest 200 mg of supplemental magnesium glycinate twice daily for long-term heart protection.

●**L-carnitine.** This supplement helps to fuel heart cells. Studies have found that L-carnitine minimizes damage to heart cells after a heart attack by strengthening the heart muscle and can reduce the likelihood of a repeat heart attack. I recommend L-carnitine in combination with CoQ10. Together, these supplements can maintain normal heart energy levels. For most people, taking 2,000 mg of L-carnitine daily helps strengthen the heart.

●**D-ribose.** During a heart attack, heart muscle cells are deprived of oxygen, and afterward they require large amounts of energy to repair damaged tissue and restore blood flow. D-ribose helps to generate energy in heart cells. I often recommend that heart attack patients take 5 grams two to three times daily.

Work Out Harder to Heal Your Heart

Trine Tegdan Moholdt, PhD, physiotherapist, postdoctoral fellow, K.G. Jebsen Center of Exercise in Medicine, Department of Circulation and Medical Imaging, and Department of Public Health and General Practice, Norwegian University of Science and Technology, Trondheim, Norway.

Extended bed rest is a thing of the past for post–heart attack care, and today we know it's by far in your best interest to get up and move around again as soon as possible. Yet a recent study suggests that *intense* exercise may be the best way to recover, as an increasing number of physicians say that a stepped up workout regimen is just what your heart needs.

LATEST RESEARCH

In a randomized, controlled trial at the Norwegian University of Science and Technology, 107 heart attack patients began to work out just two to 12 weeks after a myocardial infarction. Investigators, including postdoctoral fellow Trine Moholdt, PhD, physiotherapist, randomly assigned the participants to a 12-week program on one of two different exercise regimens—twice weekly conventional cardiac rehabilitation or more intense interval training on the treadmill. *Dr. Moholdt explained the two approaches to me…*

●**Conventional cardiac rehab.** The conventional rehab group performed aerobic workouts for about 60 minutes per session at moderate intensity under the guidance of a physical therapist. Their heart rates rose to 70% to 80% of the maximum.

●**Aerobic interval training.** A second group started with a 10-minute warm-up followed by 28 minutes on the treadmill jogging or walking uphill. Workouts included four-minute high-intensity intervals at 85% to 95% of maximum heart rate (to the point where participants couldn't say more than a few words while carrying on a conversation, but not to the point where they had chest or leg pain), interspersed with three-minute recoveries and capped off with a final cool down. Both groups were also encouraged to do an additional workout of the same type and intensity at home.

GREATER INTENSITY = GREATER OXYGEN UPTAKE

At the end of the 12-week period, Dr. Moholdt and her team found that more intense aerobic interval training was better at raising participants' peak oxygen uptake—the capacity of the body to transport and use oxygen during exercise, which is a key indicator of cardiorespiratory endurance and physical fitness. *Specifically, they discovered that…*

In people who exercised at moderate intensity, VO2peak (peak oxygen uptake) increased from 32.2 at baseline to 34.7 mL/kg per minute, demonstrating that any exercise is better than none. But in the high-intensity interval group,

VO2peak rose more significantly—from 31.6 mL/kg per minute to 36.2.

Over time, once the workout program was completed and the patients were no longer exercising at the same levels, VO2peak declined in both groups—but less so in the high-intensity group, which appeared to retain some health benefits. Thirty months after completing the program, VO2peak dropped to baseline in the aerobic interval trainees, but significantly below baseline in the conventional cardiac rehab group.

At 30 months, only 4% of the high-intensity group reported being physically inactive, in comparison with 20% of the conventional group. Although the reason for this is unclear, it could be that those who had performed at high intensity under medical supervision were more confident about continuing to work out vigorously on their own. (This might also account for their higher VO2peak at 30 months.)

Dr. Moholdt and her colleagues presented these results at the annual congress of the European Society of Cardiology in Stockholm, Sweden in 2010.

SAFETY FIRST

Of course, not all physicians yet agree about the merits of high-intensity exercise post-heart attack, and Dr. Moholdt acknowledges that further research is necessary—noting, however, that in her experience, it is well-tolerated and emphasizing that strict measures need to be put in place to ensure patient safety. In her program, doctors first check all patients' heart function with electrocardiograms during maximum-effort exercise, and patients wear heart rate monitors throughout aerobic sessions. Trained staff members are on hand to operate emergency equipment as needed in exercise labs—which are located within hospitals.

If you have suffered a heart attack, Dr. Moholdt warns that the single most dangerous thing you can do afterward is remain sedentary. Consult your cardiologist, and together you can design the exercise program that is safest and most effective for you.

Can Testosterone Help Your Heart?

Mark A. Stengler, NMD, naturopathic medical doctor in private practice, Encinitas, California…adjunct associate clinical professor at the National College of Natural Medicine, Portland, Oregon…author of *The Natural Physicians Healing Therapies* and coauthor of *Prescription for Natural Cures* (both from Bottom Line Books).

As we get older, our levels of testosterone (the "male" hormone) decline. Because of this decline, some men and women experience loss of libido, fatigue, reduced mental sharpness and increased body fat. And now there seems to be even more reason to make sure that your body has the testosterone it needs—heart health.

NEWEST FINDINGS

Most studies (but not all) demonstrate that low levels of testosterone increase the risk for heart disease. And in a study published in *Heart*, researchers found that men with heart disease whose testosterone levels were low were almost twice as likely to die over a seven-year period as those with heart disease but normal levels of testosterone.

Low levels of testosterone also have been associated with cardiovascular risk factors, including increased levels of total and LDL (bad) cholesterol…heightened risk for insulin resistance…and blood-vessel wall dysfunction.

CAN YOU BENEFIT?

Recent research suggests that the prevalence of abnormally low testosterone levels may be more widespread than was previously thought. In one study, from the New England Research Institutes in Watertown, Massachusetts, researchers analyzed data from 1,500 men and discovered that 24% had low total testosterone. They estimate that in about 15 years, as the population ages, as many as 6.5 million American men will have a testosterone deficiency.

Testosterone levels can be tested with either a saliva test for free testosterone or a blood test for both total and free testosterone. Both tests work equally well.

MY TESTOSTERONE PROTOCOL

For my patients with low testosterone, I prescribe a bioidentical transdermal testosterone in gel or cream form.

For men: I usually prescribe a gel or cream containing 50 mg to 100 mg, to be applied each morning. If men don't respond within a few weeks to the gel or cream, I often prescribe a once-weekly injection.

For women: Women need much lower amounts of testosterone than men. I often recommend applying a daily dose of a gel or cream containing 0.5 mg to 2 mg of testosterone (depending on the patient's testosterone level). Women usually experience symptom relief (including increased libido and enhanced energy) within four to eight weeks of starting to take testosterone.

If your doctor prescribes topical testosterone for you, make sure that it doesn't come in contact with anyone else (including pets).

Taking testosterone can occasionally cause side effects in men and women, including acne, fluid retention, tender breasts and facial hair growth in women and prostate growth in men. The most common side effect I see is acne breakouts, and this only rarely.

Both men and women can take testosterone indefinitely as long as they are closely monitored.

ER Test Spots Heart Trouble Faster

Judd Hollander, MD, professor and clinical research director, department of emergency medicine, University of Pennsylvania, Philadelphia.
Gregg C. Fonarow, MD, director, Ahmanson-UCLA Cardiomyopathy Center, and codirector, UCLA Preventative Cardiology Program.
New England Journal of Medicine, online

Most people who go to the emergency room with chest pain aren't having a heart attack, but it can take hours or days to make a definitive diagnosis.

However, a recent study finds that a special kind of CT scan given in the emergency room seems to identify a heart attack faster than traditional methods, so patients can be sent home safely sooner.

Chest pain is one of the most common reasons people go to the emergency room in the United States, accounting for as many as 8 million visits each year, at a cost of several billion dollars, the researchers noted.

"You can go to an emergency department with chest pain, be concerned it might be a heart attack—get a CT scan, like we do for everything else in the emergency department—and we can say it's not your heart and you can go home, within a couple of hours," said researcher Judd Hollander, MD, clinical research director of the department of emergency medicine at the University of Pennsylvania, Philadelphia.

Using the CT scan is faster than traditional methods, Dr. Hollander said, noting it can take 25 hours to get the results of blood tests that indicate whether a patient has had a heart attack.

An EKG (electrocardiogram) may accurately show larger heart attacks, but it can miss smaller ones, according to Dr. Hollander. "Two-thirds of heart attacks will have an EKG that's not diagnostic," he added.

For every 100 patients who go to an ER with chest pain, only 10 or 15 have cardiac disease specific to heart failure, Dr. Hollander said. Many of those who don't have heart disease have minor problems such as bad indigestion. In addition, ERs are busy and crowded, and this is a way to move patients out faster and increase the ability to see more patients sooner, he said.

STUDY DETAILS

For the study, Dr. Hollander's team randomly assigned more than 1,300 patients with chest pain, but no previous history of heart disease or risk factors such as high blood pressure or diabetes, to CT scans or regular care.

The scans generate three-dimensional images of the heart and the blood vessels surrounding it, the researchers noted.

Among those with a normal scan, none died or had a heart attack within a month after being seen in the ER. In addition, more of these patients were sent home than those who received usual care—about 50% versus 23%, the researchers found.

Those who received scans spent less time in the hospital and had heart problems diagnosed faster.

The findings were published in the *New England Journal of Medicine*.

CT SCANS SAVE MONEY

Scans are also cost-effective, Dr. Hollander said. The tests, which are like a standard CT scan, cost about $1,500. Patients who have a normal scan can be sent home within a few hours. A patient who is admitted to the hospital can run up bills of more than $4,000 for stress tests and monitoring alone, the researchers noted.

Many patients with chest pain are suffering from anxiety, pneumonia or indigestion that can cause the same symptoms as a heart attack, the researchers explained. Yet, more than half of patients with chest pain are admitted to the hospital for observation or testing such as cardiac catheterization or a stress test.

WHAT EXPERTS SAY

Commenting on the study, Gregg Fonarow, MD, director of the Ahmanson-UCLA Cardiomyopathy Center and codirector of the UCLA Preventative Cardiology Program, said that the trial demonstrated that these scans may be useful in screening low- to moderate-risk patients.

There has been great interest in developing strategies that efficiently evaluate these patients and identify which ones can be safely discharged, he said.

"However, further studies are needed to evaluate the cost-effectiveness of this strategy and how it compares to protocols using high-sensitivity troponin tests," he added.

A troponin test measures the levels of one of two proteins, troponin T or troponin I, in blood, Dr. Fonarow explained. These proteins are released when the heart has been damaged, such as during a heart attack. However, this test is usually repeated over 12 to 16 hours, so the results are not determined as quickly as a CT scan.

info For more on heart attacks, visit the American Heart Association Web site at *www.heart.org*.

Shorter Stays Send Heart Attack Patients Back to the Hospital

Manesh Patel, MD, assistant professor, medicine, division of cardiology, Duke University, Durham, North Carolina.

Suzanne Steinbaum, DO, preventive cardiologist, Lenox Hill Hospital, New York City, and spokesperson, American Heart Association.

Journal of the American Medical Association

People who have heart attacks in the United States are far more likely to be readmitted to the hospital within 30 days than people in 16 other countries, a recent study indicates.

Researchers suspect that the average length of stay in the hospital, which was just three days in the United States compared with at least six days in other countries, is the main reason for the higher readmission rates. When they completed an analysis that adjusted the data for length of stay, they found that location was no longer a predictor of readmission.

"We found two striking predictors of 30-day readmission. Having multi-vessel disease (more than one coronary artery is blocked) and being in the US. This difference is probably multifactorial, but the length of stay is the shortest in the US. It was three days here and six, seven or more in other countries," said study senior author Manesh Patel, MD, an assistant professor of medicine in the division of cardiology at Duke University in Durham, North Carolina.

"When we adjusted for the length of stay, the difference went away. We're really good at opening up their arteries, but our systems of care may not be as integrated as they are in other countries. We need to make the link from the hospital to the primary care doctor to ensure that patients are getting set up in cardiac rehab and that they're following up with a cardiologist," Dr. Patel said.

And, while the study found that US patients had higher readmission rates after a heart attack, Dr. Patel noted that mortality rates weren't higher in the United States.

STUDY DETAILS

The study looked at people who were hospitalized for a specific type of heart attack called an ST-segment elevation myocardial infarction (STEMI). This type of heart attack accounts for up to 38% of all heart attacks, according to background information in the article, and the coronary artery is completely blocked by a clot in these cases.

The study included 5,745 people from 296 hospitals in 17 countries who were admitted for a STEMI. Most of the patients (5,571) survived to be discharged from the hospital. Of those, 11.3% of patients overall ended up being readmitted within 30 days.

Thirty-day readmission rates in the United States were 14.5%, but just 9.9% in the other countries in the study. The average length of stay was three days in the United States compared with eight days in Germany, the country with the longest average length of stay.

People who had multi-vessel disease were almost twice as likely to be readmitted to the hospital within 30 days, according to the study.

The other significant predictor of readmission within 30 days was being in the United States. After excluding people returning to the hospital to have additional elective procedures, people admitted in the United States had a 53% greater chance of being readmitted within 30 days versus people in other countries.

After adjusting the data to account for differences in the patients, such as age and underlying health conditions, the researchers found a 14.4% readmission rate in the United States versus a 9.3% rate for all of the other countries. Italy had the lowest readmission rates at 4.4%, followed closely by Germany at 4.8%. Canada had a 5.6% adjusted readmission rate, according to the study.

Results of the study are published in the *Journal of the American Medical Association*.

IMPLICATION

"This study compared the US against 16 other countries and asked how do we [the US] measure up? And, their findings were a little disturbing. About 60% of patients with major heart attacks were discharged in three days or less. And, our readmission rates were higher than in other countries. We have the technology and the ability to provide quality care, but we're just not doing well. Even for the sickest patients, we're not doing well," said Suzanne Steinbaum, DO, a preventive cardiologist at Lenox Hill Hospital in New York City, and a spokesperson for the American Heart Association.

"We're not sure that staying in the hospital longer would keep you from being readmitted. We know we provide good initial care. But, how well is that care transferred from the hospital to the home? We have to make sure patients know how they need to follow up," Dr. Patel said.

info To learn more about what type of care is necessary after a heart attack, visit the Web site of the US National Heart, Lung, and Blood Institute, *www.nhlbi.nih.gov*, and search "Life After a Heart Attack."

■ ■ ■ ■

Aspirin Before Heart Surgery Saves Lives

Cardiac patients on aspirin therapy who continued taking aspirin—instead of stopping one week before surgery, as many doctors recommend—had a significantly lower risk for death in the month after surgery than patients who stopped taking aspirin. The aspirin users had a lower risk for kidney failure and major postsurgical cardiac problems, and they spent less time in intensive care.

Jian-Zhong Sun, MD, associate professor of anesthesiology at Thomas Jefferson University Hospital, Philadelphia, and leader of a study of cardiac patients published in *Annals of Surgery*.

Your Heart Races or Skips a Beat—How to Tell If It's Serious

Jennifer Cummings, MD, associate professor of medicine at Northeastern Ohio Universities College of Medicine, Rootstown, Ohio, and a cardiologist with City Cardiology Associates, Akron, Ohio.

Has your heart ever "skipped" a beat? Or have you noticed that your heart was racing or fluttering?

Occasional irregularities in the heart's rhythm, known as *arrhythmias*, generally are harmless for people without underlying heart problems. But some arrhythmias indicate a serious disruption in the heart's electrical pathways.

Example: More than 325,000 Americans die from sudden cardiac arrest each year. The impulses that regulate the heartbeat become too rapid, too chaotic or both—and the heart simply stops.

What you need to know now about arrhythmia…

TRANSMISSION ERRORS

The heart beats in an on-off rhythm, a cycle that allows the heart to fill with blood and then pump the blood through the body.

How it works: Each heartbeat originates in the *sinoatrial node*, a cluster of cells in the *atria*, the top chambers of the heart. Signals from the sinoatrial node cause the atria to contract and pump blood into the ventricles beneath. When the ventricles are full, that electrical signal crosses over a "bridge" to the bottom chambers, causing them to contract and push blood outward into the body.

When you feel as though your heart has "skipped" a beat, what most likely has happened is that either the atria or the ventricles pulsed prematurely. These are *premature atrial contractions* (PACs) or *premature ventricular contractions* (PVCs). This type of arrhythmia may not cause symptoms and doesn't need treatment—although anyone who gets it frequently should undergo testing to make sure that his/her heart is healthy.

Other common arrhythmias that can be more serious…

ATRIAL FIBRILLATION (AF)

This is the most common serious arrhythmia in adults. It is suspected that nearly 50% of patients either have no symptoms or aren't bothered by the symptoms that they do experience.

What happens: Rather than producing a single, forceful beat, the atria "quiver" for a few minutes to more than an hour and can beat faster than 300 times a minute.

During these episodes, eddies of blood can cause a clot—the trigger of most strokes. Depending on other risk factors, the risk for a stroke in people with AF can be from 5% to 25% higher than in people without this condition.

Symptoms: Sensation of irregular or racing heartbeats…sometimes fatigue and shortness of breath.

Treatment: Anticoagulant therapy to lower the risk for stroke. A daily low-dose aspirin —81 milligrams (mg)—is enough for many patients. Those with a higher risk for stroke will need stronger anticlotting agents, such as *warfarin* (Coumadin) or *dabigatran* (Pradaxa). Other treatments…

•**Medications that slow the heart rate,** including beta-blockers, such as *propranolol* (Inderal), or calcium-channel blockers, such as *verapamil* (Isoptin). Some patients may need stronger antiarrhythmics.

•**Cardioversion,** an outpatient procedure in which surface electrodes shock the heart back into normal rhythm. This can restore a normal heartbeat for months or even years, especially if combined with antiarrhythmic medication.

•**Ablation therapy,** in which one or more catheters are threaded through blood vessels into the heart. The tips of the catheters are positioned near the areas of the heart that are causing arrhythmias. Heat from the catheter tips destroys (ablates) small patches of heart tissue and blocks irregular electrical signals. Ablation therapy can reduce or eliminate arrhythmias in 70% to 80% of cases. The procedure, usually done under general anesthesia in a hospital, can take four to six hours.

BRADYCARDIA

This is an umbrella term that refers to a slow heartbeat. Anyone whose heart beats less than 60 times a minute has *bradycardia*, but this doesn't always mean that he/she has a dangerous condition.

Example: Many healthy adults have a normal heart rhythm of 40 to 60 beats a minute—in athletes, the heart can beat as slowly as 30 times a minute. Bradycardia is a problem only when the heart beats so slowly that it causes symptoms.

Symptoms: Low blood pressure, dizziness, light-headedness, fatigue.

Drug side effects are the main cause of symptomatic bradycardia. This often happens when medications used to lower blood pressure, such as calcium-channel blockers or beta-blockers, slow the heart too much. Bradycardia also can be caused by a number of conditions, including inadequate levels of thyroid hormone, an electrolyte imbalance (such as low levels of calcium or magnesium) or kidney disease.

Treatment: A medication review. In some cases, patients need to stop taking certain medications, or take a lower dose, to see if the heart rate increases—this should be done only under a doctor's supervision. Or patients may be prescribed medications that don't have this effect (such as diuretics for hypertension).

Another option: A pacemaker, a device surgically implanted under the skin near the collarbone with electrodes that run to the heart. The pacemaker detects when the heart is beating too slowly and delivers a series of electrical signals that speed up the heart.

In cases where a medical condition is causing brachycardia, treating the underlying problem will correct the heart rate.

VENTRICULAR TACHYCARDIA/FIBRILLATION

These are among the most serious arrhythmias. When you hear that someone "dropped dead" from a heart attack, a ventricular tachycardia/fibrillation most often is the cause.

What happens: Electrical signals in the ventricles are so rapid and chaotic that the heart is unable to pump blood.

Result: A rapid drop in blood pressure cuts off circulation to the brain and other organs. Patients will collapse within seconds—most will die without emergency treatment.

Many patients who experience these arrhythmias have underlying heart disease, damage from a previous heart attack or electrical and/or valve abnormalities that have a genetic origin.

Symptoms: Racing heartbeat, loss of consciousness.

Treatment: Call 911 immediately. If an *automated external defibrillator* (AED) is available, it should be used. This portable device analyzes the heart's rhythm. If arrhythmias are present, the machine will instruct the operator to press a "shock" button. The heart rhythm will again be analyzed to determine if additional shocks are needed. The machine won't deliver a shock if the heart rhythm is normal.

Patients with cardiac risk factors, including a previous heart attack, should ask their doctors if they should buy an AED.

If an AED is not available and the heart has stopped, cardiopulmonary resuscitation (CPR) should be done until an ambulance arrives. To learn how to do CPR, go to the American Heart Association Web site, *www.heart.org* (put "CPR" in the search box).

Other treatment options: Patients who have survived a heart attack but have a weakened heart muscle may be advised to get an *implantable cardioverter defibrillator* (ICD), a device that continuously analyzes the heart and administers electrical shocks, as needed, to treat ventricular fibrillation. The procedure takes about an hour and often can be done on an outpatient basis.

In some cases, radiofrequency ablation can be helpful. Your doctor can decide what is right for you.

SUPRAVENTRICULAR TACHYCARDIA (SVT)

These originate in the area above the ventricles, causing a burst of rapid beats that begin suddenly and can last up to an hour. SVTs usually occur in young adults. They're uncomfortable but rarely dangerous in people without other heart disorders.

Symptoms: Rapid heartbeat that starts and stops suddenly. It may be associated with dizziness, chest pressure and/or shortness of breath. Some people have no symptoms.

Treatment: Patients may be taught how to do a *vagal maneuver*, such as coughing or holding their breath while bearing down. This stimulates the vagus nerve and slows the electrical impulses that cause rapid beats. If that doesn't work, radiofrequency ablation can eliminate the problem in most patients. Or patients may be advised to take a beta-blocker or other anti-arrhythmic medications that will reduce the frequency of these episodes.

■ ■ ■ ■

Antidepressants Speed Stroke Recovery

Both depressed and nondepressed stroke patients who were given antidepressant medication daily for three months following their strokes showed greater physical recovery than patients given a placebo.

And: Improvements continued even nine months after the patients stopped taking the medication.

Theory: Antidepressants may block inflammatory proteins released during a stroke that inhibit cellular growth and can promote growth of new cells in the brain.

Robert Robinson, MD, professor of psychiatry at University of Iowa City and leader of a study published in *American Journal of Geriatric Psychiatry.*

■ ■ ■ ■

NSAIDs Increase Heart Risk

NSAID use linked to increased risk for second heart attack.

Recent study: Researchers examined data on 83,677 heart attack survivors (average age 68) to study the effects of nonsteroidal anti-inflammatory drugs (NSAIDs), such as *ibuprofen* (Advil), *diclofenac* (Voltaren) and *celecoxib* (Celebrex).

Result: Regularly taking NSAIDs after a heart attack increased the risk for a second heart attack or death by 45% after just one week, and by up to 55% after three months.

If you've had a heart attack: Talk to your doctor before regularly using an NSAID. Earlier research has linked regular use of an NSAID to an increased risk for a first heart attack.

Anne-Marie Schjerning Olsen, MD, research fellow, Copenhagen University Hospital, Hellerup, Denmark.

■ ■ ■ ■

Heart Bypass Surgery and Blood Type

Researchers examined data on more than 15,000 patients (ages 60 and older) who had undergone coronary artery bypass graft (CABG) surgery.

Result: Patients with AB blood type were 20% less likely to die in the eight years after surgery than those with type O, A or B.

Theory: People with AB blood have the highest levels of certain blood-clotting proteins and, as a result, receive fewer blood transfusions after surgery. Blood transfusions have been linked to higher risk for death.

Ian Welsby, MD, associate professor of anesthesiology, Duke University Medical Center, Durham, North Carolina.

The Vitamin That's Better Than Statins

Steven Nissen, MD, chairman of the Robert and Suzanne Tomsich Department of Cardiovascular Medicine at the Cleveland Clinic main campus. He is coauthor of *Heart 411* (Three Rivers). *www.heart 411book.com*

Niacin, a B vitamin, has been known as the best way to raise HDL "good" cholesterol, thus helping to reduce risk for heart attacks. But a recent study has called this into question—which has made many patients and doctors wonder just how effective niacin is. *What you need to know…*

NEW CONTROVERSY

A government study, reported last year in *The New England Journal of Medicine*, involved 3,414 patients who were randomly assigned to receive either niacin or a placebo. All of the patients already were taking a cholesterol-lowering statin medication.

The study was stopped early when investigators concluded that patients getting niacin did not have fewer heart attacks or other cardiovascular events, even though they did have increases in HDL. The study, taken in isolation, suggests that increasing HDL with niacin isn't protective.

However, most authorities believe that the study, called AIM-HIGH, was seriously flawed. It involved a relatively small number of patients— the most authoritative cardiovascular studies typically include tens of thousands of patients. Also, patients in the control group were given small amounts of niacin to mimic the side effects of full-dose therapy. This prevented them from knowing they were taking a "placebo," but it could have skewed the results.

This study's findings were sufficiently different from previous research that they have to be viewed with caution. We'll need additional, larger studies to determine how much (if any) benefit patients will get from combining niacin with a statin.

Here's what we do know: Niacin alone is effective at raising HDL and, based upon older studies, probably reduces the risk for heart attack.

A PHARMACOLOGICAL VITAMIN

Most people with undesirable cholesterol are advised to take one of the statin medications, such as *atorvastatin* (Lipitor) or *simvastatin* (Zocor). These medications are very effective at lowering LDL "bad" cholesterol, but they have only a modest effect on HDL.

Niacin works both ways. It increases HDL by 15% to 35%. At the same time, it slightly lowers LDL (by about 10% to 12%) and triglycerides, blood fats that have been loosely linked to heart disease.

Like other B vitamins, niacin (vitamin B-3) is naturally present in foods, such as meats, leafy vegetables, legumes and whole grains. It also is in multivitamins and B-complex supplements.

WHEN TO USE IT

Some patients with low HDL who are at moderate risk for heart disease and who don't need statins to lower LDL may be advised to take niacin to reduce their risk. Men with an HDL level substantially below 40 milligrams per deciliter (mg/dL) and women with an HDL below 45 mg/dL might be candidates for treatment. For both men and women, an HDL of 60 mg/dL or higher is ideal.

Important: Niacin is recommended only when these patients have tried, without success, to significantly increase HDL with lifestyle changes.

Examples: Not smoking, regular exercise and eating a healthful diet. When combined, these factors can increase HDL by 10% to 15%. That's enough for some patients—but not for everyone.

Modest amounts of alcohol—no more than two alcoholic beverages a day for men or one alcoholic beverage for women—also have been shown to cause slight increases in HDL.

People who already are taking a statin to reduce LDL may be advised to take niacin to boost HDL. We usually wait for a few months after starting statin therapy before adding niacin because statins slightly increase HDL, which can affect the niacin dose.

Niacin is sometimes used as an alternative treatment for patients who can't tolerate statins (because of muscle pain, for example). Niacin doesn't reduce LDL anywhere near as much as statins, but it can help patients with slightly high LDL who also have low HDL and high triglycerides.

HOW TO USE IT

The standard dose of nicotinic acid (the form of niacin used to raise HDL) is one gram to three grams daily. Patients usually are advised to start with the lower dose, increasing it as needed to achieve the recommended HDL level.

In these doses, niacin almost always causes side effects. The main one is flushing, in which the skin (often on the face) reddens and feels hot. Flushing can last anywhere from a few minutes to several hours. It usually becomes less bothersome after patients have taken niacin for several weeks or months.

Other side effects may include an upset stomach, headache or, in rare cases, liver damage. Patients who take niacin or other medications for cholesterol usually are advised to get regular blood tests.

Over-the-counter (OTC) niacin supplements may be just as effective as prescription drugs. However, supplements are more loosely regulated than medications—it's difficult to know if the OTC product that you're taking has the amount of niacin listed on the label. But whether you get it OTC or by prescription, don't take high-dose niacin without a doctor's supervision.

TO REDUCE FLUSHING

To alleviate this common side effect, I recommend the following...

•**Use extended-release niacin,** such as prescription Niaspan. This is the only form of niacin I prefer because it causes somewhat less flushing than immediate-release niacin.

Warning: Do not take any product labeled "no flush niacin"—these products do not raise HDL at all.

•**Take it at bedtime.** You still will experience flushing, but you probably will sleep through it.

Also helpful: Don't drink alcohol within an hour of taking niacin. It increases the intensity of flushing.

•**Take one aspirin, wait an hour and then take niacin.** It's an effective way to reduce flushing.

Important: Take 81-mg to 325-mg regular aspirin. Be aware that enteric-coated forms will reduce the antiflushing benefit. Aspirin can cause bleeding and stomach ulcers, so always check with your doctor.

Lightheaded? You Could Be at Risk For Heart Failure

Robert Myerburg, MD, professor, cardiology, University of Miami Miller School of Medicine.
Christine DeLong Jones, MD, preventive medicine resident, University of North Carolina, Chapel Hill.
Stephen Green, MD, chief, cardiology, North Shore University Hospital, Manhasset, New York.
Tara Narula, MD, cardiologist, Lenox Hill Hospital, New York City.
Hypertension

If your blood pressure drops suddenly when you stand up, leaving you feeling lightheaded or woozy, you may be at greater risk for developing heart failure, a recent study suggests.

This condition is known as *orthostatic hypotension*. According to the study, people with orthostatic hypotension were 54% more likely to develop heart failure than their counterparts who did not develop low blood pressure upon standing. This risk was reduced to 34% when the researchers teased out those who also had high blood pressure.

"Multiple risk factors can increase a person's risk for developing heart failure, including high blood pressure, coronary heart disease and diabetes," explained study author Christine DeLong Jones, MD, a preventive medicine resident at the University of North Carolina at Chapel Hill. "Orthostatic hypotension may also increase this risk."

HEART FAILURE AND ORTHOSTATIC HYPOTENSION

Heart failure occurs when the heart can no longer pump strongly enough for blood to reach the rest of the body. About 5.7 million people in the United States have heart failure, and about 300,000 people die from it each year, according to the US National Heart, Lung, and Blood Institute.

Exactly how orthostatic hypotension could lead to heart failure is not fully understood. "We speculate that orthostatic hypotension and high blood pressure may contribute to the risk of heart failure through a similar pathway, such as through high blood pressure that happens primarily when a person is laying down," she added.

To test for orthostatic hypotension, your doctor will measure your blood pressure while lying down and shortly after standing up. Orthostatic hypotension is defined as a drop of 20 mmHg or more in systolic (the top number) blood pressure or a decrease of 10 mmHg or more in diastolic (bottom number) blood pressure upon standing.

Some people with orthostatic hypotension might not have symptoms and may not require treatment. Others may experience dizziness, and others may even pass out, Dr. Jones said. "If one passes out or has severe dizziness, they should see a provider urgently."

People with orthostatic hypotension who also have high blood pressure should take steps to control blood pressure, and make sure their heart is healthy, she said.

STUDY DETAILS

For the study, researchers looked at more than 12,000 people between the ages of 45 and 64 from four US counties. Close to 11% of people who developed heart failure during about 17.5 years of follow-up had orthostatic hypotension at the start of the study, compared with only 4% of those who did not go on to develop heart failure. This link was most pronounced among people ages 45 to 55, according to the findings, published in *Hypertension*.

THEORY

The study authors speculated that orthostatic hypotension might be an indicator of early atherosclerosis—a buildup of plaque in the arteries—brought on by high blood pressure.

However, the study does not show that orthostatic hypotension causes heart failure, merely an association between the two.

EXPERT COMMENTARY

Robert Myerburg, MD, a professor of cardiology at the University of Miami Miller School of Medicine, said it is way too premature to say that orthostatic hypotension is a risk factor for heart failure based on this study.

"Orthostatic hypotension can cause unpleasant symptoms and if they lead to loss of consciousness or near loss of consciousness, it can lead to accidents, but this is not something that will lead to cardiac arrest," he said. His advice is to drink plenty of fluid if you have low blood pressure upon standing. "If it doesn't bother you or cause any significant symptoms, you don't have to treat it," he said.

Stephen Green, MD, chief of cardiology at North Shore University Hospital in Manhasset, New York, agreed. "If you get lightheaded, see your doctor and they should see if you have orthostatic blood pressure, which is a common source of lightheadedness or dizziness when you change positions," he said.

"It doesn't mean you will die of heart failure if you have it, but over time, we can keep an eye on any signs or symptoms for heart failure," Dr. Green added.

Tara Narula, MD, a cardiologist at Lenox Hill Hospital in New York City, said that anything that helps diagnose heart failure earlier could be beneficial. "This is an interesting paper, and if orthostatic hypotension proves to be a cause or leads to heart failure in future studies, we could possible identify heart failure earlier than we can now."

info To learn more about heart failure and how to treat it, visit the National Heart, Lung, and Blood Institute's Web site, *www.nhlbi.nih.gov*, and search "heart failure."

Drug-Free Ways to Fight Killer Blood Clots

Decker Weiss, NMD, naturopathic medical doctor who specializes in integrative cardiology. He is the founder and owner of Weiss Natural Medicine, in Scottsdale, Arizona, *www.weissnaturalmedicine.com*, and author of *The Weiss Method: A Natural Program for Reversing Heart Disease and Preventing Heart Attacks* (Shannake).

Millions of Americans take anticlotting medications, or "blood thinners," including aspirin and *warfarin* (Coumadin), to prevent clots and reduce the risk for such conditions as heart attack and stroke.

These drugs are extremely effective. Daily aspirin, for example, can reduce the risk for a first heart attack by 44%, according to data from the Physicians' Health Study.

The downside: Even at low doses, every anticlotting agent can cause bleeding—often from the stomach, gums or intestines—as a side effect. Sometimes, gastrointestinal bleeding can occur even without causing noticeable symptoms.

In addition, warfarin, one of the leading blood thinners, doubles the risk for *intracerebral hemorrhage* (bleeding in the brain).

NATURAL BLOOD THINNERS

The good news is that certain herbs and other supplements can be used for their anticlotting properties—and may have a reduced risk for side effects, such as bleeding.

This approach is not intended to replace medications—patients with a high risk for clotting need to take such drugs. Under a doctor's supervision, these supplements can be combined with blood-thinning medications to boost the drugs' effectiveness and potentially allow you to take a lower dose, thus reducing the risk for bleeding.

Those with only a slight risk for clots (due to family history, for example) may want to consider using natural anticoagulants alone, under a doctor's supervision, to promote better circulation.

Bonus: Natural blood thinners usually have anti-inflammatory properties. This is important because most chronic diseases, including heart disease, rheumatoid arthritis and stroke, are caused in part by inflammation.

The supplements below can be taken alone or in combination, depending on the degree of protection that's required.

Some of these supplements may interact with prescription medications, so consult a doctor who is knowledgeable about supplement use.* *Best choices…*

•**Fish oil.** Studies of large populations show that people who eat a lot of cold-water fish, such as salmon and mackerel, tend to have lower heart attack death rates than people who don't eat fish.

The omega-3 fatty acids in cold-water fish are strong anticlotting agents. Fish oil is thought to inhibit platelet aggregation (clumping), part of the clotting process. One report, published in *The Annals of Pharmacotherapy,* found that taking fish oil along with warfarin caused an increase in anticlotting activity.

Typical dose: Depending on other risk factors, such as elevated cholesterol and high blood pressure, one tablet twice daily of Vectomega's Whole Food Omega-3 DHA/EPA Complex—it provides 292 mg of omega-3s (DHA and EPA balanced) in a phospholipid peptide complex, in which the fish oil is bound to peptides to increase absorbability. Or one teaspoon twice daily of Nordic Naturals' Ultimate Omega Liquid, which provides 1,626 mg of EPA and 1,126 mg of DHA.

•**Ginger and curcumin.** Ginger reduces levels of fibrinogen, a precursor to fibrin, a protein that is a major component of blood clots. Curcumin has only modest effects on coagulation but is a stronger anti-inflammatory agent. That's why I advise patients to take these herbs together. Studies have shown that both ginger and curcumin can reduce inflammation in the body. An Australian study found that substances

*To find a doctor who has experience treating patients with supplements, consult the American Association of Naturopathic Physicians, 866-538-2267, *www.naturopathic.org.*

in ginger inhibited the activity of arachidonic acid, part of the chemical sequence involved in clotting. In the study, ginger compounds were more effective than aspirin at blocking platelet activity.

Typical dose: Twice daily, 50 mg to 100 mg of ginger and one or two 375-mg capsules of curcumin.

Good products: Gaia Herbs' Ginger Supreme Phyto-Caps and EuroPharma's Cura Med curcumin complex.

•**Nattokinase.** Extracted from soybeans, nattokinase is an enzyme that helps prevent clot formation—it also makes platelets less likely to clump together. Unlike warfarin, which only prevents clots, nattokinase appears to break down clots that already have formed.

Typical dose: Depending on other risk factors, one to two capsules or tablets (2,000 fibrin units per 100 mg) twice daily.

Important: I recommend taking nattokinase between meals. The anticlotting properties are strongest when it is taken without food.

•**Vinpocetine.** This supplement is extracted from periwinkle. It's extremely important to take vinpocetine under a doctor's supervision. Vinpocetine is the most potent natural substance for preventing clots—and, like prescription anticlotting agents, it can cause internal bleeding in some patients. For this reason, I recommend it mainly for high-risk patients who are unable to take warfarin because of side effects and/or complications.

Typical dose: 2 mg total—in divided doses twice daily. Higher doses (5 mg total in divided doses) might be needed, but don't increase from the starting dose without talking with your doctor. Should be taken without food.

•**Ginkgo.** The extract from the dried leaves of the ginkgo biloba tree has traditionally been used to treat intermittent claudication, leg pain caused by insufficient blood flow, as well as cognitive impairments (such as memory problems) due to poor blood circulation in the brain.

Ginkgo is effective at reducing clots and also acts as a vasodilator that helps improve blood flow to the brain, heart and other parts of the body. I don't recommend it as often as other anticoagulants because it has little effect on inflammation. If you use ginkgo, ask your doctor about combining it with curcumin or other anti-inflammatory herbs/supplements.

Typical dose: About 40 mg, three times daily.

•**Garlic.** Studies have shown that patients who take garlic supplements have a lower risk for clots. Use only those products that list a high allicin content—the main active ingredient in garlic. This can be found frequently in fresh garlic supplements.

Typical dose: The optimal dose for garlic hasn't been definitively established. However, some studies indicate that you need at least 180 mg of allicin twice daily.

Good brand: Allimax.

Important: In general, natural therapies should be started at low doses that are slowly increased, under a doctor's supervision, over time. I recommend that the supplements described in this article be used at least twice daily to ensure that adequate levels of the therapeutic compounds are maintained in the body.

■ ■ ■ ■

Tall People at Higher Risk for Blood Clots

In taller people, blood must be pumped a longer distance, so there may be reduced blood flow in the legs—raising clot risk. Clot risk is greatest in men who are tall and heavy. Obese men who are five feet, 11 inches tall have five times the risk of normal-weight men who are about five feet, seven inches tall or less. In obese, tall women—more than five feet, six inches—the risk is 2.9 times greater than in normal-weight women, who are five feet, 2.6 inches tall or less.

Sigrid Braekkan, PhD, researcher, Hematological Research Group, University of Tromsø, Norway, and investigator of a study of 26,714 Norwegian people, published by the American Heart Association in *Arteriosclerosis, Thrombosis and Vascular Biology.*

■ ■ ■ ■

White-Fleshed Fruits Fight Strokes

White-fleshed fruits and vegetables may protect against stroke.

Recent finding: The more apples, bananas, cauliflower, cucumbers, pears and other white-fleshed produce people ate, the more their stroke risk was reduced—by up to 52%. Other fruits and vegetables did not affect stroke risk, but they have health benefits as well.

Linda Oude Griep, MSc, postdoctoral fellow in human nutrition at Wageningen University, the Netherlands, and lead author of a study of 20,069 people, published in *Stroke.*

■ ■ ■ ■

High Radiation Risk

Post–heart attack cardiac imaging can pose high radiation risk. Cancer risk rises with cumulative exposure to radiation from catheterization, angioplasty and nuclear scans—and some of these tests may not be necessary.

Self-defense: Ask your doctor which tests you really need.

Louise Pilote, MD, PhD, MPH, professor of medicine—James McGill Chair and director, division of general internal medicine, McGill University, Montreal. She led an analysis of data on 82,861 people, published in *Canadian Medical Association Journal.*

New Ways to Prevent a "Brain Attack"

Bruce Ovbiagele, MD, professor of neurosciences at the University of California, San Diego. He is the lead author of a recent study on the role that systolic blood pressure plays in stroke prevention, published in *The Journal of the American Medical Association.*

For many people, stroke—a major cause of disability and the third-leading cause of death in the US (behind heart disease and cancer)—is one of the most feared medical emergencies.

Now: There's reason to be optimistic as recent research zeros in on the best ways to prevent and treat stroke. *Important findings you should know about...*

DON'T IGNORE ATRIAL FIBRILLATION

Nearly three million Americans have atrial fibrillation (AF)—a common type of irregular heartbeat that increases stroke risk substantially by promoting the formation of tiny clots that can travel through the body and lodge in blood vessels of the brain. This risk can be reduced with medication, such as blood thinners, to prevent blood clots.

Recent scientific finding: Research conducted by the American Heart Association found that half of people with AF are unaware of their increased risk for stroke. What's more, a significant number of people with AF don't even know that they have the condition, perhaps because AF doesn't always cause noticeable symptoms.

What you can do: During your next checkup, ask your doctor whether you should be tested for AF. The condition is diagnosed with tests that include an electrocardiogram. If you experience any AF symptoms, such as heart palpitations, chest pain, dizziness, shortness of breath or lack of energy, see your doctor as soon as possible—or call 911 if symptoms are severe.

BLOOD PRESSURE—DANGER BEGINS BEFORE IT'S "HIGH"

High blood pressure (hypertension)—defined as 140/90 mmHg or above—is the leading risk factor for stroke. But growing evidence suggests that even at "prehypertensive" levels, stroke risk increases more than previously believed.

Recent scientific finding: A 2011 analysis of data on more than 500,000 people found that those with prehypertension—blood pressure that is above the "normal" reading of 120/80 but still below the "high" threshold of 140/90— were 55% more likely to suffer strokes in the next five to 10 years than those with normal blood pressure. The increased risk was particularly striking when blood pressure was at or above 130/85 and among people under age 65 when the study began.

What you can do: If you have prehypertension, talk to your doctor about healthy lifestyle changes—for example, lose weight if you're overweight...cut back on salt and saturated fats...quit smoking...and exercise for at least 30 minutes daily.

Important: Your ideal blood pressure may vary based on your specific medical profile, so be sure to ask your doctor for advice on your target blood pressure.

SMALL STROKES ARE A BIG DEAL

A transient ischemic attack (TIA), or "ministroke," causes stroke symptoms (such as sudden numbness on one side of the body, dizziness, severe headache or difficulty speaking) that go away within minutes or hours, causing no lasting damage. TIAs are known to greatly increase risk for a full-blown stroke in the months to come, but recent research shows that the danger from a TIA is greater than once thought.

Recent scientific finding: A study conducted by Australian researchers found that people who had a TIA were 13% more likely to die in the next five years than others of the same age and 20% more likely to die in the next 10 years.

Research presented at the 2011 Canadian Stroke Congress shows that even in the short run, TIAs are more serious than they appear— nearly one-fourth of 200 people studied were clinically depressed six weeks after a TIA, and vision and thinking problems were common.

What you can do: Seek emergency care even if your stroke symptoms subside within a few minutes. The average duration of a TIA is about one minute. If you suffer a TIA, medication, such as blood thinners, can be prescribed to reduce your risk for a full-blown stroke.

CARDIAC REHAB WORKS FOR STROKE, TOO

Cardiac rehabilitation—which typically includes exercise, nutrition education, smoking cessation and counseling for stress, anxiety and depression—has long been recommended after a heart attack. Now research shows that such a rehab program could be useful for people who have suffered a ministroke.

Recent scientific evidence: A hundred people who had suffered TIAs during the previous year were enrolled in a traditional cardiac rehabilitation program. Seven months later, the participants had significantly reduced their risk for stroke—for example, average total cholesterol decreased by almost 12 mg/dL…and average waist circumference was cut by one inch.

What you can do: If you suffer a TIA, talk to your doctor about enrolling in a cardiac rehab program. To find such a program near you, visit the American Association of Cardiovascular and Pulmonary Rehabilitation Web site, *www.aacvpr.org.* Under "Resources," click on "Resources for Patients," then "Cardiovascular Rehab Patient Resources," then "AACVPR Program Directory."

DEPRESSION—TREATMENT IS CRUCIAL

Depression has long been linked to increased heart attack risk, but its relation to stroke has been unclear.

Recent scientific finding: In an analysis of more than 300,000 adults published in *The Journal of the American Medical Association,* researchers found that those who were depressed when first tested were 45% more likely than others to have a stroke at follow-up periods of two to 29 years.

It's unclear whether depression actually leads to stroke—for example, through chemical changes that promote blood clots or by making people less likely to exercise, quit smoking or take needed medication. Nor do researchers know whether relieving depression will reduce stroke risk.

What you can do: Now that the association between depression and stroke has been discovered, it's another compelling reason to seek treatment if you believe that you may suffer from depression.

EAT WHITE FRUITS AND VEGGIES

As part of a healthy diet, fruits and vegetables reduce the likelihood of stroke, according to several large studies. Now, recent research suggests that certain kinds of produce may be better than others.

Recent scientific finding: In a study published in the journal *Stroke,* researchers asked more than 20,000 men and women about their consumption of various fruits and vegetables that were categorized based on the color of the edible portion.

Result: The more white-colored fruits and vegetables people ate, the less likely they were to have strokes in the next 10 years.

What you can do: More research will be conducted to confirm these findings. Meanwhile, it makes sense to go ahead and include plenty of apples, pears, bananas, cauliflower, cucumbers and other white-fleshed fruits and vegetables in your diet.

FACTS ABOUT STROKE

A stroke occurs when blood flow to the brain is interrupted by a blocked artery (ischemic stroke)…or bleeding (hemorrhagic stroke). Ischemic stroke accounts for about 90% of strokes.

Stroke symptoms occur suddenly and may include: Numbness or weakness of the face, arm or leg (especially on one side of the body)…confusion, trouble speaking or understanding…difficulty seeing in one or both eyes…trouble walking, dizziness, loss of balance or coordination…and/or severe headache with no known cause.

When Drugs Are Better Than Surgery For Stroke Patients

William J. Powers, MD, H. Houston Merritt Distinguished Professor and Chairman of Adult Neurology, University of North Carolina School of Medicine, Chapel Hill.

Joseph P. Broderick, MD, Chair of Neurology, University of Cincinnati College of Medicine.

Ralph Sacco, MD, Chairman of Neurology, University of Miami Miller School of Medicine.

Journal of the American Medical Association

To prevent stroke in certain high-risk patients—those with a blocked neck (carotid) artery who have already had a so-called "mini-stroke"—drug treatment appears as effective and far less risky than bypass surgery, researchers find.

Their study evaluated nearly 200 patients, about half of whom had carotid artery bypass surgery. In the 30 days after surgery, patients had a 14% risk of having a stroke, compared with a 2% risk among those treated medically, the study found.

The study was published in the *Journal of the American Medical Association*.

ABOUT CAROTID ARTERY BYPASS SURGERY

The surgical procedure is called *extracranial-intracranial* arterial bypass surgery. It involves drilling a hole in the head and attaching a blood vessel from the scalp to one of the blood vessels of the brain, bypassing the blockage in the neck, explained lead researcher William J. Powers, MD, chairman of adult neurology at the University of North Carolina School of Medicine, at Chapel Hill.

STUDY DETAILS

In the trial, called the Carotid Occlusion Surgery Study, Dr. Powers' team randomly assigned 195 patients to carotid bypass surgery or medical management. The patients were at a high risk of having a stroke, with a 23% risk of having one within two years, according to Dr. Powers.

Based on early findings, the trial was stopped. Over a two-year period, the researchers found that 21% of the patients who had surgery died or had a stroke, compared with 22.7% of those on medical therapy alone—which is not a significant difference, Dr. Powers said.

Moreover, at 30 days after surgery, 14.4% of the surgical patients had a stroke, compared with 2% of those on medical therapy. That's a 12.4% difference, the study group noted.

IMPLICATION

"We were trying to figure out a way of taking people who were at high risk of having stroke and prevent that from happening," said Dr. Powers. "The unfortunate part is that we didn't do that," he added. "If you made it through the surgery, your risk of having a stroke was 6%, but, unfortunately, the risk of having a stroke from surgery was 15%," he said. "This procedure should not be used for this purpose."

Dr. Powers added that despite this failure, they are still looking for a safer way to get blood to the brain in patients who have a completely blocked carotid artery, the large blood vessel in the neck. "We are hoping to take what we learned and take the same type of patients and try a catheter stent-based approach," he said.

EXPERT COMMENTARY

Commenting on the study, Ralph Sacco, MD, chairman of neurology at the University of Miami Miller School of Medicine and past president of the American Heart Association, said "medical therapy with anti-clotting drugs, blood pressure and cholesterol-lowering drugs has improved over the years, which makes it more effective.

"Current guidelines would say there is no indication for pursuing a bypass in these patients," Dr. Sacco added. "The Heart Association says the procedures should be done with less than a 6% perioperative risk in symptomatic patients and 3% in asymptomatic patients." Perioperative refers to the period of hospitalization for surgery.

Looking at a larger picture, Joseph P. Broderick, MD, chair of neurology at the University of Cincinnati College of Medicine and coauthor of an accompanying journal editorial, said the effectiveness of any new therapy needs to be demonstrated before it can be used.

"Potential new therapies, particularly surgical procedures that use devices to reopen blocked arteries, need to be tested against the standard proven approach of intravenous tPA [a drug that breaks up clots and is standard therapy for stroke]," he said.

Yet, these devices are already being used in clinical practice since they have been cleared by the Food and Drug Administration (FDA) for use and are currently reimbursed by Medicare for acute stroke treatment despite a lack of evidence that they improve outcomes as compared to standard therapy, Dr. Broderick said.

This happens because the rules for FDA approval and Medicare reimbursement of devices are different from the rules for approving drugs, he said. This makes it harder to get people to take part in clinical trials of devices, because they are in use before they are clinically proven to work, he added.

info For more information on stroke, visit the Web site of the American Stroke Association, *www.strokeassociation.org*.

Stroke Patients Undergo Unnecessary Tests

University of Michigan, news release

Most stroke patients undergo both CT and MRI brain scans, an unnecessary duplication that contributes to the rising costs of stroke care in the United States, a recent study indicates.

MRI BEST TEST FOR STROKE

University of Michigan researchers analyzed data from more than 600,000 patients diagnosed with stroke between 1999 and 2008 in 11 states, and found that 95% of the patients who had MRI scans also had CT brain scans.

"Compared with CT, MRI is a more accurate test for stroke. But our results showed that MRI is not replacing CT as the primary stroke neuroimaging study—instead, patients are getting both," said study author James Burke, MD, a clinical lecturer in the medical school's neurology department.

"Minimizing the use of multiple studies could be a viable strategy to reduce costs," he added.

The researchers noted that the costs of inpatient stroke care rose 42% between 1997 and 2007, an increase of $3,800 per stroke case. Brain scans were the largest contributor to the increased costs, they found.

"The data shows that neuroimaging practices in stroke are neither standardized [nor] efficient," Dr. Burke said. "This represents an area where we have an opportunity to substantially reduce the cost of care without adversely affecting the quality of care."

The study was published in the *Annals of Neurology*.

The US National Institute of Neurological Disorders and Stroke has more about stroke at *www.ninds.nih.gov/disorders/stroke/stroke_needto know.htm*.

Better Treatment for Weekend Strokes

When researchers examined data on 134,000 hospitalizations over 12 years for stroke, patients treated at hospitals on weekends were 5% more likely to die over the next 90 days than those admitted during the week. However, this "weekend effect" was not present for patients admitted to comprehensive stroke centers, which have 24/7 availability of acute stroke teams.

Self-defense: Contact your state's department of health to learn the location of the nearest comprehensive stroke center (known as "primary stroke centers" in most states) or go to *www.stroke.org* and click on "Emergency Stroke Center Locations."

James McKinney, MD, assistant professor of neurology, Robert Wood Johnson Medical School, University of Medicine and Dentistry of New Jersey, New Brunswick.

Citrus Fruits May Cut Women's Stroke Risk

Researchers studied the health records of 69,622 women, who reported their food intake every four years for 14 years.

Result: Women whose diets contained high levels of flavanones (found in oranges, grapefruit and other citrus fruit) had a 19% lower risk for ischemic stroke (caused by a blood clot) than those who ate the least amount of flavanones.

Theory: Flavanones are thought to improve blood vessel function and have anti-inflammatory qualities.

Caution: Because grapefruit can interact with some medications, speak to your doctor before increasing your intake.

Aedin Cassidy, PhD, professor of diet and health, Norwich Medical School, University of East Anglia, Norwich, United Kingdom.

Longevity, Brain Health & Optimum Aging

How to "Reset" Your Genes to Live Longer

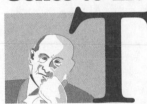

The life span of the average American has increased by more than 60% in the last 100 years, and some experts believe that's just the beginning. It might be possible for people living today to extend their lives to 120 years or even more. How is this possible?

Two landmark discoveries: Genetic researchers have identified structures, known as telomeres, that appear to control how long cells live and how healthy they remain. Along with that, researchers have identified an enzyme, called telomerase, that maintains the integrity of these structures. These two discoveries could be the key to a much longer life.

What you need to know...

WHAT ARE TELOMERES?

Telomeres are structures on the ends of chromosomes that help keep these strands of gene-carrying DNA intact. Chromosomes, which are found in the nucleus of every human cell, control the cellular division and replication that are necessary for human life. As people age, telomeres shorten—a process that is believed to play a fundamental role in the development of genetic diseases and age-related conditions, including heart disease, cancer and Alzheimer's disease.

TELOMERES AND LONGEVITY

Every cell in the human body contains 46 strands of DNA. These strands (chromosomes) contain all of our genetic information—for example, the color of our hair and how tall we are as well as our propensity for certain diseases.

As a person ages and undergoes decades of cell divisions, there's a shortening of the telomeres that help keep chromosomes intact. With

Michael Fossel, MD, PhD, and David Woynarowski, MD, coauthors of *The Immortality Edge: Realize the Secrets of Your Telomeres for a Longer, Healthier Life* (Wiley). Dr. Fossel, retired clinical professor of medicine, founding editor of the *Journal of Anti-Aging Medicine* and author of a textbook on telomeres and aging. Dr. Woynarowski, board certified in internal medicine and antiaging medicine, is in private practice in Reading, Pennsylvania.

time, the telomeres get so short that cells can no longer survive—and, eventually, we die.

Research shows that the length of a person's telomeres is crucial. For example, people who are born with (or develop) relatively short telomeres tend to have more health problems, and die sooner, than those with longer telomeres. In a study of 780 patients with heart disease, researchers found that those with the shortest telomeres had twice the risk for heart failure and death after 4.4 years as those with the longest telomeres. Shortened telomeres have also been linked to cancer, osteoarthritis and Alzheimer's.

AN ANTIAGING PLAN

When cells are damaged—due, for example, to free radicals, inflammation and excessive alcohol intake—they divide more frequently than aging healthy cells. This rapid division accelerates the rate at which telomeres shorten—and, potentially, shortens your life.

This is where telomerase, the enzyme that repairs and maintains the length of telomeres, comes into play. And the discovery of telomerase was so important scientifically that it was the basis for Carol Greider, PhD, of Johns Hopkins University School of Medicine, to be awarded the 2009 Nobel Prize in Physiology or Medicine, along with two other researchers.

Although telomerase won't keep cells alive forever, it does seem to greatly extend their lives. For example, in a laboratory study, scientists inserted a telomerase-producing gene into skin cells with short telomeres. These cells were then grafted onto the skin of mice, while untreated skin cells were grafted onto different mice.

Result: The skin grown from telomerase-containing cells looked young…skin grown from cells without telomerase was wrinkled and looked old.

Fortunately, a growing body of evidence suggests that you may be able to slow the rate at which your telomeres shorten—and, in some cases, slightly increase their length—by minimizing cell damage with certain nutrients.*

•**Fish oil.** A study in *The Journal of the American Medical Association* that followed 608 heart patients for five years found that those

*Consult your doctor before starting the following regimen. Some of these supplements may interact with blood-thinning, diabetes or other medications.

who consumed the most fish oil had the longest telomeres. This may be the reason that people who routinely take fish oil supplements have lower rates of heart disease, arthritis and other chronic diseases.

What's behind fish oil's health-promoting effects? As an adaptogen, fish oil is a substance that helps maintain the body's normal functions. It has different effects in different parts of the body and on different cells. For example, fish oil inhibits telomerase in cancer cells (which shortens the life span of the disease-causing cells) but increases it in healthy cells (which helps them live longer).

Antiaging dose: 1,500 mg of omega-3 twice daily with meals. Within this total, aim for 900 mg of *eicosapentaenoic acid* (EPA) and 600 mg of *docosahexaenoic acid* (DHA).

•**Acetyl-L-carnitine (ALCAR).** This supplement reduces free-radical damage to cells. It also repairs *mitochondria*, the structures within cells that produce energy. This is important because damaged mitochondria produce large amounts of free radicals, which accelerate cell turnover and damage to telomeres.

Every cell in the body has mitochondria, but cells that require the most energy to function, such as those in the brain, have the most—about 1,000 mitochondria per cell. ALCAR supplements may reduce mental declines from aging and from Alzheimer's disease or chronic cerebral ischemia, a condition that reduces blood flow to the brain.

Antiaging dose: 1,000 mg twice daily.

•**Anthocyanidins.** A type of flavonoid derived from berries, such as blueberries and bilberries, anthocyanidins have a higher antioxidant capacity than either vitamin E or vitamin C. Reducing oxidation is among the most effective ways to reduce cell damage and telomere shortening.

Antiaging dose: 80 mg of bilberry extract twice daily.

•**N-acetylcysteine (NAC).** This amino acid is metabolized in the body into a substance that's used to manufacture the "master" antioxidant, glutathione. Glutathione improves the body's ability to remove damaged/dying cells. When this process is working well, there's a slower shortening of the telomeres.

Antiaging dose: 600 mg twice daily.

•**Vitamin D.** It's among the most important nutrients for health and longevity. Some researchers speculate that it increases levels of telomerase—and it clearly reduces telomere shortening.

British researchers who studied more than 1,000 sets of female twins (whose average age was 49 and whose telomeres had been the same lengths at birth) found that those with higher levels of vitamin D had longer telomeres. The difference was dramatic—the telomeres in women in the higher vitamin D group showed the equivalent, in length, of five years less aging.

Antiaging dose: 2,000 international units (IU) to 5,000 IU daily, depending on your starting blood level. A blood test for vitamin D is recommended before taking these supplements. Work with your doctor to determine the optimal vitamin D level for you.

SHOULD YOU GET TESTED?

Your doctor can order a blood test, called polymerase chain reaction (PCR), that will determine the length of your telomeres and compare it to what's normal for your age. The test can be used to track, over time, how much your telomeres are shortening.

Typical cost: About $350. Insurance will not cover the cost.

However, telomere testing is not routinely used because there's not a lot you can do with the information beyond improving your lifestyle, which you should do anyway. In the future, as more products and medications are developed that can significantly lengthen telomeres, the test could be used to determine whether the dose/medication that you're using is right for you.

Why Some People Live to 110

Boston University Medical Center, news release

People who live 110 years or longer have as many disease-associated genes as those in the general population, but they may also be blessed with protective genes that help them live so long, researchers report.

A team of US scientists noted that supercentenarians, as they are called, are extremely rare, with only one per five million people in developed nations. There is growing evidence that genetics play a major role in living to such an old age.

STUDY RESULTS

In what they describe as a first-of-a-kind study, the researchers analyzed the whole genome sequences of a male study participant and a female participant who both lived past the age of 114 and found that they had as many disease-associated genes as other people.

For example, the man had 37 genetic mutations associated with increased risk for colon cancer.

"In fact, he had an obstructing colon cancer earlier in his life that had not metastasized and was cured with surgery. He was in phenomenal cognitive and physical shape near the time of his death," said study senior author Thomas Perls, MD, director of the New England Centenarian Study.

The woman had numerous genetic variations associated with age-related disease, such as heart disease, cancer and Alzheimer's disease. She did develop congestive heart failure and mild cognitive impairment, but these conditions didn't become evident until she was more than 108 years old.

The study was published in the journal *Frontiers in Genetics* and researchers will be able to access the information at the US National Institutes of Health data repository.

VARIANTS CANCEL OUT DISEASE GENES

"The presence of these disease-associated variants is consistent with our and other researchers' findings that centenarians carry as many disease-associated genes as the general population," Dr. Perls said.

"The difference may be that the centenarians likely have longevity-associated variants that cancel out the disease genes. That effect may extend to the point that the diseases don't occur—or, if they do, are much less pathogenic or markedly delayed toward the end of life, in these individuals who are practically living to the limit of the human life span."

ⓘ **info** To learn more about good health habits at age 60 and older, visit the Web site of The American Academy of Family Physicians at *http://familydoctor.org/familydoctor/en/seniors/staying-healthy/good-health-habits-at-age-60-and-beyond.html*.

Intelligence Is Genetic... But You Can Control Memory Loss

Ian Deary, PhD, professor, differential psychology and director, University of Edinburgh Centre for Cognitive Ageing and Cognitive Epidemiology, Scotland.

US National Human Genome Research Institute.

S. Duke Han, PhD, assistant professor, department of behavioral sciences and clinical neuropsychologist, Rush University Medical Center, Chicago.

Nature, online

Some 65-year-olds aren't as "with it" as they once were, and some 90-year-olds are still sharp as a whip.

What accounts for the differences? Using a genetic analysis and intelligence tests given to a group of people in childhood and old age, researchers from Scotland concluded that both genes and environmental factors play a role in whether you'll maintain your level of intelligence throughout your lifespan.

Maintaining brain health into old age is key to aging well, including the ability to do everyday tasks and stay independent, according to background information in the report. Plenty of prior research has found that how smart you are in adolescence generally carries over into adulthood and old age.

"We estimated that about a quarter of the lifetime changes in intelligence test scores might be due to genetic factors," said lead study author Ian Deary, PhD, a professor of differential psychology and director of the University of Edinburgh Centre for Cognitive Ageing and Cognitive Epidemiology, in Scotland. In other words, around three quarters of mental decline may be linked to factors you can change, such

as how much you exercise, the quality of your diet, and how much you stimulate your brain with a variety of activities.

And yet, "some people's intelligence ages better than others," Dr. Deary and colleagues noted.

STUDY DETAILS

In the study, investigators used genome-wide association data on 1,940 unrelated people in Scotland, along with information from intelligence tests participants took when they were about age 11, and then again between 54 and 68 years later, when they were 65, 70 or 79.

Genome-wide association research "involves rapidly scanning markers across the complete sets of DNA, or genomes, of many people to find genetic variations," the US National Human Genome Research Institute explains.

Dr. Deary's team looked specifically for differences in bits of DNA called SNPs (single nucleotide polymorphisms) associated with people whose intelligence either declined or stayed stable.

"We were able to make estimates of the genetic contribution to intelligence differences in childhood and old age, and the change between these times, in the same people," Dr. Deary said. "What was novel about these estimates was that they were made from actual testing of DNA, not from twin or adoption studies."

The study appears in the online edition of *Nature.*

EXPERT PERSPECTIVE

S. Duke Han, PhD, an assistant professor in the department of behavioral sciences and a clinical neuropsychologist at Rush University Medical Center, in Chicago, said the study is unique in that it was able to measure intelligence in the same group of people over such a long period of time.

"What this is saying is something many researchers have accepted for a long time, that intelligence seems to be very much influenced by genetic makeup but also environmental factors, such as education," Dr. Han said.

In analyzing the data, the researchers were able to make broad inferences about how much genetics played a role in maintaining intelligence over the life span, but they weren't able to identify specific genes or gene variants that might contribute.

In general, there's a "paucity of data about genetic influences on lifetime cognitive change," with a few exceptions, the study authors noted. The APOE4 mutation, for example, is a risk factor for severe cognitive decline associated with Alzheimer's disease.

info For more information on aging, visit the US National Institute on Aging Web site at *http://www.nia.nih.gov/*.

■ ■ ■ ■

Walk to Prevent Alzheimer's

Walking just six miles weekly may prevent Alzheimer's.

Recent finding: In a study of 426 adults with or without cognitive decline, those who walked at least six miles weekly were half as likely to develop Alzheimer's disease over 13 years as nonwalkers. Among those with cognitive impairment, walking five miles a week reduced cognitive decline by more than half.

Theory: Exercise improves blood flow to the brain, which helps keep neurons healthy.

To help preserve brain health: Aim to walk at least three-quarters of a mile daily.

Cyrus Raji, MD, PhD, physician-scientist, department of radiology, University of Pittsburgh.

■ ■ ■ ■

Dietary Choline and Sharper Memory

Researchers examined dietary and memory-test data on nearly 1,400 adults (average age 61) over a three- to 10-year period.

Result: People whose diets contained the highest levels of the nutrient choline performed better on memory tests than those who consumed the least amount.

Theory: Choline is a precursor to a brain chemical called *acetylcholine*, which plays a key role in cognition.

Good sources of choline: Eggs, poultry, saltwater fish, liver and kidney beans.

Rhoda Au, PhD, associate professor of neurology, Boston University School of Medicine.

Retrain Your Brain

Rebecca Gladding, MD, staff psychiatrist with the Veterans Administration California Healthcare System. She is coauthor of *You Are Not Your Brain: The 4-Step Solution for Changing Bad Habits, Ending Unhealthy Thinking, and Taking Control of Your Life* (Avery).

Habits are hard to break because of the way the brain is wired. Each time you repeat a harmful behavior—overeating, overspending, procrastinating or something else—the brain circuits involved in that action become stronger. The brain associates the action with the situation that gave rise to it, such as being under stress. Over time, the brain becomes hardwired to choose that behavior automatically any time a similar situation arises.

That's the bad news. The good news: You can rewire your brain to choose constructive habits...

STEP 1: RELABEL

Negative habits are triggered by deceptive brain messages—thoughts, beliefs and impulses that run counter to your positive, healthy intentions. These thoughts and urges are accompanied by unpleasant emotions or physical sensations such as anger, sadness, anxiety or fatigue. Because the discomfort is so intense, you are driven to get rid of it as fast as you can, usually by indulging in an unhealthy habit.

Relabeling means recognizing your impulses and negative thoughts as deceptive brain messages and calling them what they are, such as, *My boss just yelled at me, and because of that, now I need some chocolate.* The more you are aware of these habits, the more opportunities you have to stop acting on them.

Becoming aware of these messages can be challenging at first. *To develop your ability to relabel...*

•**Practice making mental notes.** Any time you feel "off" or uneasy in some way, notice what is going on in your body or mind, and pick a simple word or phrase to describe it. For example, if you notice that you are thinking about a conversation with a friend that went awry—when you really need to be working— say to yourself, *Mind wandering*. The key is to snap yourself back into awareness—which is the first step toward doing something about the situation in a healthy, productive way.

•**Focus on your breathing.** One way to enhance your ability to notice what's happening in a moment-to-moment way is by focusing on your breath. For five minutes, sit in a quiet place, close your eyes and simply pay attention to your breath as you inhale and exhale. Whenever you realize that you have become lost in thought, say to yourself, *Thinking* or *Planning* or *Wandering*, then gently turn your focus back to your breathing.

Do this focused breathing exercise once a day, and gradually extend the length of time to 20 or 30 minutes.

STEP 2: REFRAME

As you become aware of deceptive brain messages, you can begin changing your perception of their importance. You do this by reframing—challenging your default response.

Reframing does not mean denying the existence of a thought or judging yourself for having it. Instead, you look at the thought from a new perspective and diminish its importance.

Example: I feel upset right now, but that doesn't mean I have to have a cigarette (or that I am a bad person because I am craving one).

To change your perspective…

•**Use distancing phrases.** When you notice a deceptive brain message, say to yourself, *That's not me, it's just my brain*…or *Oh, that's just mental chatter.*

•**Look for thinking errors.** We often make inaccurate assumptions about difficult situations and painful feelings. To uncover these erroneous, unhelpful thoughts, ask yourself nonjudgmental questions, such as, *What is it about this situation that is upsetting me? What am I telling myself about what is happening? What are some other interpretations?*

Common thinking errors include…

All-or-nothing thinking: Seeing situations and people in extremes, such as perfect or hopeless, all good or all bad.

Worst-case thinking: Assuming that something terrible inevitably is going to happen.

Discounting the positive: Ignoring your good qualities and failing to take seriously other people's positive reactions toward you.

•**Be compassionate with yourself.** Write down the deceptive brain message that is bothering you. Then ask yourself what a kindhearted friend would advise or think.

•**Use the 15-minute rule.** When you experience an especially powerful impulse, try to wait 15 minutes before you act. Then if you still cannot resist the urge, slowly and mindfully engage in the activity that your deceptive brain message is insisting upon.

Important: Do not try to talk yourself out of an uncomfortable feeling. Simply examine it. You are training yourself to be less frightened of discomfort, to learn that it will pass and that it is not such a big deal.

STEP 3: REFOCUS

Once you have relabeled and reframed a deceptive brain message, you may find it surprisingly easy to actively shift your attention to a healthy, constructive activity—even as your deceptive thoughts are urging you to act in your old, habitual way. By refocusing repeatedly, you weaken the brain circuits associated with your cravings and retrain your brain to choose healthier responses.

The best refocusing activities are ones that engage and interest you. If they require strategy or learning something new, they will be even more effective, but any wholesome activity that you enjoy is fine.

Examples: Do a crossword puzzle, read, exercise, call a friend, play with a pet…

If you are at work, refocus on a task that you can accomplish quickly or easily.

STEP 4: REVALUE

The final step is really about gaining perspective and the strength to believe in yourself. Each person gets there at his/her own pace, and when you do, you can look at the deceptive brain message and unhelpful impulses and simply say to yourself, *This is nothing more than the feeling of a deceptive brain message. I do not have to act on it, and it does not define me.* The more you are able to relabel, reframe and refocus, the more empowered you will be to dismiss those deceptive brain messages and move on with your life in a positive direction—one that you define. That's the essence of revalue and the goal of the four steps.

How Nicotine Patches May Help Get Your Memory Back

Paul Newhouse, MD, director, Vanderbilt Center for Cognitive Medicine, Vanderbilt University School of Medicine, Nashville.

Jennifer Rusted, PhD, professor, experimental psychology, Sussex University, Brighton, UK.

Recent research suggests that the nicotine patches used by people trying to quit smoking could serve an unexpected purpose. They appear to counteract mild memory loss in older patients.

The research is preliminary and only involved a few dozen subjects.

There's also the matter of expense: While they're available over the counter, patches can cost several dollars a day.

Still, "nicotine treatment may be a way to improve people's symptoms and maybe extend their ability to do all of those cognitive things we need to do," said study author Paul Newhouse, MD, director of the Center for Cognitive Medicine at Vanderbilt University School of Medicine. "We're hoping to pursue this with a much larger group."

This isn't the first time researchers have tried to analyze connections between the brain and nicotine. In the 1980s, Dr. Newhouse and others discovered through autopsies that the brains of patients with Alzheimer's disease lacked certain "receptors" that help the brain's chemicals work properly, he said. Nicotine appears to stimulate these receptors, which revs up the system involved in attention, learning and memory skills.

However, it appears that nicotine isn't a huge help if someone already has a well-functioning ability to pay attention, he said.

STUDY DETAILS AND RESULTS

In the study, researchers recruited 74 non-smoking seniors with mild cognitive problems and watched what happened to 34 who received treatment with nicotine patches (15 milligrams a day) and 33 who got placebo patches for six months. Another seven didn't finish the study.

The people in the study weren't in bad enough shape to be diagnosed with Alzheimer's disease. However, they did have moments of memory loss that the people around them noticed, Dr. Newhouse said.

"They might repeat themselves, tell the same thing several times over or not remember something they've been told," he explained, "or make a mistake in calculations for their checkbook." Their losses in cognitive function were beyond those of normal aging, he added.

After testing cognition and memory at the start of the study and again at three and six months, the researchers found that those who used the real patches did better in terms of attention and memory, although the differences weren't huge and their doctors didn't notice them. The nicotine patch group regained 46% of their long-term memory loss, while the placebo patch group saw a 26% further decline in memory. Also, "people subjectively thought they were doing better," Dr. Newhouse said.

The only consistent side effect was weight loss, he said, and it's not clear if that stabilizes over time.

The participants who got the real patches didn't suffer withdrawal symptoms when they went off them, Dr. Newhouse said. "There's no worries about becoming dependent on it or wanting to take nicotine even though you shouldn't take it."

The patches seem to boost memory by affecting the brain's chemicals and allowing a person to pay attention more easily, he said. "Attention is necessary for memory to work."

However, Dr. Newhouse said he can't recommend the nicotine treatment for memory loss at this time. "If you want to think about it, discuss it with your physician," he said.

The study appeared in the journal *Neurology*. The researchers received federal funding for the research and the pharmaceutical company Pfizer contributed the nicotine patches.

EXPERT RESPONSE

Jennifer Rusted, PHD, a professor of experimental psychology at Sussex University in England, said the study was well done but it doesn't address the effectiveness of using nicotine patches in the long term. Also, Dr. Rusted said, there's debate about who should qualify as having mild cognitive problems in studies like this one.

As for the idea of taking nicotine patches to keep sharp mentally, she said that "realistically, the benefits even in this careful test were so small as to be indiscernible in the general scheme of daily activities. More important, there are many, many other ways of achieving much bigger improvements—exercise, diet, social and cognitive engagement and interaction."

info For more about cognitive impairment, visit the Web site of the US National Library of Medicine at *http://www.nlm.nih.gov/med lineplus/mildcognitiveimpairment.html*.

Forgetful at 45? Here's Why

Archana Singh-Manoux, PhD, research director, INSERM, Center for Research in Epidemiology and Population Health, Paul-Brousse Hospital, Paris.

Francine Grodstein, ScD, associate professor, medicine, Brigham and Women's Hospital, Boston.

Heather M. Snyder, PhD, senior associate director, medical and scientific relations, Alzheimer's Association, Chicago.

BMJ (British Medical Journal)

Sorry, Boomers, but a recent study suggests that memory, reasoning and comprehension can start to slip as early as age 45.

This finding runs counter to conventional wisdom that mental decline doesn't begin before 60, according to researchers.

"Cognitive function in normal, healthy adults begins to decline earlier than previously thought," said study author Archana Singh-Manoux, PhD, research director at INSERM's Center for Research in Epidemiology and Population Health at the Paul-Brousse Hospital in Paris. "It is widely believed that cognitive ability does not decline before the age of 60. We were able to show significant cognitive decline even in individuals aged 45 to 49 years."

These findings should be put in context of the link between cognitive function and the dementia, Dr. Singh-Manoux said.

"Previous research shows small differences in cognitive performance in earlier life predict larger differences in risk of dementia in later life," she said.

The report was published in the medical journal *BMJ*.

STUDY DETAILS

For the study, Dr. Singh-Manoux and colleagues collected data on nearly 5,200 men and 2,200 women who took part in the Whitehall II cohort study. The study, which began in 1985, followed British civil servants from the age of 45 to 70.

Over 10 years, starting in 1997, the participants' cognitive function was tested three times. The researchers assessed memory, vocabulary, hearing and vision.

Dr. Singh-Manoux's group found that over time, test scores for memory, reasoning and vocabulary skills all dropped. The decline was faster among the older participants, they added.

Among men aged 45 to 49, reasoning skills declined by nearly 4%, and for those aged 65 to 70 those skills dropped by about nearly 10%.

For women, the decline in reasoning approached 5% for those aged 45 to 49 and about 7% for those 65 to 70, the researchers found.

SIGNIFICANCE OF FINDINGS

Understanding cognitive aging might enable early identification of those at risk for dementia, Dr. Singh-Manoux said.

In addition, knowing when cognitive decline is likely to start can help in treatment, because the earlier treatment starts the more likely it is to be effective, the researchers noted.

"Greater awareness of the fact that our cognitive status is not intact until deep old age might lead individuals to make changes in their lifestyle and improve [their] cardiovascular health, to reduce risk of adverse cognitive outcomes in old age," Dr. Singh-Manoux said.

Research shows that "what is good for the heart is good for the head," which makes living a healthy lifestyle a part of slowing cognitive decline, she said.

Targeting patients who have risk factors for heart disease such as obesity, high blood pressure and high cholesterol might not only protect their hearts but also prevent dementia in old age, the researchers said.

"Understanding cognitive aging will be one of the challenges of this century," especially as people are living longer, Dr. Singh-Manoux added.

EXPERT COMMENTARY

Francine Grodstein, ScD, an associate professor of medicine at Brigham and Women's Hospital in Boston and author of an accompanying editorial, said more research is needed into how to prevent early cognitive decline.

"If cognitive decline may start at younger ages, then efforts to prevent cognitive decline may need to start at younger ages," she said.

"New research should focus on understanding what factors may contribute to cognitive decline in younger persons," Dr. Grodstein added.

"This is consistent with what we have seen in other studies and the cognitive changes that occur as we age," said Heather M. Snyder, PhD, senior associate director of medical and scientific relations at the Alzheimer's Association.

These changes do not mean that all these people will go on to develop Alzheimer's disease or another dementia, Dr. Snyder noted. "It is important to remember that the cognitive changes associated with aging are very different from the cognitive changes that are associated with Alzheimer's disease," she stressed.

Although some of these people may go on to develop Alzheimer's disease there is currently no way to tell who is at risk, Dr. Snyder said. "This is why it is so important to continue to investigate biological changes that occur in the earliest stages, because it is difficult to [determine] the cognitive changes that are associated with Alzheimer's disease," she said.

Dr. Snyder also noted that Alzheimer's disease can start 15 to 20 years before symptoms are apparent, which makes finding a biological marker so important.

info To learn more about cognitive decline, visit the Web site of the US National Library of Medicine at *http://www.nlm.nih.gov/medlineplus/mildcognitiveimpairment.html*.

Type of PET Scan That Can Detect Alzheimer's

Gil Rabinovici, MD, attending physician, Memory and Aging Center, University of California, San Francisco.
Catherine Roe, assistant professor, neurology, Knight Alzheimer's Disease Research Center, Washington University School of Medicine, St. Louis.
American Academy of Neurology news release

In the vast majority of cases, researchers can distinguish between Alzheimer's and another form of dementia with shared symptoms by using a specific type of PET (positron emission tomography) scan that looks for evidence of plaque in the brain, recent research suggests.

Known as the "PIB PET" scan, this type of scan appears to be more accurate in telling apart the two types of dementia than the more commonly used "FDG PET" scan.

"These two types of dementia share similar symptoms, so telling the two apart while a person is living is a real challenge, but important so doctors can determine the best form of treatment," study author Gil Rabinovici, MD, of the University of California, San Francisco Memory and Aging Center, explained in a university news release.

The study was published in an online issue of *Neurology*.

HOW THE SCAN WORKS

The PIB PET scan harnesses a "PIB marker" to uncover signs of brain plaque (known as amyloid). The presence of such plaque is a telltale sign of Alzheimer's, but is not a signal of another type of dementia called frontotemporal lobar degeneration (FTLD).

In FTLD, the frontal and temporal lobes of the brain atrophy. It's less common than Alzheimer's, but equally as devastating. People with FTLD can develop erratic behavior, emotional problems, trouble communicating and difficulty with walking and other basic movements.

To gauge the effectiveness of PIB PET scans, the team focused on 107 patients who either had early onset Alzheimer's or FTLD.

All the patients underwent both the PIB PET scan and the FDG PET scan. The latter looks for signs of metabolic changes in the brain.

THE RESULTS

While the FDG PET scan was found to accurately differentiate between the two forms of dementia nearly 78% of the time, PIB PET scans did so nearly 90% of the time.

Although the study found that FDG PET resulted in fewer false positives in select situations, overall, PIB PET appeared to perform better.

"While widespread use of PIB PET scans isn't available at this time, similar amyloid markers are being developed for clinical use, and these findings support a role for amyloid imaging in correctly diagnosing Alzheimer's disease versus FTLD," Dr. Rabinovici noted.

EXPERT REACTION

Catherine Roe, PhD, an assistant professor of neurology with the Knight Alzheimer's Disease Research Center at Washington University School of Medicine in St. Louis, said that currently PIB PET technology is impractical to deploy outside of specialized research institutions. But that, she noted, is about to change.

"The authors are correct in saying that new amyloid marking technology is being developed right now that will be easier to use in a clinical setting," she said. "Testing is under way. So based on their findings, their support for the use of this type of scan makes really good sense to me. Because 90% sensitivity in correctly identifying disease is a lot better than 78%."

info For more on Alzheimer's, visit the Web site of the Alzheimer's Association, *www.alz.org.*

Folks Who Feel Health Is "Poor" Have Greater Risk for Dementia

Christophe Tzourio, MD, PhD, neuroepidemiology unit, Victor Segalen Bordeaux II University, France.
Heather M. Snyder, PhD, senior associate director, Medical & Scientific Relations, Alzheimer's Association, Chicago.
Neurology online

Older adults who think they're not in tip-top health may have a greater risk of developing dementia than folks who believe they're healthy, French researchers reported in the journal *Neurology.*

Someday, "having people rate their own health may be a simple tool for doctors to determine a person's risk of dementia, especially for people with no symptoms or memory problems," said Christophe Tzourio, MD, PhD, of the neuroepidemiology unit at the Victor Segalen Bordeaux II University.

Still, not everyone was convinced by the research.

"It is one of the first studies to look at this correlation and we really don't know what that means," said Heather M. Snyder, PhD, senior associate director for Medical & Scientific Relations at the Alzheimer's Association. She was not involved in the study.

STUDY DETAILS

In their report, published online in *Neurology,* Dr. Tzourio's team suggest that doctors might use a patient's self-rated health to predict the potential for mental decline.

They collected data on almost 8,200 people aged 65 years and older who were asked to rate their health at the start of the study.

During roughly seven years of follow-up, 618 people developed dementia. For those who said their health was poor, the risk for developing dementia was 70% higher than for those who rated their health as good. For those who rated their health as fair, the risk was 34% higher, they noted.

ZEROING IN ON THE ASSOCIATIONS

Of course, health problems such as heart disease have been strongly linked to increased odds for dementias—including Alzheimer's disease—in prior studies. But the French team note that the increase in risk for dementia tied to poor self-reported health stuck even after they accounted for heart disease and other chronic ailments.

Furthermore, the association between fair and poor health ratings and dementia was even greater among those who had no memory or thinking skill problems at the time, Dr. Tzourio's group found.

For these symptom-free people who rated their health as poor, the risk of developing dementia was almost twice as high compared with those who rated their health as good, the researchers found. In the absence of a full assessment of their mental skills, their self-reported health was therefore the only indicator of a possible decline in brain functioning, the authors said.

CONTRIBUTING FACTORS

What factors might be contributing to the effect? "We know that having a large social network and social activities are associated with a decreased risk of dementia," Dr. Tzourio noted in the news release. "Therefore, it's possible that rating one's health as poor might be associated with behaviors that limit social interaction and in turn accelerate the dementia process," he speculated.

However, before the findings can be taken as fact, they need to be replicated, Dr. Snyder said. "We would really need to have a much larger study in a more diverse population to assess and figure out what this correlation means," she said.

What is known is that Alzheimer's, the most common form of dementia, starts to develop 10 to 20 years before symptoms show, Dr. Snyder said. So, these feelings about general health might indicate that a person senses something has changed before the disease is evident, she added.

info For more on dementia, visit the Web site of the US National Library of Medicine, *http://www.nlm.nih.gov/medlineplus/dementia.html.*

Dementia/Sepsis Connection

Dementia may be linked to sepsis. Sepsis, a life-threatening blood infection, kills about one-third of those affected.

Recent study: Elderly patients who survive severe sepsis are more than three times as likely as other elderly patients to experience long-term cognitive impairment. Talk to your doctor about steps to prevent and treat sepsis.

Theodore J. Iwashyna, MD, PhD, assistant professor of internal medicine, University of Michigan Medical School, Ann Arbor, and lead author of a study of 5,093 patients, published in *The Journal of the American Medical Association.*

Marriage and Dementia

Did you know that spouses of people with dementia are six times more likely to develop the illness? Increased risk may be caused by the stress associated with caring for a loved one struggling with dementia. Shared environmental factors such as diet also may be responsible.

Maria C. Norton, PhD, associate professor, department of family, consumer and human development, Utah State University, Logan, and leader of a study of 1,221 couples, published in *Journal of the American Geriatrics Society.*

Secrets to Improve Your Running at 60+

Timothy Quinn, PhD, associate professor, exercise science, University of New Hampshire, Durham.
Jeff Galloway, Olympian and marathon training director, author of *Running Until You're 100* (Meyer & Meyer). *Journal of Strength and Conditioning Research*

For runners lacing up their jogging shoes at age 60 and beyond, there's encouraging news and not-so-encouraging news, according to recent research.

"The good news is that as we age, we maintain good running economy," said study leader Timothy Quinn, PhD, an associate professor of exercise science at the University of New Hampshire.

BACKGROUND

Running economy refers to how efficiently your body uses oxygen at a specific pace. The less this "oxygen cost," the longer you can run.

When it comes to oxygen cost, Dr. Quinn found that runners past age 60 "are no different than the 22-year-old runners, which is kind of amazing."

Yet, as runners age, they typically slow down, Dr. Quinn said. Based on his study of runners ages 18 to 60-plus, he said this decline could result from loss of strength, muscle power and flexibility, rather than running economy differences. And these declines can be addressed, he said.

STUDY DETAILS

For the study, Dr. Quinn and his team evaluated 51 men and women, all strong runners. One group was 18 to 39 years old, another 40 to 59 and the third 60 and older. All had finished first, second or third place in their age categories in local running events. They logged, on average, from 40 to nearly 70 miles a week.

On average, the men 60-plus ran a 5K race (about 3.1 miles) in 20 minutes; the women 60-plus in nearly 27 minutes.

For perspective, the 5K New Hampshire state record for men 60-plus is about 18 minutes; for women, about 23.

The study appears in the *Journal of Strength and Conditioning Research.*

OTHER CONCERNS

Besides looking at each runner's use of oxygen, the researchers also tested the runners' upper and lower body strength, flexibility and muscle power and their "VO2 max"—maximum oxygen capacity. In those areas, the older runners fell short of the younger ones. "What we found was there is a big difference in strength, especially in the upper body," Dr. Quinn said.

Runners need upper-body strength, he said, because the arms provide a lot of the "drive," especially when running uphill.

The upper-body strength in the 60-plus runners was about half what the younger groups had, Dr. Quinn said. The older runners also had about half the flexibility of the younger runners.

Less flexibility can affect stride length and step frequency, accounting for slower times.

The muscle power of the older group was lower, too.

WHAT IT MEANS FOR YOU

The shortcomings can be addressed, Dr. Quinn said. Weight training for a half hour or so twice a week could build strength, he said. Engaging in plyometrics—also called jump training—could help with muscle power. Plyometrics stretches the muscles, then contracts them, to strengthen them.

He also suggested stretching after running, which could help maintain flexibility.

EXPERT REACTION

The finding that older runners maintain their "running economy" doesn't surprise Jeff Galloway, a 1972 Olympian who directs marathon training programs. He wrote the book, *Running Until You're 100* and estimated he has helped train more than 50,000 runners who are 60-plus.

Galloway said he is not too concerned about the lack of flexibility and other declines noted in the study. Even younger distance runners lose flexibility, he said, citing other studies.

With age, Galloway said, "the body finds intuitive ways of running more efficiently." For instance, he said, younger runners have a tendency to bounce because they have more muscle power. With age, as muscle power declines, older runners adapt by running lower to the ground, taking more steps per minute and other measures, he said.

Overall, Dr. Quinn's findings are good, Galloway said. "The one caution I have among the age group over 50 or 60 is, if you try to change Mother Nature too much by doing intense work, bad things can happen." He cites cases of runners doing intense weight work and suffering injuries that benched them from running for a time.

info To learn more about plyometrics, visit the Web site of the American Council on Exercise, *www.acefitness.org/fitfacts/fitfacts_display. aspx?itemid=73.*

Boost Your Brain Health: Learn a Second Language

Kira Gor, PhD, associate professor of second-language acquisition and director of its PhD program at the University of Maryland's School of Languages, Literatures, and Cultures in College Park, Maryland.

Learning a second language is one of the best ways to achieve the type of mental stimulation that many experts believe can help us stave off neurodegenerative diseases such as Alzheimer's.

But if it's been decades since you've called yourself a student—or if you consider yourself just "not good" at languages—how should you embark upon this brain-boosting goal?

We spoke with Kira Gor, PhD, a leading authority on how adults acquire second-language skills.

Here are her secrets…

Secret 1: **Choose wisely.** Learning a second language is a popular way to promote brain health because it activates the brain's capacity for "neuroplasticity"—that is, the brain's ability to "rewire" itself by creating new connections among brain cells.

But it's important for an English speaker to realize that trying to learn Chinese or Arabic, for example, will be far more difficult than, say, a romance language, such as Spanish, French or Italian. That's because the grammar, spelling systems and sounds of Chinese and Arabic are so different from those of English.

My advice: Pursue a second language that will challenge you—but not be overwhelming. The more difficult a language is, the longer the route to its mastery. To determine the difficulty and time it takes to learn a particular language, visit the Effective Language Learning Web site, *www.effectivelanguagelearning.com* and click on the "Language Guide" tab. (*Note:* These Foreign Service Institute estimates are for intensive classroom instruction, not self-instruction.) Motivation is also important when deciding on a language—for example, are you drawn to the culture of people who speak that particular language?…do friends and/or family members speak it?

Secret 2: **Uncover your learning style.** Just as some people are athletic and others artistic, each of us has a learning style that works best for us—whether visual, auditory or kinesthetic (movement based). For example, if you wanted to remember a new phone number, consider which is easier for you—to read it, hear it or write it down. Those who are visual might rely on flash cards, while auditory learners depend on recordings of the language. A kinesthetic learner would be wise to write out words and phrases many times.

Note: There is always an advantage to having an instructor, but a motivated adult can learn a language on his/her own.

My advice: Particularly in our Internet-dominated culture, most adults need a significant amount of visual input—it tends to be relied upon more heavily than auditory or kinesthetic input. For this reason, you should make sure that you spend at least some time, preferably every day, reading in the foreign language. Internet sites chosen based on your personal interests are excellent resources.

Secret 3: **Make it personal.** Language is meaningless if you're practicing rote, impersonal words and phrases. Good language instruction often relies on simple conversational formulas that help students personalize their speech even at low proficiency levels. For example, you may learn to discuss your preferences—say what your favorite foods are or your favorite season in the language you are studying.

My advice: As much as possible, incorporate personal information, such as small facts about yourself, family members, friends or even your pets, when learning a second language. This keeps you motivated and helps you turn what could be a mechanical drill into something personal and fun.

Secret 4: **Trick your brain.** New research helps explain why adults sometimes have difficulty learning a second language. Adult brains, scientists have discovered, are accustomed to ignoring unfamiliar sounds or grammatical features so that one's full attention can be given to the speaker's native language—a process that often makes it tougher to learn a second language.

Fortunately, we can retrain our brains to focus on specific sounds or grammatical structures of the language we are trying to learn. But we first must become familiar with the unique elements of that language, including letters and symbols that may sound alike for a speaker of English, but differentiate words in the foreign language.

My advice: Once you've started learning a new language, make a chart of phonological units (using words that sound alike) in the language you're learning. In English, for example, this could include such words as "bad" and "bed"…or "big" and "pig." In French, such words would include "tu" (which means "you" informally) and "tout" (meaning "every"), that in pronunciation differ only by the vowel sound—the "t" being the same and the final consonant silent.

Frequently reading and speaking those words together, ideally for 10 minutes every day—whether alone, in class or listening to a recording—is the most efficient way to retrain your brain to identify and produce new sounds.

Secret 5: **Practice, practice, practice.** By far the most important factor in determining your ability to learn a second language is how much time you spend immersed in it. Without consistent practice, you won't retain what you've learned.

While listening is important, it is the most passive form of learning—speaking and writing engage more active parts of the brain. Repeating words and sentences over and over helps your mouth get used to pronouncing unusual sounds and sequences of words.

My advice: Several times a week—or even better, every day—listen to the language you're learning (for example, on CDs). When listening, do so at a proficiency level that's only slightly above your own—it will stretch your abilities without overwhelming you. (You will know the level is right when you understand almost everything and can guess the rest.) Even more importantly, speak, read and write in the language. The key is consistency and frequency—30 minutes every day is better than two hours twice a week. Language is very much a "use it or lose it" skill—ignore it, and it will go away.

Suggestion: Find a conversational partner using teleconferencing—for example, on Skype or foreign language Internet chat rooms.

Fish Oil May Pump Up Muscles

Older adults who took high doses of omega-3 fatty acids daily for eight weeks showed an increase in muscle protein synthesis and improved muscle-cell growth. Study participants took Lovaza—a prescription-strength omega-3 that is approved by the FDA for treating high triglycerides. One dose of Lovaza has 1.86 grams of EPA and 1.5 grams of DHA—significantly more than is found in typical fish oil supplements. Dietary omega-3 fatty acid supplementation may provide a safe, low-cost way to fight *sarcopenia*, a loss of lean muscle mass, strength and function associated with aging, but further research is needed.

Bettina Mittendorfer, PhD, research associate professor in medicine, Washington University, St. Louis, and author of an eight-week study published in *American Journal of Clinical Nutrition*.

Cool Brain, Better Sleep

A refrigerated cap worn by insomnia patients caused them to fall asleep in 13 minutes (faster than those who also wore caps but didn't have insomnia). Cooling the frontal cortex, an overactive area in those with insomnia, restores restful sleep—a finding that may lead to the development of brain-cooling caps.

University of Pittsburgh School of Medicine

Alzheimer's Disease: Myths and Truths

Alzheimer's Association, 225 N. Michigan Ave., Chicago 60601, *www.alz.org*.

Alzheimer's disease is a frightening diagnosis—one that we all hope never to face. Unfortunately, there are many myths about what can cause Alzheimer's or increase your risk for the disease.

Here, we set the record straight…

Myth: Use of aluminum is linked to the disease.

Truth: No study has confirmed any link between Alzheimer's and aluminum.

Myth: The low-calorie sweetener aspartame causes memory loss.

Truth: There is no scientific evidence of this.

Myth: Flu vaccinations raise Alzheimer's risk.

Truth: Several studies show the opposite—that flu shots reduce risk for Alzheimer's. Past exposure to specific types of vaccines may be related to a lower risk for Alzheimer's because aging and Alzheimer's may involve changes in immune responses.

Myth: Amalgam tooth fillings raise Alzheimer's risk.

Truth: There is no evidence that these fillings—which contain 50% mercury—are linked to Alzheimer's disease.

■ ■ ■ ■

Better Antidepressant Choice For Older Adults

Researchers analyzed the use of antidepressants in 60,746 depression patients (age 65 and older).

Result: Those who took selective serotonin reuptake inhibitors (SSRIs), such as *citalopram* (Celexa), were at increased risk for several adverse events (including death, stroke, falls and fractures) compared with those who took older tricyclic antidepressants (TCAs), such as *amitriptyline* (Elavil).

If you're 65 or older and your doctor prescribes an SSRI: Be sure to ask about the risks and benefits—and discuss perhaps taking a lower dose.

Carol Coupland, PhD, associate professor, medical statistics, The University of Nottingham, UK.

■ ■ ■ ■

Sharks, Alzheimer's and ALS

Scientists took tissue samples from the fins of seven species of sharks to measure their levels of the neurotoxin BMAA, which is linked to

human neurological disorders such as Alzheimer's disease and amyotrophic lateral sclerosis (ALS), also known as Lou Gehrig's disease.

Result: The average single shark fin contained a similar level of BMAA as that found in the brains of humans with Alzheimer's or ALS.

Implication: Eating shark fin soup, an Asian delicacy, or taking shark cartilage supplements, used by some people as an unproven cancer treatment or for osteoarthritis, may pose a risk for degenerative brain diseases.

Neil Hammerschlag, PhD, research assistant professor, University of Miami, Florida.

■ ■ ■ ■

What to Do When You No Longer Drive

Avoid social isolation after you are no longer able to drive by taking advantage of public, private and volunteer programs to help you get where you want to go. Some volunteers offer to drive seniors around…and there are transportation programs such as ITNAmerica (*www.itnamerica.com*), to which people can donate vehicles and obtain credits for rides in the future.

USA Today

■ ■ ■ ■

Cold Sores May Be Linked To Alzheimer's Disease

Research has shown that a herpes simplex infection—the virus that causes cold sores—increases the amount of amyloid precursor protein, the parent protein of the plaque associated with Alzheimer's disease.

Self-defense: Treat cold sores quickly with an antiviral agent to minimize the amount of time that the virus remains active.

Elaine Bearer, MD, PhD, Harvey Family Professor and vice-chair for research, departments of pathology and neurosurgery, University of New Mexico School of Medicine, Albuquerque, and principal investigator in a study published in *PLoS One*.

■ ■ ■ ■

Diagnosing Alzheimer's

New diagnosis guidelines for Alzheimer's may double the number of people defined as having the disease. The guidelines create two new stages—the preclinical stage, when there are no symptoms but brain changes are occurring...and mild cognitive impairment (MCI), with mild symptoms.

Guy M. McKhann, MD, professor of neurology and neuroscience, department of neurology, Johns Hopkins University, Baltimore, and coauthor of new Alzheimer's diagnostic guidelines, published in *Alzheimer's & Dementia*.

Best Ways to Connect With Alzheimer's Patients

Beth Kallmyer, MSW, senior director of Constituent Services, Alzheimer's Association, Chicago.

Empathy is especially important when interacting with people who have Alzheimer's disease.

Example: If an Alzheimer's patient starts talking about his/her long-dead mother as if she were still alive, the caregiver should not try to correct him. Instead, say something like, "It sounds as if you really miss your mom." Learning how Alzheimer's progresses and how to handle it can help family members develop empathy—go to *www.alz.org* for details. Paid caregivers can be taught to have more empathy, too. Tell caregivers what the patient is used to doing—share his interests and patterns with them.

Example: If the person with Alzheimer's is used to taking showers only at night, he/she may become distressed if caregivers try to help him shower in the morning.

Helpful: Fill out the "Personal Facts and Insights" form at *www.alz.org* (search for "Personal Facts and Insights"). The form, which asks questions about the person with Alzheimer's, can be given to all caregivers.

■ ■ ■ ■

New Device Keeps Alzheimer's Patients Safe

An innovative walking shoe has a global positioning device implanted in the heel. A caregiver can specify a zone in which his/her loved one can move around freely. When a patient goes outside the designated area, a message alerts the caregiver.

Cost: $300 plus $35 to $40 a month for tracking services. Aetrex Worldwide, 800-526-2739, *www.aetrex.com*.

Aetrex.

■ ■ ■ ■

Falls Can Indicate Alzheimer's

Early sign of Alzheimer's that often is ignored...frequent falls.

Recent finding: Older people with preclinical Alzheimer's, as measured by brain scans that showed signs of amyloid plaques, are twice as likely to fall as people without preclinical Alzheimer's.

What to do: Everyone over age 65 should evaluate his/her fall risk. If you have had a fall, or a loved one has fallen, consult a physician.

Susan Stark, PhD, assistant professor, program of occupational therapy and department of neurology, Washington University in St. Louis, and lead author of a study of 125 adults, presented at the Alzheimer's Association's annual International Conference in Paris, France.

Secrets to Preventing Falls

Hylton Menz, PhD, deputy director of the Musculoskeletal Research Centre at La Trobe University in Victoria, Australia. He is author of the textbook *Foot Problems in Older People* (Churchill Livingstone) and a coauthor of *Falls in Older People: Risk Factors and Strategies for Prevention* (Cambridge University).

Each year, about one in every three people over age 65 suffers a fall, a mishap that is far more dangerous than most people realize.

Important research: In a 20-year study of nearly 5,600 women ages 70 and older, breaking a hip doubled the risk for death in the following year. Men who suffer a broken hip after a fall are also at increased risk for an untimely death.

Most people know the standard recommendations to reduce their risk for falls—get medical attention for balance and vision problems…improve the lighting in and around their homes…and eliminate loose carpets, cords and other obstacles.

What often gets overlooked: Painful feet…foot deformities such as bunions…weak foot and ankle muscles…and improper footwear also can significantly increase one's risk for falls.

Recent scientific evidence: In a 2011 study in the *British Medical Journal,* a comprehensive program of foot care reduced falls by one-third among a group of older people with assorted foot problems.

GET A FIRM FOUNDATION

With age, the muscles that support our ankles and feet often become weak—a common problem that contributes to foot pain and reduced activity levels. Structural abnormalities in the feet, such as bunions and hammertoes, undermine stability. And conditions that blunt sensations in the feet, such as nerve damage commonly caused by diabetes, may impair the ability of one's feet to react quickly and adjust to potentially hazardous conditions.

BASIC FALL-PREVENTION WORKOUT

Stretching and strengthening exercises can reduce foot pain—and lower your risk for falls. Basic exercises to perform daily…

To help increase your ankles' range of motion: Sit in a chair with one knee extended. Rotate your foot in a clockwise, then counterclockwise direction. Repeat 10 times with each foot, in each direction.

To strengthen your toe muscles: Place small stones or marbles on the floor in front of you. While seated, pick up the stones with your bare toes and place them in a box, one by one. Pick up 20 stones with each foot, then repeat.

To stretch your calf muscles: Stand about two feet from a wall, then lean into it with one leg slightly bent at the knee about three inches in front of the other. Then reverse the position of your feet and lean forward to stretch the muscles of the other calf. Hold the stretch for 20 seconds, three times for each leg.

PROPER FOOTWEAR

The right shoes are essential for everyone, but especially those with problem feet.

Most women know to avoid high heels, which make it more difficult to maintain balance. But many people opt for flimsy slip-on footwear, such as flip-flops, which may be comfortable but often become loose or come off the foot altogether, creating a balance hazard. It's far better to wear shoes that fasten to your feet with laces, Velcro or buckled straps.

Surprising fact: Most people assume that thick, cushiony soles, such as those found on most sneakers, help prevent falls because they tend to provide good support for your feet. But thinner, harder soles, such as those on some walking shoes, are safer because thin-soled shoes allow your feet to feel the sensations that help you maintain balance. A trade-off between comfort and safety may be necessary—you may have to wear less cushiony shoes that optimize balance.

Also, be sure that your shoes are the right size. Your feet may slide around in shoes that are too loose, while tight footwear won't allow your toes to respond to variations in the ground to help maintain stability while walking.

Remember: Shoe size often changes with age, as feet swell and spread. So have your feet measured every time you buy shoes.

Slightly more falls occur indoors than outdoors, and the proportion increases with age. Therefore, even when you're at home, proper footwear is crucial.

Important recent finding: When researchers at Harvard's Institute for Aging Research followed a group of older adults for more than two years, they found that more than half of those who fell indoors were barefoot, in their stocking feet or wearing slippers. These injuries tended to be more serious than those of people who were wearing shoes when they fell.

Best to wear at home: Sturdy, thin-soled shoes that have more structural integrity than the average slipper.

DO YOU NEED ORTHOTICS?

Many adults over age 65 could benefit from wearing orthotics—inserts that fit inside the shoe—to help prevent falls by providing additional support.

Properly made orthotics may improve the way your feet move as you walk, distribute your weight more broadly to reduce pressure on sensitive spots and help convey sensory information to your feet, all of which may lessen the risk for falls.

If you have structural foot problems due to diabetes or rheumatoid arthritis, you may need customized orthotics from a podiatrist.

Typical cost: About $400. Insurance coverage varies. But over-the-counter versions (made with firm material, not just a soft cushion) may work as well if your feet are relatively normal and your foot pain is fairly mild. Good brands include Vasyli and Langer. Usually, you will be able to transfer orthotics between shoes.

Most people find that full-length orthotics are less likely to slip inside the shoe than the half-length variety. Full-length orthotics also may feel more comfortable, especially if you have corns or calluses under the toes or on the ball of your foot.

GETTING HELP

If you have foot problems, seek care from a podiatrist or other health professional—and be sure to mention any concerns about falling. Also ask for exercises, in addition to the ones described here, to address your specific foot issues.

■ ■ ■ ■

Conquer Your Fear of Falling

Did you know that fear of falling raises risk of falling? Recent research revealed that older people who overestimated their risk of falling were more likely to fall than those who perceived their risk accurately.

Stephen Lord, PhD, professor, Falls and Balance Research Group, Prince of Wales Medical Research Institute, University of New South Wales, Australia, and leader of a study of 500 people, published online in BMJ.

Dangers of Ignoring Hearing Loss

Virginia Ramachandran, AuD, audiologist at Henry Ford Hospital in Detroit. She is coauthor of Basic Audiometry Learning Manual *(Plural) and an adjunct professor and clinical education coordinator at the audiology program in the department of communication sciences and disorders at Wayne State University, also in Detroit.*

For most people, age-related hearing loss, also known as *presbycusis*, happens so slowly that they don't notice it at first.

In fact, hearing loss actually begins in our late 20s and early 30s, when we lose the ability to hear high pitches, such as that of a buzzing mosquito. And by the time we reach our 70s, about half of us have diagnosable hearing loss.

What you may not know: Despite the high incidence of hearing loss, only about two in every five adults over age 65 with hearing loss use hearing aids. Plenty of people resist getting a hearing aid because they fear that it will make them look old, be too complicated to use and/or cost too much money.

Now: Based on recent research, people with untreated hearing loss have more reason than ever before to consider getting a hearing aid.

HEALTH HAZARDS

While most people consider hearing loss a mere annoyance, researchers are now discovering that it may increase one's risk for...

•**Dementia.** In a study of 639 men and women (ages 36 to 90) published in the *Archives of Neurology,* the risk of developing dementia was two, three and five times higher in those with mild, moderate and severe hearing loss, respectively, than in those with normal hearing.

Researchers do not have an explanation for the association between hearing loss and dementia—and they point out that the link does not prove cause and effect.

However, it's possible that damage to the cells involved in hearing may be a sign that damage has also occurred to nerve cells that are responsible for cognitive functions, including memory. Hearing loss also can cause social isolation, which contributes to the risk for dementia.

•**Depression.** Significantly more older adults with hearing loss who did not wear hearing aids reported feelings of sadness and depression for two or more weeks during a one-year period than their peers who wore hearing aids, according to a study from the National Council on Aging.

Possible reason: Depression may be caused or worsen in people with hearing loss who withdraw from social interactions.

•**Injury.** Hearing loss is a safety hazard, especially for pedestrians who may have trouble hearing oncoming traffic and for drivers who rely on their ability to hear to prevent collisions. It also affects a person's ability to hear a phone, doorbell and smoke detector alarm.

DO YOU NEED A HEARING AID?

If you have hearing loss, a loved one may be the first to notice it. *In addition, if any of the statements below applies to you, it may mean that you have hearing loss…*

•**You frequently ask, "What?" in conversations.**

•**You have trouble following conversations.**

•**Everyone around you seems to mumble.**

•**You're always turning up the volume on the TV.**

•**You can hear someone talking, but not what the person is saying.**

•**It's especially difficult for you to hear women and children,** both of whom have higher-pitched voices and generally speak with a lower volume than men. Higher-pitched voices are the most difficult to hear.

BEST HEARING AID OPTIONS

Many of today's hearing aids are highly sophisticated. *For example…*

Cutting-edge product: One of the newest hearing aids available is the SoundBite Hearing System, which allows sound to travel via the teeth to the inner ear. A small microphone in the ear canal transmits sounds to a wireless unit behind the ear, which sends a signal to a device that fits over the back teeth. The device converts the signals into vibrations, rerouting sound to the inner ear. SoundBite is especially helpful for people with hearing loss in one ear or who have conductive hearing loss—a problem in the middle or outer ear.

Main types of hearing aids…

•**Behind-the-ear (BTE) hearing aids,** which are generally larger than other types of hearing aids, are the traditional kind that hooks over the top of your ear and sits behind it. The hearing aid picks up sound, amplifies it and carries the amplified sound to an ear mold that fits inside your ear canal. The large size allows for directional microphones and easier adjustment of volume and battery changing.

The BTE hearing aid is appropriate for almost all types of hearing loss and does the best job of amplifying sound for people with severe hearing loss. Siemens offers a couple of rechargeable BTE hearing aids for mild-to-moderately severe hearing loss.

Typical cost: $500 to $2,000 per ear.

•**Open-fit models are among the newer aids available today.** They are smaller than 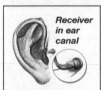 BTE aids and suitable for mild-to-moderate hearing loss. Generally placed behind the ear, these aids leave the ear canal mostly open and are less visible than BTE models. Sound travels from the open-fit hearing aid through a small tube or wire to a tiny dome or speaker in the ear canal.

Receiver in ear canal

Typical cost: $1,000 to $2,500 per ear.

•**In-the-ear (ITE) hearing aids are custom-made to fit in the outer ear.** ITE devices may pick up background sounds such as wind, since the microphone sits at the outermost portion of the ear. But the batteries tend to last longer than other types of hearing aids and are easier to change, especially if you have arthritis in your fingers.

Typical cost: $1,200 to $2,500 per ear.

•**In-the-canal (ITC) hearing aids fit farther into the ear canal than ITE aids.** This style is best for mild-to-moderate hearing loss. It is hardly visible and is easy to use with the telephone. The small size makes adjustments, including battery changes and volume control, difficult for some people. The device may not fit well in smaller ears.

Typical cost: $1,300 to $2,500 per ear.

•**Completely-in-the-canal hearing aids are custom-molded and best for mild-to-moderate hearing loss.** This is the least no-

ticeable type of hearing aid and the least likely to pick up background noises such as wind. It also works well with telephones. But the small batteries require frequent replacement.

Typical cost: $1,300 to $3,000 per ear.

Main hearing aid manufacturers: Oticon, Phonak, Starkey, ReSound, Widex and Siemens.

Important: There are many over-the-counter devices that simply amplify sound. However, hearing aids are usually preferable because they are customized for an individual's specific degree and type of hearing loss, allowing them to be programmed for optimal hearing improvement.

If you are having difficulty hearing: See an audiologist. You can find one at the American Academy of Audiology consumer Web site at *www.howsyourhearing.org*. An audiologist can help you select the best hearing aid for you and explain how to properly use and maintain it. If the audiologist suspects that you may have an undetected medical condition that is causing your hearing loss, you will be referred to a physician.

WHAT ABOUT COST?

Some individuals put off purchasing hearing aids because of their high cost—about $500 to $3,000 per ear.

Recent research finding: People who have insurance plans that cover the entire cost of hearing aids purchased them seven years earlier, on average, than those who had partial or no insurance, according to a study conducted at Henry Ford Hospital in Detroit.

But only about one-third of health insurance policies cover the cost of hearing aids. Medicare

does not. Health insurance from the Veterans Administration does cover the cost, and the Lions Club has a program that provides hearing aids to people who can't afford them.

You can use a health savings account or flexible spending account to pay for hearing aids with pretax funds, or you can deduct the cost on your tax return (check with your tax preparer for details).

Illustrations: Courtesy of NIH Medical Arts.

Now Available: Invisible Hearing Aid

Lynn Sirow, PhD, audiologist and adjunct assistant professor, City University of New York, and director, Port Washington Hearing Center, Port Washington, New York.

The Lyric hearing aid is professionally inserted deep into the ear canal. It is placed four millimeters from the eardrum and is worn continuously for three to four months, then removed and replaced with a new one. The Lyric eliminates common problems people have with hearing aids, such as losing them, battery insertion and poor hearing at night when hearing aids are removed, including not hearing the phone or an alarm while sleeping. Some people find that the Lyric provides better sound than conventional hearing aids. It is invisible and can be worn while showering or bathing, but it cannot be worn when swimming under water and must be removed for MRI testing or ear exams—and it must be reinserted only by a professional. It comes in a number of sizes but does not fit everyone comfortably. A subscription for two ears costs about $3,300 to $3,400 a year, which includes a year's worth of devices—new ones are provided at each follow-up visit, every three to four months. (Conventional hearing aids cost from $600 to more than $2,000.) For information, go to *www.lyrichearing.com*.

Best Phones for Seniors

Jim Miller, an advocate for senior citizens, writes "Savvy Senior," a weekly information column syndicated in more than 400 newspapers nationwide. Based in Norman, Oklahoma, he also offers a free senior news service at *www.savvysenior.org.*

For people with hearing loss, weak vision or arthritis, using a standard telephone can be challenging. Fortunately, there are phones on the market today that can help. *Here are some of the best...*

For fast help in adjusting the phone: Clarity Professional XL45. This phone offers 50 decibels (dB) of sound amplification (in addition to the standard phone dB level of 12 to 15). It also has large "talk back" buttons that speak the numbers and a very large caller-ID display screen. The phone not only helps seniors with hearing and vision problems, it also is ideal for those who struggle with technology. The XL45 offers a unique feature called "ClarityLogic" that, at the press of a button, connects you with a customer service representative who can remotely adjust your phone's settings anytime for optimal sound quality. The representative even can program in the names and numbers of people you call often. 800-426-3738, *www.clarityproducts.com* (and click on "Products").

For emergencies: Geemarc Ampli-600. This remote-controlled emergency response phone comes with a neck pendant and SOS buttons on a wristband that you press to automatically dial the phone's preprogrammed emergency numbers if you can't get to the phone. It offers 50 dB of amplification, caller ID, a speakerphone and one-touch emergency dial buttons. 888-515-8120, *www.teltex.com.*

For owners with soft voices: Serene HD-40S. For seniors with difficult-to-hear voices, the HD-40S can amplify the outgoing voice by as much as 40 dB. This phone also provides photo-memory dialing (you simply press a picture of the person you wish to call) and 18-dB amplification for incoming calls. 800-825-6758, *www.harriscomm.com.*

For limited mobility: Clarity RC200. This remote-controlled speakerphone provides hands-free conversations from up to 15 feet away. It has voice-activated answering capabilities that allow you to answer incoming calls by just saying "hello," and it disconnects when the caller hangs up and the dial tone returns. It also comes with a wireless remote control that will let you make and receive calls from a distance. 800-426-3738, *www.clarityproducts.com* (and click on "Products").

For severe hearing loss: CapTel 800. This captioned phone lets you listen to the caller and read word-for-word captions of what he/she is saying on the phone's display window. It is sold through the manufacturers Weitbrecht Communications. Many states have programs that offer these phones for free to qualified residents. Visit *www.captel.com*, and click on your state to learn more, or call 888-269-7477.

Cordless phone: Serene CL-60A. The CL-60A offers big "talk-back" buttons that announce the numbers you dial, up to 50 dB of amplification, tone controls, amplified talking caller ID and an amplified slow-play answering machine that makes messages easier to understand. 800-825-6758, *www.harriscomm.com.*

Free phones: Many states offer specialized programs that give free amplified telephones to residents in need. Check with your phone company.

■ ■ ■ ■

A New Treatment May Eliminate Tinnitus

Researchers were able to eliminate tinnitus (persistent ringing in the ears) in rats by stimulating the vagus nerve in the back of the neck while playing a variety of tones.

Theory: The technique releases chemicals that encourage changes in the brain and resets the brain's auditory system, eliminating tinnitus.

Michael Kilgard, PhD, professor, School of Behavioral and Brain Sciences, University of Texas, Dallas, and leader of the animal study published in the online edition of *Nature.*

Favorite Devices for Reading Small Print

Jim Miller, an advocate for older Americans, writes "Savvy Senior," a weekly information column syndicated in more than 400 newspapers nationwide. Based in Norman, Oklahoma, he also offers a free news service for seniors at *www.savvysenior.org*

With more than 25 million Americans living with some form of uncorrectable vision impairment today, more and more high-tech devices for low-vision problems are available, ranging in price from less than $40 to several thousand dollars. These devices can help you read menus, books, magazines and newspapers…make phone calls…work on your computer…and even get around your neighborhood more easily. *Here, some of the best…*

TALKING PHONES

Cell phone that speaks: The Samsung Haven from Verizon Wireless is able to "speak" everything that appears on the display screen, including caller-ID names and numbers, text messages and keypad presses when you dial a number. It also lets you make calls and send text messages by speaking the name of the person that you want to contact. The phone has extralarge, high-contrast text and big touch keys. 800-256-4646, *www.verizonwireless.com*.

Telephone that speaks: The all-purpose ClearSounds CSC1000 Amplified Freedom Phone has big buttons with a backlit keypad that "speaks" the numbers as you dial and a caller-ID that speaks and displays the name and number of the person who is calling. It also amplifies incoming speech up to 48 decibels (dB), compared with the standard 12 dB to 13 dB. It has a built-in answering machine and eight photo-memory dial buttons that let you insert pictures of family members or friends over preprogrammed buttons, so you can simply press the picture of the person you want to call to automatically dial. 800-965-9043, *www.clear sounds.com*.

BOOK READERS

Low-vision eReader: For instant access to thousands of books, the Apple iPad 2 tops the list as the best eReading device for the visually impaired. It provides a large 9.7-inch high-resolution screen and a variety of built-in accessibility features, including font magnification up to 56 points and white text on black background contrast adjustment. Its VoiceOver feature is able to read the text of books and any other text on the screen out loud. It comes with a feature that allows you to find your iPad using GPS, should you lose it. 800-692-7753, *www.apple.com*.

For a low-tech alternative, the Library of Congress Talking Books program offers a free tape player and unlimited free books on tape to the legally blind—those whose vision is 20/200 or worse in the better eye. 888-657-7323, *www.nls talkingbooks.org*.

Portable text-to-speech: The Intel Reader turns written text into spoken words. The handheld device, which includes a five-megapixel auto-focus camera and an Intel processor, weighs a little more than one pound and is about the size of a paperback book. You hold the device over a page…and shoot and capture the image, which the device can read aloud at a speed that you choose. It can store up to 500,000 pages of text. The battery lasts for more than four hours. *www.careinnovations.com*.

Alternatives: For iPhone 4 users, the new ZoomReader application developed by Ai Squared uses the built-in iPhone camera to take a picture of text and then reads it aloud. 800-859-0270, *www.aisquared.com*.

CURRENCY READER

To protect yourself from being shortchanged or making mistakes when you pay for things with cash and receive change in bills, the iBill made by Orbit Research identifies all US bills by voice or by a series of tones or vibrations for privacy. You just insert the bill into a slot in the battery-operated device, which is small enough to fit on a key ring. Most bills are identified in less than a second, and it has just two buttons for operation. 888-606-7248, *www.orbit research.com*.

Alternatives: The LookTel Money Reader, a $1.99 application for the iPad 2 and some models of the iPhone and iPod Touch, also identifies US currency out loud. It does not require an Internet connection, so it can read money from any location. *www.looktel.com*

The free EyeNote application from the Bureau of Engraving and Printing works similarly and is compatible with the iPad 2 and all iPhones and iPod Touch models that have a camera. *www.eyenote.gov.*

SMALL PRINT

Portable electronic magnifier: For reading small print, such as food labels and bills, the Ruby handheld video magnifier by Freedom Scientific provides clarity, contrast and magnification up to 14 times, far beyond an ordinary magnifying glass. It offers four high-contrast reading modes that let you change the text and background colors for comfortable reading on a 4.3-inch full-color video screen. It also has a freeze-frame option that allows you to capture an image on the screen and bring it close for better viewing and further magnification. It's small enough to fit in your pocket or purse. 800-444-4443, *www.freedomscientific.com.*

Computer magnifier/reader: To customize a Microsoft Windows personal computer for low-vision, Ai Squared offers a software application called ZoomText Magnifier/Reader that lets you magnify everything on your computer up to 36 times. It provides eight different zoom window types that allow you to choose which part of the screen is magnified. It even speaks all program controls, including menus and list views. And when you want to give your eyes a rest, ZoomText can read your documents, Web pages and e-mail to you through your computer's speakers. It also can speak each key or word that you type and read any text that you point your mouse at. These features are far superior to the Microsoft accessibility features that are built into Windows software. 800-859-0270, *www.aisquared.com.*

■ ■ ■ ■

Daily Aspirin Warning

Daily aspirin use may be linked to vision loss. Wet late-stage aging macular disorder (AMD)—also called age-related macular degeneration—is twice as common in people who take aspirin daily as in people who never use aspirin.

Caution: Do not stop aspirin therapy without talking with your physician.

Paulus de Jong, MD, PhD, emeritus professor of ophthalmic epidemiology at the Netherlands Institute for Neuroscience and Academic Medical Center, Amsterdam, and first author of a study of 4,691 people, age 65 and older, published in *Ophthalmology.*

■ ■ ■ ■

Eye Care Helps Alzheimer's Patients

One-quarter of 38 Alzheimer's patients (average age 85) who had standard cataract surgery improved in their ability to perceive, understand and respond appropriately to their surroundings. In addition, the patients' symptoms of depression eased as much as is typical when adults without dementia undergo cataract surgery. Sleep patterns also improved, while nighttime behavior problems decreased—perhaps due to normalized levels of the sleep-regulating hormone melatonin.

If a loved one has Alzheimer's: Continue to have his/her eyes regularly examined and consider cataract surgery if necessary.

Brigitte Girard, MD, chief of ophthalmology services, Tenon Hospital, Paris.

■ ■ ■ ■

Get the Shingles Vaccine

Get the shingles vaccine even if you have already had shingles if you are age 60 or older, says the Centers for Disease Control and Prevention. Shingles can recur, and the vaccine can lower the risk for recurrence. Some people develop shingles even if they have received the vaccination, but the vaccine may reduce the severity and duration of the outbreak.

Mayo Clinic's *Health Letter, www.healthletter.mayoclinic.com*

■ ■ ■ ■

New Heart-Valve Surgery for Seniors

A new heart valve may be better for older patients (see page 177 for more details). The valve, implanted through the groin, may be the only safe way to replace a heart valve in elderly patients who would not survive a standard operation. It works as well as a valve inserted through traditional surgery, but the insertion increases the risk for stroke. Discuss the options with your doctor.

Craig R. Smith, MD, chief, division of cardiothoracic surgery, New York-Presbyterian Hospital/Columbia University Medical Center, New York City, and leader of a study presented at a meeting of the American College of Cardiology in New Orleans.

Bypass Surgery May Be Better Than Angioplasty For Seniors

William Weintraub, MD, John H. Ammon chair of cardiology, Christiana Care Health System, Newark, Delaware.
Gregory Fontana, MD, chairman, cardiothoracic surgery, Lenox Hill Hospital, New York City.
New England Journal of Medicine, online.

Patients over the age of 65 who have severe coronary artery disease fare better with bypass surgery than with minimally invasive angioplasty, a large, recent study indicates.

Although there was no significant difference in mortality after one year, patients who had undergone bypass surgery had a 21% reduced risk of dying after four years compared with those who had received angioplasty, the researchers found.

The trend in cardiology more recently has been to favor angioplasty over surgery, explained study author William Weintraub, MD, John H. Ammon chair of cardiology, Christiana Care Health System, Newark, Delaware.

During angioplasty, cardiologists insert a small "balloon" into the blocked vessel via a catheter. Once in place, the balloon is inflated to widen the vessel. The procedure can be done with or without placing a stent, a wire mesh scaffold that keeps the vessel propped open.

Coronary artery bypass surgery involves grafting part of a healthy vessel onto the blocked vessel to reroute blood flow, "bypassing" the blocked part of the vessel.

But Dr. Weintraub said he did not envision an immediate sea change in clinical practice as the result of these findings.

"People will give surgery another thought, especially for sicker patients," he said. "Rather than being a huge, huge change, this may switch it back a little."

STUDY DETAILS

Dr. Weintraub and his colleagues combined information from two large databases, which included about 200,000 patients, all elderly and all with more than one blood vessel blocked.

About 86,000 underwent surgery and 104,000 had angioplasty. Of those who had angioplasty, 78% received drug-eluting stents, 16% received bare-metal stents and 6% had no stents.

Drug-eluting stents, considered state-of-the-art, ooze a drug out into the artery that prevents scar tissue from building up.

Patients undergoing surgery tended to have more complications such as diabetes, lung disease and heart failure, although the authors did adjust for these factors.

The study was published in the *New England Journal of Medicine.*

EXPERT RESPONSE

Although the study was not a randomized, controlled trial—considered the gold standard of medicine because those studies randomly assign people to different treatments and compares them with those who are untreated—it had several advantages, including the fact that it was looking at a "real-world" population in real time, said Gregory Fontana, MD, chairman of cardiothoracic surgery at Lenox Hill Hospital in New York City.

This older population is very broad and represents probably the largest proportion of individuals who need this type of treatment, Dr. Fontana said, although the results probably can be extrapolated to other groups.

info For more information on bypass surgery, visit the US National Heart, Lung, and Blood Institute Web site at *http://www. nhlbi.nih.gov/health/health-topics/topics/cabg/.*

Medical Newsmakers

Astounding Breakthrough Brings Scientists Closer To Cancer Cure

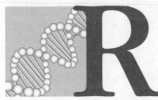Research published in *The New England Journal of Medicine* reported a long-awaited breakthrough in the fight against cancer.

Through the use of gene therapy, two patients who were dying of leukemia were seemingly cured of the disease. The results occurred after immune cells called T-cells were removed from the body, genetically engineered to attack the cancer and returned to the body, where they multiplied 1,000-fold, rapidly destroying more than two pounds of tumors in each patient. A third advanced leukemia patient went into partial remission—a lot, but not all, of the cancer was destroyed.

The research was heralded as a "huge accomplishment." Do these dramatic results mark the beginning of significant advances that may occur with other diseases?

For answers, we spoke with James Wilson, MD, PhD, one of the nation's leading experts on gene therapy...

•**What is gene therapy?** Gene therapy is a new approach for preventing, treating or curing diseases through the alteration of defective genes. Most people know that genes, which reside within the nucleus of each cell, are sequences of DNA that determine a specific trait, such as whether you have blue, green or brown eyes. There are more than 30,000 genes that make us human and make each human unique.

Genes provide the instructions for the manufacture of proteins that allow the body to function. But if genes mutate, they provide faulty instructions. Mutated genes play a role in virtually every disease. This, of course, includes so-called "genetic diseases" such as sickle-cell

James Wilson, MD, PhD, director of the Gene Therapy Program and professor of pathology and laboratory medicine at the University of Pennsylvania Perelman School of Medicine in Philadelphia and editor in chief of *Human Gene Therapy*, one of the leading journals in the field.

anemia and muscular dystrophy, which are caused by an inherited defect in a single gene, but also certain cancers such as leukemia.

Gene therapy attacks various types of disease at their roots—inserting into the cell a normal copy of the gene, which overrides the genetic mutation that causes disease.

•**How is gene therapy different from drug therapy?** When a doctor gives a drug, it treats the symptoms of the disease, not the root cause. And you must take the drug every day (or several times a day)—sometimes indefinitely.

With gene therapy, a normal gene is administered usually via injection or intravenously—sometimes multiple times—to targeted cells. Once there, it should stay active for a very long time and, in some cases, the rest of the person's life, guiding the creation of healthy cells to replace the defective ones.

•**When did gene therapy start?** In the 1980s, scientists began inserting genes into cells in petri dishes. Inserting genes into cells within the human body has proven quite difficult, however.

•**Have those challenges been solved?** The big breakthrough came when scientists realized that the shell and contents of a virus could be used to transport a normal gene into a cell. They engineered the simple genetic sequence, or genome, of a virus, removing two or three viral genes (thereby rendering them harmless), stitching in corrective human genes and then putting this encapsulated "vector" into the body. The genes were also engineered to seek out and find specific types of cells, such as lung, heart, liver or brain cells.

•**What are the risks of gene therapy?** The biggest problem is when the body recognizes the vector as a dangerous virus and mounts an immune response that can lead to inflammation, cancer or even death. Before we recognized this problem, a young man with a genetic disease of the liver died unexpectedly in a clinical trial of gene therapy in 1999. Another problem occurs when the vector inserts its genetic payload into areas of the chromosome that inadvertently activate cancer-causing genes. Needless to say, these issues prompted a search for safer vectors—and it has taken several years.

•**Have safer vectors been found?** Yes, progress has been made. The Gene Therapy Program at the University of Pennsylvania discovered and developed for gene therapy new members of an obscure family of viruses called adeno-associated viruses (AAV). Over the last few years, we have sent these vectors to approximately 1,000 scientists at 450 institutions in 30 countries—and they are now used as the principal vectors in almost all studies on gene therapy. The vectors have proven to be remarkably effective and safe, although we are still encountering and working to solve remaining problems of immune response. To prevent the inadvertent development of cancer, scientists are developing vectors that persist without perturbing our chromosomes in ways that may be harmful.

•**What are the most promising areas for gene therapy?** The most promising are the lethal genetic diseases, such as muscular dystrophy, hemophilia and Tay-Sachs disease—conditions for which there really aren't any other effective therapies. Gene therapy works well for these diseases because they are caused by a single defect in a single gene, and we know what and where that gene is.

Gene therapy is progressing in clinical trials focusing on several other diseases, presumably caused by multiple mutated genes. These diseases include Parkinson's and age-related macular degeneration.

And as the research on leukemia shows, gene therapy may also attack cancer. It works not by targeting cancer cells directly, because they are genetically diverse, but by engineering immune cells with a vector that makes them more efficient at recognizing and killing tumor cells.

•**Can my doctor prescribe gene therapy?** Gene therapy is still in clinical trials. During the next year or two, I expect to see the successful completion of Phase III clinical trials and the introduction of approved gene therapy products for genetic diseases, such as an inherited form of high lipids, hemophilia and inherited blindness. In the next decade, we may well see commercial gene therapy products for diseases such as cancer and Parkinson's.

•What's the best way to find clinical trials that use gene therapy? Check the National Institutes of Health site, *www.clinicaltrials. gov.* Search the key words "gene therapy" to see which of the more than 2,600 trials involving gene therapy are actively recruiting patients.

Doctors Explain Full-Face Transplants

Bohdan Pomahac, MD, director, plastic surgery transplantation program, Brigham & Women's Hospital, Boston.

Daniel S. Alam, MD, head, section of facial aesthetic and reconstructive surgery, Head and Neck Institute, Cleveland Clinic, Ohio.

Edwin F. Williams III, MD, facial plastic surgeon, Albany, New York, vice president, public affairs, American Academy of Facial Plastic and Reconstructive Surgery.

New England Journal of Medicine, online

Full-face transplants were once the stuff of science fiction, but not anymore. So far, 18 such transplants have been done worldwide, and US surgeons recently described the intricate procedures in the online edition of the *New England Journal of Medicine.*

The article details the stories of three face transplants that were performed at Boston's Brigham & Women's Hospital in 2011, including the much-publicized case of Charla Nash, who lost most of her face in a chimpanzee attack.

While some technical challenges remain, surgeons say they are getting better and better at performing face transplants.

"We don't know how common or rare this operation will be, but it is here to stay," said Bohdan Pomahac, MD, director of the plastic surgery transplantation program at Brigham & Women's. He was the lead surgeon on all three cases described in the journal.

WHO GETS A NEW FACE

Who is currently a candidate for a replacement face? According to the doctors, prospective recipients first undergo extensive medical and psychological evaluation. If they are deemed to be appropriate candidates, surgeons then begin their search for suitable donors and start to plan the surgery.

These lengthy and complex surgeries are reserved for individuals with severe facial traumas, but as techniques and technology improve, transplants could become an option for patients with lesser degrees of facial deformity.

OPERATIONS ARE LENGTHY AND UNIQUE

Each operation is unique and can take more than 20 hours to complete. In general, surgeons will first remove any non-viable or injured tissue from the face transplant recipient. The healthy tissue, once procured from a suitable donor, is then attached. This is not a simple task—surgeons must restore blood flow, reattach nerves, muscles and bony structures, and then reconnect each layer of the new face.

Even so, "the hardest part is the recovery of the donor face," Dr. Pomahac said. After the transplant is complete, surgeons must be on the lookout for any signs of rejection and other side effects, such as infection. These risks are highest during the first 24 hours after surgery.

"There can be clotting in the vessels that are re-connected, and we use high doses of immune suppression for a first couple of days so the patient is more susceptible to infection," he explained.

In the beginning, the patient's new face is swollen and has no motion.

"Most of the swelling goes down in six weeks and then you regain motor function in three to six months," Dr. Pomahac said. Many of these patients are eating within a few days. "They get better and better each time we see them," he said.

TRULY A BRAND NEW FACE

Unlike in the movies, the patient does not wake up with the face of the donor, Dr. Pomahac stressed. Instead, the new face is more of a hybrid between donor and recipient. "It is surprisingly easy to get used to," he said. "They have new faces, but they still have a way of speaking and have the same body language."

Another study author, Daniel S. Alam, MD, is the head of the section of facial aesthetic and reconstructive surgery in the Head and Neck Institute at the Cleveland Clinic in Ohio. He said the article in the *New England Journal of Medicine* is important because it is the first time face transplants have been reported as a series of cases.

Dr. Alam was involved with Nash's surgery, and also performed the first US face transplant on gunshot victim Connie Culp in December of 2008.

"Five years ago, we didn't know if this could be done. Full-face transplants can be done technically, they can be done safely and patients can get a lasting benefit," he said.

EXPERTS CONTINUE TO BE WARY

Full-face transplants remain a work in progress. "Surgeons have been taking gall bladders out for years [for example], but we are extremely early in our learning curve for face transplants," Dr. Alam said.

Another expert agreed.

"Face transplants are here to stay," said Edwin F. Williams III, MD, a facial plastic surgeon in Albany, New York, and vice president of public affairs at the American Academy of Facial Plastic and Reconstructive Surgery.

However, he added, "we really need to move forward carefully and they won't be something that happen in every small town and city."

info For more information on some of the issues surrounding face transplants, visit the American Academy of Facial Plastic and Reconstructive Surgery Web site page at *http://www.aafprs.org/media/media_resources/fact_pr021805.html.*

Miracle Transplant Allows Dying Man to Leave Hospital Cancer-Free

The Lancet, news release

A 36-year-old husband and father of two children with an inoperable tumor in his trachea (windpipe) has received the world's first artificial trachea made with stem cells.

A report published online in *The Lancet* described the transplant surgery, which was per-

formed June 2011 at the Karolinska University Hospital in Stockholm, Sweden.

Without the transplant, the authors of the report explained, the man from Reykjavik, Iceland, would have died. A golf ball–sized tumor on his trachea had begun to restrict his breathing. In a 12-hour procedure, doctors completely removed the affected area of his trachea and replaced it with an artificial one.

HOW TO MAKE AN ARTIFICIAL WINDPIPE

The artificial trachea was custom-made using three-dimensional imaging. First, a glass model was built to help shape an artificial scaffold. Stem cells were then inserted into the scaffold to create a functioning airway, the authors explained in a journal news release.

The scientists said their technique is an improvement over other methods because they used the patient's own cells to create the airway so there is no risk of rejection and the patient does not have to take immunosuppressive drugs.

In addition, they noted, because the trachea was custom-made it would be an ideal fit for the patient's body size and shape, and would eliminate the need to remain on a waiting list for a human donor.

"The patient has been doing great for the last four months and has been able to live a normal life. After arriving in Iceland at the start of July, he was one month in hospital and another month in a rehabilitation center," said coauthor of the study and physician who referred the patient for the procedure, Tomas Gudbjartsson, MD, Landspitali University Hospital and University of Iceland, Reykjavik.

The transplant team has since performed another transplant on a second patient from Maryland with cancer of the airway. This patient's bioartificial scaffold, however, was made from nanofibers. They now hope to treat a 13-month-old South Korean infant also using this method.

"We will continue to improve the regenerative medicine approaches for transplanting the windpipe and extend it to the lungs, heart and esophagus. And investigate whether cell therapy could be applied to irreversible diseases of the major airways and lungs," said Dr. Gudbjartsson.

EXPERT RESPONSE

Although the technique shows promise, Harald C. Ott, MD, and Douglas J. Mathisen, MD, from Massachusetts General Hospital and Harvard Medical School in Boston, cautioned that more research must be done to fully evaluate its safety and effectiveness.

"To be adjudged successful, bioartificial organs must function over a long time—short-term clinical function is an important achievement, but is only one measure of success. Choice of ideal scaffold material, optimum cell source, well-defined tissue culture conditions, and perioperative management pose several questions to be answered before the line to broader clinical application of any bioartificial graft can be crossed safely and confidently," Drs. Ott and Mathisen concluded.

info For more information on stem cells, visit the US National Institutes of Health Web site at *http://stemcells.nih.gov/index.asp*.

■ **Follow-Up Report…**

Man Survives Cancer, Thanks to Synthetic Windpipe

An American man is doing well after receiving a synthetic windpipe (trachea) that was created in a laboratory.

Christopher Lyles, 30, of Baltimore had a type of tracheal cancer that is normally considered inoperable, *The New York Times* reported.

Swedish surgeons removed the tumor and replaced Lyles' trachea with a new one made from nano-sized plastic fibers and covered in stem cells taken from his bone marrow.

"He went home in very good shape," said Paolo Macchiarini, MD, director of the Advanced Center for Translational Regenerative Medicine at the Karolinska Institute in Stockholm.

Lyles is only the second person, and the first American, to undergo this kind of procedure.

Big Medical Advances From the Tiniest Particles

Paolo Decuzzi, PhD, vice chair of the department of translational imaging and the department of nanomedicine at The Methodist Hospital Research Institute in Houston, www.methodisthealth.com. He is the director of the Center for the Rational Design of Multifunctional Nanoconstructs.

One of the biggest medical discoveries of the last few decades involves the use of the smallest imaginable particles for treating such conditions as cancer, diabetes and heart disease.

So-called nanomedicine utilizes nanoparticles that, in some cases, measure about 100,000 times narrower than a human hair. These particles are small enough to navigate safely in the circulatory system and perform a variety of crucial functions—for example, they may recognize abnormal cells, slip through cell membranes and, eventually, deliver medications precisely where they're needed, reducing side effects.

To learn how nanomedicine is now being used—and how it may affect treatments in the future—we spoke with Paolo Decuzzi, PhD, a leading authority in this emerging field…

•**Why are nanoparticles so useful in medicine?** Nanoparticles are man-made objects, measured in nanometers (nm)—that is, one-billionth of a meter.

Unlike individual drug molecules, nanoparticles can be engineered to be multifunctional. Nanoparticles can carry different molecules simultaneously, so they can be used for medication, imaging and early disease detection.

•**What are some of the most important current uses of this technology?** Though the technology itself is not widely recognized by the public, one of the first nanodrugs for treating cancer, *doxorubicin hydrochloride liposome* (Doxil), was approved by the FDA several years ago. This potent chemotherapy drug is encased by a liposome, a lipid-based nanoparticle. The drug is used to treat ovarian and breast cancers, leukemia and Kaposi's sarcoma.

Doxorubicin is carried into cells by the nanoparticle. When it's encased in a nanoparticle, more of the active ingredient stays concentrated until it is released into the tumor.

This is critical for preventing or reducing side effects. At the same time, it allows oncologists to use a higher dose because the improved bio-distribution reduces toxicity. A higher dose is more likely to kill all the cancer cells, preventing relapse. A handful of nanodrugs have been approved by the FDA, and many more are in the pipeline for clinical trials.

•**Why is a nanoparticle more "targeted" than an individual molecule?** When you take a conventional drug, the molecules enter the bloodstream and scatter in different directions. Some of the active ingredient will go where it's needed, but most of the molecules will reach and penetrate other tissues, including the liver, kidneys, heart and lungs. This scattershot effect is what causes many of the side effects of chemotherapy and other drug treatments, such as nausea and hair loss.

Currently approved anticancer nanodrugs, however, utilize the *fenestrations* (openings) in tumor blood vessels that are absent or smaller in normal tissue. Most nanodrugs are designed to pass through tumor vessel walls but are too large to enter healthy tissue.

•**Can this work with all cancers?** Potentially, yes—but in different ways. It's complicated because the size of the blood vessel openings varies depending on the type of cancer. Also, the number and/or size of the openings change over the course of the disease. They don't occur uniformly—some areas within a tumor will have these openings, and other areas do not. This limits the effectiveness of treatments. And fenestrations are characteristic in cancer but absent in other diseases.

A new strategy is to develop nanoparticles that are designed to recognize and lodge in the diseased blood vessels rather than cross into the tumor openings. The particles will stick to the outer walls of the blood vessels that supply tumors. Then, they'll release even smaller particles that pass through the blood vessels, deep into the tumor.

•**What other type of nanotreatments are available?** Much of the work is still in experi-

mental stages. Scientists have developed thermal ablation therapy nanoparticles that deliver heat instead of drugs to the diseased tissue. The nanoparticles injected into the body accumulate in tumors. When exposed to an external source of energy, the nanoparticles generate heat, increasing the temperature in the surrounding tissue. Cancer cells start to die when their temperature reaches about 115°F. Different nanoparticles and external energy sources have been proposed and tested.

For example, nanoparticles made out of gold would be warmed by an infrared laser, penetrating a few millimeters deep into the body. Magnetic fields have also been used with iron oxide nanoparticles, and this therapy is currently approved in Europe to treat *glioblastoma multiforme*, a deadly brain tumor.

•**What else can be loaded into nanoparticles?** In theory, nanoparticles can contain almost anything, including drug "cocktails" for treating cancer or other diseases, such as diabetes or heart disease.

We can also create multifunctional nanoparticles that combine imaging and treatment. For example, a nanoparticle could release drug molecules for treating a cancer. Then, it would release imaging agents to show how well the treatment is working. Such nanoparticles are now being created for experimental purposes, but it's too early to predict when the technology may be available for clinical use.

•**And what about heart disease?** It's not possible today, but one of our objectives is to develop nanoparticles that can both diagnose and treat atherosclerosis, the cause of most strokes and heart attacks.

The largest blood vessels in patients with atherosclerosis have multiple unstable plaques, areas where dangerous clots can form very quickly. These areas are difficult to detect with current imaging tools. Nanoparticles can be designed that will cling to and illuminate these areas. They can then be triggered to release drugs that will induce the regression or stabilization of the plaque.

FDA Makes Move to Help Those With Type 1 Diabetes

Charles L. Zimliki, PhD, leader, Artificial Pancreas Working Groups and Critical Path Initiative, US Food and Drug Administration.

The US Food and Drug Administration has issued new guidelines aimed at helping speed up the development of artificial pancreas systems.

If they become a reality, such technologies could make a huge difference for people with type 1 diabetes, who need insulin injections to control their blood sugar and survive.

BACKGROUND

Artificial pancreas systems combine current technologies for continuous blood sugar monitoring and pumps to deliver insulin as needed. These systems are designed to keep patients' insulin levels within normal ranges, by reacting to changes in blood sugar.

So far, however, equipment problems, computer glitches and problems with the insulin used have hampered development of these systems according to the FDA.

"We really are trying to get these devices to the market as quickly as possible," Charles Zimliki, PhD, leader of the FDA's Artificial Pancreas Working Groups and Critical Path Initiative, said during a news conference.

That's why the agency has taken the unusual step of developing a guidance for approval, something which is usually done after a device had been developed and tested, he said.

Dr. Zimliki said he has no idea when an approved device might be available. To date, the FDA has approved more than 20 clinical studies for artificial pancreas systems.

THE PURPOSE OF THE GUIDELINES

The FDA's new guidelines make designing, testing and safety and effectiveness requirements more flexible. For example, they propose more flexibility in the choice of clinical trial outcomes, number of patients needed and the length of the trial.

"We really wanted to make a push; we felt like it was a good idea to give academicians and people that aren't familiar with the regulatory process a pathway to develop these systems," Dr. Zimliki said. "We want people to move these things forward; we think this guidance will allow people to get a safe and effective product on the market quickly."

AN ARTIFICIAL PANCREAS SYSTEM

In type 1 diabetes, the pancreas produces little or no insulin, an essential hormone necessary for controlling blood sugar. People with type 1 diabetes have to monitor their blood sugar throughout the day, and calculate how much insulin they need to lower their blood sugar, which is delivered using a syringe or insulin pump.

An artificial pancreas system combines an insulin pump and a continuous glucose monitor with a sensor placed under the patient's skin. The pump and monitor work together, tracking blood sugar and automatically pumping measured doses of insulin as determined by a computer algorithm.

These systems help eliminate, or reduce the severity of dangerous drops in blood sugar by stopping insulin administration when blood sugar levels near a predetermined threshold.

The device is not a cure, but it might reduce dangerous high and low blood sugar levels, giving patients a better quality of life and reducing the risk of diabetes-related complications, the FDA said.

RECOMMENDATIONS FOR TRIALS

The new guidelines recommend a three-phase clinical study progression "so that studies may move to an outpatient setting as quickly as possible." The agency is also suggesting other ways to streamline the testing process, including ways to use existing safety and effectiveness data for the components that make up the system, and allowing data from clinical studies done outside of the United States to be used in the approval process.

In addition, those conducting the clinical trials have the option of demonstrating that the system controls blood sugar as well as standard therapies, or showing that it gives better blood sugar control when compared with other therapies.

"When final, the guidance will help manufacturers and investigators assemble submissions for clinical trials as well as product-approval submissions," the FDA said.

HURDLES TO OVERCOME

Hurdles in developing these systems include making sure the implanted sensors remain clear, the need to periodically recalibrate blood sugar monitors, problems with the software needed to operate insulin infusion pumps, problems creating algorithms to deliver insulin that take into account how long it takes the body to absorb it, the need for a faster-acting insulin and the overall development of safer and more reliable algorithms.

Another issue is the lack of a glucagon formulation that can be used in infusion pumps. Glucagon is a hormone used to treat severe low blood sugar. "There is a need for a glucagon formulation that is stable over several days and can be delivered by an infusion pump," the FDA said.

info For more on type 1 diabetes, visit the Web site of the Nemours Foundation, *http://kids health.org/parent/medical/endocrine/type1.html.*

Promising Malaria Vaccine May Save Children's Lives

Tsiri Agbenyega, PhD, principal investigator and chair, Clinical Trials Partnership Committee.

Kenneth Bromberg, MD, chairman of pediatrics and director, Vaccine Research Center, Brooklyn Hospital Center, New York City.

Andrew Witty, chief executive officer, GlaxoSmithKline plc, Middlesex, England.

Bruce Hirsch, MD, attending physician in infectious diseases, North Shore University Hospital, Manhasset, New York.

US Centers for Disease Control and Prevention news release

New England Journal of Medicine

In an important first, a new vaccine has been shown to cut the risk of malaria in young African children by about half, according to researchers.

Although the effectiveness shown in this Phase 3 trial is far less than the near-100% effectiveness often seen in childhood vaccines for other illnesses in the West, the findings are promising, given that malaria kills some 800,000 people in sub-Saharan Africa alone each year.

"This potentially translates into [the prevention of] tens of millions of cases of malaria in children," said Tsiri Agbenyega, PhD, a principal investigator of the trial.

Other experts agreed.

A VACCINE FIRST

"This is really important because it's a viable strategy against a major killer of children in the world," added Kenneth Bromberg, MD, chairman of pediatrics and director of the Vaccine Research Center at the Brooklyn Hospital Center, New York City.

This is also the first vaccine that is successful against a parasite—in this case, *Plasmodium falciparum*, which causes mosquito-transmitted malaria.

The results—the first from the Phase 3 trial—were announced at the Malaria Forum hosted by the Bill & Melinda Gates Foundation in Seattle, and published simultaneously online in *The New England Journal of Medicine.*

The trial was funded by GlaxoSmithKline (GSK) Biologicals and the PATH Malaria Vaccine Initiative, which are developing the vaccine together with African research centers.

Speaking at a news briefing, Andrew Witty, CEO of GSK, said he is "hopeful we're going to be able to bring the vaccine to children in Africa perhaps as early as 2015."

DETAILS OF THE TRIAL

The trial enrolled more than 15,400 children from seven countries in sub-Saharan Africa in two age groups: six to 12 weeks old and five to 17 months.

Children were assigned to one of two groups, one receiving the vaccine (called RTS,S/AS01) and the other receiving a placebo. Seventy-five percent of both groups also followed conventional preventive measures, namely the use of insecticide-treated bed nets in the home.

The announcement addressed only the results from 6,000 children in the older age group who were followed for a year after vaccination.

For infants five to 17 months old, three doses of the vaccine reduced the rate of severe malaria by 47% and less-severe cases, characterized by fever and chills, by 56%. Severe malaria can affect the blood, brain or kidneys and can be fatal.

EVALUATING THE RESULTS

The less impressive results in regards to the more severe malaria cases was not surprising given that similar results had been seen in the Phase 2 trial, said Dr. Agbenyega, who is also chair of the Clinical Trials Partnership Committee, a collaboration of scientists, academic partners and others engaged in malaria prevention.

"Obviously, one would want to have higher efficacy when it comes to severe disease, but we're hoping we can still improve on the vaccine as we go along," he added.

In both groups together, the vaccine cut the rate of malaria by about 35%.

"Children have a relative immune deficiency between the time they lose their antibodies from their mother until their own immune system kicks in at six to nine months," explained Bruce Hirsch, MD, attending physician in infectious diseases at North Shore University Hospital in Manhasset, New York. "A vaccine like this could help bridge that gap."

While noting that the results were "gratifying," Dr. Hirsch also cautioned that "the efficacy rate is not 100% and…these are preliminary results."

SIDE EFFECTS OF THE TREATMENT

Side effects were about the same in both groups and "were what you might typically see with other childhood vaccines—low-grade fever and some swelling at point of injection," said Dr. Agbenyega.

Seizures in participants were attributed to malaria.

FURTHER DATA AWAITED

Data on the six- to 12-week age group should be available by the end of 2012, said Dr. Agbenyega.

The authors are also awaiting 30-month follow-up safety and efficacy data by the end of 2014.

Calling the trial results a "promising advance," the US Centers for Disease Control and Prevention said the vaccine builds on already successful efforts to beat back malaria in poorer countries.

"The vaccine provided this protection in settings where there is ongoing use of other effective malaria prevention and treatment interventions: bed nets, antimalarial drugs, indoor residual insecticide spraying to prevent mosquito-borne transmission, and drugs to protect pregnant women and their fetuses from malaria's adverse effects," the CDC said in a news release.

Efforts to help prevent malaria in these ways are working, the agency said, and "many countries have seen decreases of up to 50% in deaths of children younger than five years."

The final results of the vaccine trial will eventually be submitted to health regulators in Europe and elsewhere for approval. There are no plans to file for approval from the US Food and Drug Administration at this point.

According to Witty, GSK plans to make the vaccine available "at the lowest price possible," with only a 5% profit margin, which will be reinvested into research into malaria and "other neglected tropical diseases."

info Learn more about malaria at the US Centers for Disease Control and Prevention Web site, *www.cdc.gov/MALARIA/.*

■ ■ ■ ■

Measles on the Rise

Did you know that the largest measles outbreak in 15 years is due to unvaccinated travelers from Europe? In 2011 there were more than 10,000 cases of measles and at least six deaths in France alone…and thousands more cases have been reported in 38 European countries. According to the Centers for Disease Control and Prevention, 222 cases of measles were reported in the US alone (the average is 60 per year). The CDC advises that all adults and children update their measles vaccinations.

William Schaffner, MD, infectious disease expert, professor and chair of preventive medicine, Vanderbilt University School of Medicine, Nashville.

Centers for Disease Control and Prevention.

■ ■ ■ ■

Important Test for Boomers

Everyone born between 1945 and 1965 should be tested for hepatitis C. Most people with the virus acquire the infection 20 to 40 years before having any symptoms. If an infection is detected, drug treatment reduces the likelihood of serious consequences, such as cirrhosis and liver cancer, by about 97%. Universal testing would detect 800,000 new cases of hepatitis C and prevent 82,000 deaths.

One reason baby boomers are at increased risk: They may have had transfusions before the blood supply was fully monitored.

Robert G. Gish, MD, professor of medicine and codirector of Center for Hepatobiliary Disease and Abdominal Transplantation, University of California, San Diego School of Medicine.

■ ■ ■ ■

New Lyme Disease Defense

Delays in the diagnosis and treatment of Lyme disease can lead to muscle, nerve and organ damage.

Self-defense: An experimental antibiotic gel, applied soon after a tick bite, kills bacteria before it can spread and cause infection, according to German researchers.

Fraunhofer Institute for Cell Therapy.

How Your "Body Clock" Affects Your Health

Steve A. Kay, PhD, dean and Richard C. Atkinson Chair in the division of biological sciences at the University of California, San Diego, where he is also a Distinguished Professor of Cell and Developmental Biology.

For most of us, our bodies need a day or two to adjust when we travel across time zones or change the clock.

But increasing evidence now shows that chronic (or even occasional) interruptions in our circadian rhythms—the 24-hour cycles that regulate sleep and wakefulness—may affect our health more than we thought.

What's new: The brain used to be considered the body's only biological "clock." Now researchers are finding that many cells in the body have "clock genes" that regulate their activity—for example, organs such as the liver also have cycles.

WHAT IS CHRONOBIOLOGY?

Chronobiology is the study of circadian rhythms—the body's 24-hour cycles of physical, mental and behavioral changes. Light and darkness are the main factors that influence one's circadian rhythms, affecting the body's temperature, sleep-wake cycles, hormone release and other key bodily functions.

WHEN BODY CLOCKS FALTER

Exposure to light is one of the main factors for maintaining, or changing, our daily rhythms. And our modern society has essentially turned night into day with near-constant exposure to lights, TVs, computers and other electronic gadgets. In many cases, our bodies haven't adapted, and it's putting us at increased risk for health problems.

Age is also a factor. Older adults tend to have a weaker circadian orchestration of physiology, which means the body's clocks are less able to work together—a problem that has been linked to heart disease.

What you can do: Here's how to help manage your body's internal clocks so that you minimize your risk for health problems, such as…

DEPRESSION

Seasonal affective disorder (SAD), in which episodes of depression increase in the fall and winter when there are fewer hours of daylight, is thought to be caused in part by changes in the circadian cycles.

Simple self-defense: Light therapy, which involves the use of indoor light that mimics sunlight.

Light boxes, available at many pharmacies and online retailers for about $100 to $400, are typically used for a half hour or longer each morning. Exposure to the light increases alertness, and repeated exposure can help fight SAD.

Caution: If you have cataracts, glaucoma or another eye condition…or take medications that increase your skin's sensitivity to light, be sure to consult a doctor before using a light box. In addition, light boxes may trigger mania in people with bipolar disorder.

HEART ATTACK

More than half of heart attacks occur in the six hours between about 6 am and noon. The greater frequency probably is due to several circadian factors, including body position—most people experience about a 10-to-25-point increase in systolic (top number) blood pressure when they rise from bed in the morning. What's more, people who have a heart attack in the morning are likely to suffer more damage to the heart than those who have heart attacks later in the day.

Recent finding: In a study published in *Heart*, researchers analyzed data from 811 patients who had suffered heart attacks. Those whose attacks occurred in the morning were found to have about a 20% larger infarct, an area of dead tissue, than those whose attacks happened later in the day. It's not known why morning heart attacks are more severe.

Caution: In most people, blood pressure rises in the morning, then dips slightly in the afternoon and falls during sleep. However, some people don't have these periodic declines. Known as "non-dippers," they're more likely to have a heart attack than those who experience normal cycling.

Simple self-defense: Get out of bed slowly. In addition, because high blood pressure is a leading risk factor for heart attack, people who take blood pressure–lowering medication may benefit from timing it so that they get the greatest reduction in the morning.

Example: The blood pressure medication *verapamil* (such as Verelan PM) is meant to be taken at bedtime. The active ingredient isn't released during the first hours of sleep (when blood pressure is already low)—more is released in the morning, the time when blood pressure rises. Other drugs that are designed to provide greater benefit when taken at night include timed-release versions of *diltiazem* (Cardizem LA) and *propranolol* (InnoPran XL). If you take blood pressure medication, ask your doctor about timed-release drugs—or if you could take your current medication at night.

ASTHMA

People with asthma are more likely to need emergency treatment between 10 am and 11 am than at other times of the day, research has shown. The use of rescue inhalers also increases during the morning.

Reason: Lung movements are reduced during sleep and soon after waking up. This impairs the elimination of mucus, which can lead to congestion and difficulty breathing several hours later.

Simple self-defense: If you have asthma and use a bronchodilator, such as one containing *theophylline* (Uniphyl), talk to your doctor about taking your last dose of the day a few hours before bedtime. This allows the active ingredients to increase through the night and reach peak levels in the morning.

DIABETES

Several studies have shown that people with poor sleep habits (especially those who sleep five or fewer hours per night) are more likely to be overweight—and have a higher risk for diabetes. Now researchers are speculating that disruptions in circadian rhythms may be to blame.

Recent research: In lab studies, mice with a genetic mutation in the part of the brain that synchronizes circadian rhythms ate all day instead of just in the evening, the time that they're normally active. They were more likely to be obese and also had high blood sugar.

Why does this occur? A protein called *cryptochrome* stimulates the production of *hepatic glucose*, a sugar used for energy. In humans, cryptochrome is normally suppressed during the day, when energy is supplied by eating, and increased at night to provide energy while we're sleeping. Research has shown that a disruption in sleep-wake cycles causes a prolonged elevation of cryptochrome and an increased risk for obesity and diabetes.

Simple self-defense: To help minimize your risk for weight gain and diabetes, be sure to keep a regular sleep schedule. Go to bed at the same time every night, and get up at the same time in the morning. Aim for seven to eight hours' sleep each night, and don't change your routine on weekends. If you work at night, use heavy curtains to block sunlight, and turn off telephones so that you can sleep during the day.

DROWSINESS

Feel drowsy after lunch? Blame your circadian rhythms. It's normal for body temperature, blood pressure, metabolism and cognitive abilities to decline in the afternoon.

The peak mental hours for most adults are from about 7 am or 8 am until early afternoon. This is followed by a brief (one- to two-hour) dip, after which energy rises again until later in the evening.

Simple self-defense: If your job and lifestyle allow it, take a brief (20- to 30-minute) nap in the afternoon. Or, if that's not possible, try to schedule less demanding tasks during the "dip" period.

Melatonin: New Help For Heartburn

Mark A. Stengler, NMD, licensed naturopathic medical doctor in private practice, Stengler Center for Integrative Medicine, Encinitas, California…adjunct associate clinical professor at the National College of Natural Medicine, Portland, Oregon…author of many books, including *The Natural Physician's Healing Therapies* and coauthor of *Prescription for Natural Cures* (both from Bottom Line Books).

We tend to think of melatonin, often called the "sleep hormone," in terms of—you guessed it—sleep. So what does melatonin have to do with your digestion? The answer is a lot, according to new research. It turns out that this hormone, in addition to regulating our sleep/wake cycle, also can help gastroesophageal reflux disease (GERD). This is very good news!

Known for its symptoms of acid reflux or heartburn, GERD is a very common condition that occurs when the lower esophageal sphincter—the valve between the esophagus and the stomach—relaxes at the wrong time, allowing gastric acid to escape from the stomach into the esophagus. The result is pain and a burning sensation in the chest and throat. Over time, the acid exposure from GERD can damage the esophagus, even causing cancer and other serious conditions.

Melatonin as an effective treatment is exciting news because there are many possible dangerous side effects (such as bone fractures and stomach disorders) that can occur with popular medications for GERD—namely, proton-pump inhibitors (PPIs) and H2 receptor antagonists, which work by suppressing stomach acid production. One study even suggests that their long-term use may increase risk for cognitive decline.

THE MELATONIN BREAKTHROUGH

Melatonin is a naturally occurring hormone that is made in various parts of the body. When produced by the brain's pineal gland (which happens whenever you're exposed to darkness), melatonin has a strong influence on circadian rhythms and encourages sleep. It also has many other beneficial effects. Preliminary studies show that it is an effective treatment for migraine, obesity and seasonal affective disorder.

What many people don't know: The gastrointestinal (GI) tract secretes up to 500 times as much melatonin as the pineal gland. Researchers have determined that the hormone plays an important role in the GI system by preventing oxidative stress on GI cells…regulating cholesterol uptake by the intestinal wall…helping to heal damage to the lining of the GI tract…and promoting the secretion of other hormones that aid digestion and elimination. Studies have shown that supplementing with melatonin can help to treat esophageal ulcers, dyspepsia (upset stomach) and irritable bowel syndrome.

Now there is evidence that melatonin supplements also alleviate GERD symptoms.

One possible reason: Melatonin has been found to reduce gastric acid secretion (although not to the degree of PPIs) and to normalize pressure of the lower esophageal sphincter, allowing it to close more effectively.

In one study, published in *Journal of Pineal Research,* GERD patients received a daily supplement of 6 milligrams (mg) of melatonin, along with L-tryptophan, vitamin B-6, folic acid, vitamin B-12, methionine and betaine (the additional nutrients were administered for their anti-inflammatory and analgesic effects). An equal number of subjects were treated with daily 20-mg doses of the PPI *omeprazole.* Remarkably, after 40 days, 100% of the melatonin group reported no noticeable GERD symptoms, compared with just 65% of the omeprazole group.

My advice: I recommend that patients with GERD take 3 mg to 6 mg daily of melatonin 30 minutes before bedtime. I recommend the sublingual form for those who have trouble falling asleep or the time-release form if they tend to wake up during the night. If you have no obvious sleep problems, take a close look at your sleep pattern and determine if you have a tendency to either struggle when falling asleep or wake at night—and take the form accordingly. Melatonin is not recommended for children or for women who are pregnant.

Chin Up! Why These Implants Are on the Rise

American Society of Plastic Surgeons, news release

The number of American women and men having cosmetic chin surgery increased drastically in 2011, according to the American Society of Plastic Surgeons.

The growth in chin augmentation procedures was greater than breast augmentation, Botox injections and liposuction combined.

Reasons for the boom in chin augmentation may include increased use of video-chat technology, an aging baby boomer population and a desire to improve work success, suggested a society news release.

VIDEO CHATS CREATE PUSH FOR CHIN FIXES

"The chin and jaw line are among the first areas to show signs of aging," said Malcolm Roth, MD, president of the society. "We also know that as more people see themselves on video-chat technology, they may notice that their jaw line is not as sharp as they want it to be. Chin implants can make a dramatic difference."

There were nearly 21,000 chin augmentations last year, a 71% increase from 2010, according to the release. Women had nearly 10,100 procedures, a 66% increase, and men had almost 10,600 procedures, a 76% increase.

Among younger adults, ages 20 to 29, 2,750 underwent augmentations, representing a 68% increase. Among those ages 30 to 39, nearly 2,600 had the procedure, a 69% increase.

Numbers increased with age: There were more than 5,000 chin surgeries in adults ages 40 to 54, marking a 77% increase. For those 55 and older, nearly 8,500 procedures were performed, a 70% increase.

Other cosmetic procedures that increased in 2011 were: Lip augmentations (49%), cheek implants (47%), laser skin resurfacing (9%), soft-tissue fillers (7%) and facelift (5%).

info The US Department of Health and Human Services Office of Women's Health has more about cosmetic surgery at its Web site *www.womenshealth.gov.* Click on "A-Z Health Topics," then "Body Image."

Amazing Device Helps Paralyzed Walk

Steven Kirshblum, MD, medical director and director, Spinal Cord Injury Services, Kessler Institute for Rehabilitation, West Orange, New Jersey.

Kim Anderson-Erisman, PhD, education director, Miami Project to Cure Paralysis, University of Miami Miller School of Medicine.

Mike Rhode, Monmouth Beach, New Jersey.

Veteran ski patrol member Mike Rhode was speeding down a snowy slope at Hunter Mountain in New York when his ski unexpectedly popped off.

Rhode, then a member of the ski patrol for 13 years, could not regain his balance before hitting a fence. Now, tragically, he is paralyzed from the chest down.

But in October 2011, 10 months after the accident, Rhode was able to walk again with the assistance of Ekso, a robotic "exoskeleton" that he and five other testers "wore" on their body during an initial trial, enabling them to stand up and even take steps.

"I was upright for an hour and 10 minutes and was actually walking for 31 minutes," said Rhode. "It was such a positive feeling."

ROBOTIC MECHANICS PROVIDE MOBILITY

Ekso is one of just a few robotic "exoskeletons" giving paraplegics and quadraplegics something they may never have dreamed of before: the ability to stand and walk on their own again.

With the Ekso that Rhode tested, "the therapist controls the sit-to-stand and moving forward," explains Steven Kirshblum, MD, medical director and director of Spinal Cord Injury Services at the Kessler Institute for Rehabilitation in West Orange, New Jersey.

All Rhode had to do was start pushing out of his wheelchair as he had done many times before and the Ekso, as manipulated by the therapist, did the rest.

MODEL FOR HOME USE DUE OUT SOON

A clinical model is due out "very soon," said Dr. Kirshblum. It will be modified for home use and will have the ability to negotiate stairs.

The updated model will also allow the individual patient to control the device, he said.

"This will occur via wireless communication between the crutches and the sensors on the exoskeleton, assuring the individual is in the appropriate position and is safe to undertake the movements," explained Dr. Kirshblum.

Ekso improves on other exoskeletons in that it doesn't use electrodes to stimulate the muscles. The problem with electrodes, Dr. Kirshblum said, is that the energy expenditure to get a muscle to contract is enormous.

With less energy required, Ekso's developers hope users can travel farther on their own.

Right now, Ekso is mainly intended for use in therapy settings, and researchers at the Kessler Institute and elsewhere will study its impact on bone strength, muscle, bowel and bladder function, blood pressure and quality of life.

EXPERTS WEIGH IN

Kim Anderson-Erisman, PhD, education director for the Miami Project to Cure Paralysis at the University of Miami Miller School of Medicine, envisions exoskeletons one day helping other types of patients, such as stroke survivors and people with traumatic brain injury or multiple sclerosis. "Anything that would lead to muscle weakness," she explained.

"This could potentially be something that they could use to help train and strengthen their muscles so that they might be able to eventually walk on their own," said Dr. Anderson-Erisman.

Of course, more research is needed first to see if exoskeletons could actually help build up muscle, she added.

RECOVERY AND MONEY

Ekso can help people move, but will it prompt neurological recovery?

Dr. Kirshblum couldn't say. But whatever its use, the price will have to come down considerably, said Dr. Anderson-Erisman.

Dr. Kirshblum also wouldn't say how much Ekso will cost, but one estimate put the price at $100,000.

"This would have to be something insurance would pay for and I don't think that's in the immediate future," said Dr. Anderson-Erisman.

In 2012, the Kessler Institute embarked on a clinical trial with Ekso, a trial Rhode hopes to join.

"Hopefully, I'll be able to use it again," said Rhode, who has not used Ekso since October 2011, when he was one of six adults, and the only quadriplegic, to test the device.

"I think it's going to be a great tool for therapy right now, to get people up and walking and weight-bearing," Rhode said. "Until possibly they do come up with a cure, it will keep people's legs strong."

info The National Spinal Cord Injury Association (*www.spinalcord.org*) has more information on spinal cord injuries and disorders.

Technology May Help You Kick The Habit

Jed E. Rose, PhD, medical research professor, department of psychiatry, Duke Center for Nicotine and Smoking Cessation Research, Durham, North Carolina.
Biological Psychiatry news release

In smokers, stimulating the brain in certain ways can manipulate their cravings for cigarettes, researchers have found. The finding could lead to new treatments to help people kick the habit, according to the authors of the study published in the journal *Biological Psychiatry*.

BRAIN IMAGING TECHNOLOGY AT WORK

Using brain imaging technology, researchers from Duke University Medical Center identified several regions of the cerebral cortex and the limbic system, which is involved in emotion, that are activated during cravings. Based on these studies, they used noninvasive magnetic stimulation of these areas of the brain in an attempt to manipulate these cravings.

"We directly stimulated a frontal brain region using magnetic fields and showed that it exaggerated smokers' craving for cigarettes when they viewed smoking-related cues. By gaining a better understanding of how the brain influences craving responses, strategies for blocking these responses can be devised and ultimately, more effective smoking cessation treatments may be developed," explained one of the study authors, Jed Rose, PhD, in a journal news release.

HIGH-FREQUENCY STIMULATION

Although low-frequency stimulation did not reduce smokers' cravings, high-frequency stimulation did have this effect when participants were viewing nonsmoking cues, the researchers found. They also noted that high-frequency stimulation reduced the ability of cigarettes to satisfy smokers' cravings, an effect that helps keep them addicted.

More research is needed to explore how this could lead to new treatments to help smokers quit, the authors pointed out.

"This elegant study implicates the superior frontal gyrus in controlling the activity of the craving circuit," John Krystal, MD, editor of *Biological Psychiatry*, said in the news release. "Additional research will be needed to determine the potential value of repetitive [transcranial magnetic stimulation] as a treatment for smoking."

info The Web site of the US Centers for Disease Control and Prevention has more about the health effects of smoking at *http://www.cdc.gov/tobacco/basic_information/index.htm*.

■ ■ ■ ■

Pain-Free Injections?

Researchers are developing tiny, silk-based needles that incorporate precise doses of medication. The needles penetrate the skin without reaching the nerves, which could eliminate discomfort.

Advanced Functional Materials.

■ ■ ■ ■

Safer Spinal Surgery

Spinal surgery and certain chest surgeries have serious potential complications such as paraparesis (partial paralysis of lower limbs), paraplegia (paralysis of the legs and/or trunk) and quadriplegia (paralysis of the arms and legs).

Latest development: The American Academy of Neurology recently issued guidelines recommending that electrical functioning of the spinal cord be monitored during surgery so that the surgeon can address problems before damage occurs.

Marc Nuwer, MD, PhD, chief of clinical neurophysiology, University of California, Los Angeles.

Drug Helps Seriously Ill Enjoy Their Last Months

Roland R. Griffiths, PhD, The Johns Hopkins University School of Medicine, Baltimore.

Could a drug help dying people arrive at a place of serenity and acceptance so they truly enjoy their last months and are able to say their goodbyes and leave loved ones feeling peaceful, too?

Researchers at Johns Hopkins University—along with others at New York University and University of California, Los Angeles—are making great progress with a drug that can be used to help produce intense, mystical insights that almost always create a spiritually uplifting, transcendent experience and put seriously ill patients at ease about facing their mortality.

SOUNDS LIKE...?

If you're thinking this sounds something like what used to be called "dropping acid," you're not far off. The drug is called *psilocybin* and it is indeed the active agent in "magic mushrooms." It produces effects quite similar to those of LSD, mescaline and ayahuasca. Lead study author Roland R. Griffiths, PhD, a psychopharmacologist at Johns Hopkins, has spent the last decade studying how psilocybin might be put to good use not only for end-of-life care but also for those who are deeply distressed over a cancer diagnosis.

It's important to note that we're not talking about recreational use of this (or any) potent drug. Psilocybin is being explored in scientific clinical trials in which the drug is administered under carefully controlled and medically supervised conditions, Dr. Griffiths said. The doses administered are precise, and volunteers are supervised by trained professionals who provide reassurance and guidance if negative side effects (such as anxiety, panic or paranoia) arise. And this can sometimes happen. Equally important, people with a history of schizophrenia (their own or a family member's) are screened out, because in rare cases psilocybin may trigger a psychosis.

GETTING IT RIGHT

This latest study, published in the online medical journal *Psychopharmacology*, explored the effects of several different doses of psilocybin on healthy adults. The study showed that the best effects occurred when participants received lower psilocybin doses before the higher doses. These participants were more likely to have long-lasting positive changes in attitudes and behavior—such as improved relationships with family and others, increased physical and psychological self-care, and increased devotion to spiritual practice.

Explaining that the insights and their meaning vary from person to person, Dr. Griffith said that some patients are able to see their experience of life as more sacred and meaningful… others understand their life experiences as part of a larger story and feel a sense of continuity with what will happen after they're gone. "In some instances," he said, "a person might say that though he or she doesn't know what happens at death, he now has a sense of a larger picture and a feeling that all of life is beautiful and working just as it should."

A NEW VISION OF THE END OF LIFE

In Dr. Griffiths's view, psilocybin has the potential to literally transform our culture's approach to death and dying. "I am convinced," he said, "that there is an important, replicable phenomenon here that is remarkable—and it has important implications on many levels."

info You can learn more about this clinical trial at *www.cancer-insight.org,* or call 410-550-5590 for more information.

Men's Health

New Prostate Cancer Treatment Plan

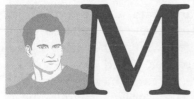

More than 33,000 American men die from prostate cancer annually. But this type of cancer can also be relatively harmless, growing slowly, if at all, and never spreading beyond the gland itself.

This poses a dilemma: While a life-threatening condition requires aggressive action, the standard treatments for any form of prostate cancer—including the slow-growing kinds—are surgery and/or radiation, and these treatments can result in impotence and/or incontinence in a significant number of men.

For cancer confined to the prostate when diagnosed, one strategy has been watchful waiting—doing nothing unless a patient develops symptoms indicating that the cancer has spread. This was usually reserved for men with limited life expectancy (typically less than 10 years) and those who have significant other health problems or whose medical condition made surgery or radiation inadvisable. *But there are two newer, more effective, approaches...*

•**Active surveillance,** which is for men of any age whose cancer looks unlikely to progress quickly. With this strategy, the situation is closely monitored with regular tests—beyond digital rectal exams and prostate-specific antigen (PSA) tests. If the cancer seems to be growing, treatment is initiated.

•**Active holistic surveillance,** which adds diet and lifestyle changes to optimize the odds that a minor prostate cancer will stay that way.

NOT FOR EVERYONE

In December 2011, a panel of experts convened by the National Institutes of Health (NIH) reviewed available research and endorsed active surveillance as "a viable option that should

Aaron E. Katz, MD, chairman of urology at Winthrop University Hospital in Mineola, New York. He is author of *The Definitive Guide to Prostate Cancer: Everything You Need to Know About Conventional and Integrative Therapies* (Rodale).

be offered to patients with low-risk prostate cancer."

According to the NIH committee, 100,000 of the 240,000 American men diagnosed annually with prostate cancer might be candidates for active surveillance. (Right now, only 10% of them are treated this way. The other 90% go on to some form of treatment, usually surgery or radiation.)

Active surveillance may be considered an option if the cancer is confined to the prostate, and lab tests and biopsy results indicate the tumor is unlikely to become dangerous. This calculation takes into account the concentration of PSA circulating in the blood...the Gleason score, which is based on the pathologist's reading of the cells and estimates of how aggressive the tumor will be...and the amount of cancerous tissue in the biopsy.

Ultimately, it's a decision for you and your doctor to make together. If you have other chronic diseases that make surgery or radiation especially risky, this can weigh in favor of active surveillance. But if the idea of leaving cancer in your body makes you unbearably anxious despite the low risk that it will progress, the approach is not for you.

ACTIVE-SURVEILLANCE STRATEGIES

PSA testing every few months is part of active surveillance. A marked increase in PSA indicates the need for more extensive tests.

Many doctors also repeat the prostate biopsy periodically, sometimes as often as every year, to see if the cancer has become more aggressive. But because biopsy is invasive and carries a small risk for infection and inflammation, some opt for an annual MRI or ultrasound instead, performing a biopsy only when rising PSA, MRI findings and/or symptoms, such as increased difficulty urinating, suggest the situation may have worsened. If this is the case, standard treatments for prostate cancer are usually necessary.

ACTIVE HOLISTIC STRATEGIES

In addition to keeping tabs on your cancer, you can enhance the body's natural defenses and attack the processes that support the growth of cancer by...

•**Fighting free radicals.** These highly active molecules, produced in the course of normal metabolism and increased by toxic chemicals and certain foods, damage healthy cells and allow cancer to flourish. Diet improves the body's own antioxidant system.

•**Reducing chronic inflammation.** The immune system produces chemicals and mobilizes cells to attack infection and heal injury. But when inflammation becomes chronic, it creates a steady stream of free radicals that damage cells and promote cancer growth.

PROTECTIVE DIET

The eating plan to subdue low-risk prostate cancer includes elements of the Mediterranean diet and traditional Japanese diet that are recommended for cardiovascular and brain health as well.

Key elements...

•**Consume plenty of fruits and vegetables.** Cruciferous vegetables (such as broccoli and cauliflower), highly colored fruits (especially berries), and garlic and onions are particularly rich in antioxidants and other cancer-fighting chemicals.

•**Include nuts and seeds,** which appear to reduce prostate cancer risk.

•**Avoid saturated fats,** which promote inflammation, and eliminate or limit red meat, which is associated with higher rates of advanced prostate cancer. Cured meats (such as bacon or salami), processed meat (such as cold cuts) and—especially—grilled, charred meats increase cancer risk and should be avoided.

•**Eat fatty fish** (such as wild-caught salmon or sardines) at least one or two times a week for its inflammation-fighting omega-3 fatty acids.

•**Substitute whole grains for foods with refined flour and sugar** (they promote inflammation).

•**Limit dairy products**—high dairy intake corresponds to higher risk for prostate cancer, probably due to its fat and calcium content.

•**Watch your weight**—obesity promotes oxidation and inflammation and alters hormones in a way that increases risk for aggressive prostate cancers.

SUPPLEMENT POWER

In addition to diet, nutritional and herbal supplements add protective power. *The most important...*

•**Vitamin D.** Most people don't get enough of this nutrient, which normalizes cell activity and thus may reduce the risk for cancer. Ask your doctor to test your blood level of vitamin D. If it is below 50 ng/ml, take a supplement.

•**Fish oil.** It can be hard to get enough omega-3 fatty acids in the diet. Therefore, some men may benefit from fish oil supplements (1 g to 4 g daily). Check with your doctor first if you take a blood thinner.

•**Anti-inflammatory herbs.** Certain herbs—such as turmeric, rosemary and holy basil—and green tea have strong anti-inflammatory effects. The supplement products Zyflamend (New Chapter) and ProstaCaid (EcoNugenics), which combine these herbs and others, have been shown to fight prostate cancer. Both products are available online and at health-food stores.

AN OUNCE OF PREVENTION

Men with low-risk prostate cancer who followed a program of exercise and stress reduction combined with a low-fat, plant-based diet were significantly less likely to need conventional treatment within the next two years, compared with a control group, according to recent research.

It's not surprising. Exercise reduces inflammation and enhances immune protection. Reducing stress lowers inflammation and promotes cellular repair. *What to do...*

•**Exercise at least a half hour a day—** brisk walking, biking or swimming—at a pace that seems comfortable. Add strength training three times a week to build muscle.

•**Incorporate a stress-reducing activity into your daily schedule.** Relaxation exercises, such as yoga or meditation, are ideal, but anything that releases tension (reading, listening to music) will be helpful.

IS IT SAFE TO WAIT?

Delaying treatment does not seem to risk a worse outcome. Results from a 2011 multicenter study of 731 men diagnosed with early-stage prostate cancer showed that those who had no initial treatment were no more likely to die in the next 12 years than those who had surgery.

Additionally, in a recent study at Johns Hopkins University, none of 769 participants in an active-surveillance program died of prostate cancer in the 15 years after being diagnosed, and 41% had no need for surgery or radiation.

The Truth About Life After Prostate Cancer

Arnold Melman, MD, professor of urology at Albert Einstein College of Medicine in New York City, where he also has a private practice. A former president of the Society for the Study of Impotence, he specializes in prostate surgery and the diagnosis and treatment of male sexual dysfunction. He is author, with Rosemary E. Newnham, of After Prostate Cancer: A What-Comes-Next Guide to a Safe and Informed Recovery *(Oxford University).*

Roughly two million American men are now living with prostate cancer or the aftereffects of treatment.

That's largely because the ability to detect and treat prostate cancer has greatly improved. Now, about 90% of the nearly 250,000 American men who are diagnosed with the disease each year are alive at least 15 years after treatment.

The downside: Surgery and radiation, the main treatments, can cause serious side effects, including erectile dysfunction (ED) and incontinence.

Important recent study: Nearly half of men who had surgery for prostate cancer expected to have a better recovery than they actually did.

WHAT TO REALLY EXPECT

The complications of surgery (which typically involves total removal of the prostate gland) and radiation vary widely, depending on a man's age, the presence of other diseases (such as diabetes) and the specific type of treatment he receives. For example, a 50-year-old who had good erections prior to surgery will probably have them again within a year or two. An older man with a history of health problems won't do as well.

COPING WITH ED

Some of the nerves that control erections are invariably damaged during prostate removal surgery. This occurs even with so-called nerve-sparing procedures that are designed to minimize damage to nerves that supply the penis. In many cases, a man's ability to have erections can return within about 18 months, but there's no guarantee of a full recovery. In fact, recovery varies widely depending on the age and health of the patient—overall, 50% to 60% have permanent ED.

Men who are treated with radiation may retain their ability to have erections initially, but damage to nerves and blood vessels from radiation increases in the weeks and months after treatment.

Even so, prostate cancer survivors and their partners can still have satisfying sex lives (though the man may have a somewhat lower level of performance). *Here's how...*

•**Consider injections.** The average man is unwilling to stick a needle in his penis when he wants to have sex. But I encourage my patients to consider this treatment because it is the most effective—and always the least expensive—approach.

The drugs that are injected, *papaverine, prostaglandin* and *phentolamine*, are often combined in one solution. The injection usually produces an almost immediate erection even when a man isn't sexually aroused. The erection can last anywhere from about 10 minutes to four hours, depending on the dose.

The needle is so small that the injections are virtually painless. Once a man learns how to inject himself, he's given a prescription for enough medication to provide at least 50 doses.

Cost per shot: About $3.

Drawbacks: Apart from the fear of injections, the only likely side effect is an erection that lasts too long. This might not sound like a problem, but an overly persistent erection is painful and dangerous, potentially leading to permanent dysfunction. It can be prevented by reducing the dose.

•**Take a pill.** For those patients who are unwilling to try injections, *sildenafil* (Viagra), *vardenafil* (Levitra) and *tadalafil* (Cialis) promote blood flow to the penis when a man is sexually aroused and improve erections in about 60% of prostate cancer survivors who use the medications.

These medications work best in men who are in relatively good physical shape, don't have other serious health problems and have had nerve-sparing surgery or radiation alone. They're least effective in older men or men with low testosterone or complications from diabetes—and usually not effective at all for men who have had total removal of the prostate and surrounding tissue because they may have suffered nerve damage. Viagra, Levitra and Cialis can produce an erection in 30 to 60 minutes, and it typically lasts two to four hours.

Drawbacks: The medications cost $12 to $20 per pill (sometimes covered by insurance) and often cause headaches, dizziness, nasal congestion and other side effects. These drugs can also be dangerous or even deadly when combined with nitroglycerine medications, taken for heart problems.

•**Use a vacuum device.** This can be a good choice for men in long-term relationships who are comfortable "tinkering" before intercourse.

What happens: Just before intercourse, a man places a plastic sheath over his penis. Then, a motor (or a plastic crank, in less expensive models) creates a vacuum inside the sheath, which pulls blood into the penis. Once a man has an erection, he slips a rubber band around the base of the penis to hold the blood in place for 30 minutes.

Cost: $95 to $550, depending on the model.

Important: Use a vacuum device that has FDA approval and is prescribed by a doctor—the devices sold at "adult" stores may lack safety controls and generate too much pressure.

Drawbacks: Some men experience bruising on the penis. Also, many couples find the mechanical aspect of the devices unromantic.

•**Ask your doctor about surgical implants.** Men who can't get an erection any other way or prefer not to use the ED treatments described earlier may opt for a surgical implant.

Main choices: Semirigid, rodlike devices that are implanted in the penis and can be bent, like a pipe cleaner, into the proper position for intercourse…or a hydraulic device, controlled by a small bulb implanted in the scrotum, that pushes fluid into hollow tubes in the penis, causing them to inflate.

Most men who have these devices like them because they don't need pills or injections or require the steps that are necessary to use a vacuum device. As a result, they can have sex whenever they want.

Drawbacks: Postsurgical infection is the main risk. This occurs in about 3% of nondiabetic men. In men with diabetes, the infection rate is about 8%. The devices are expensive but often partially covered by insurance. Out-of-pocket costs are about $5,000 for the semi-rigid device and $8,000 for the inflatable one.

URINARY INCONTINENCE

Lack of urinary control is the second most common complication of prostate cancer treatments.

Reason: The prostate gland helps control/block the flow of urine. When the gland is removed or damaged, the urinary sphincter (the muscle that controls urine) has to work alone—and often fails. Most men eventually regain bladder control, but this can take two years or more.

Surgery—to implant an artificial sphincter, for example—may be needed if a man accidentally voids or "leaks" large amounts of urine. *My advice…*

•**Expect some leakage.** Most men who are treated with surgery and/or radiation for prostate cancer will experience some degree of stress incontinence—the leakage of a few drops of urine when they cough, sneeze, laugh, etc. It can be embarrassing, but as long as the amounts of urine are small, it's usually nothing to worry about. It will probably improve with time. Some men who have radiation may also have urge incontinence—a strong, sudden need to urinate.

When men are leaking large amounts of urine or when they're so embarrassed that they feel they can't leave the house, over-the-counter pads can help.

•**Do Kegel exercises.** Apart from surgery, this is the most effective way for men to regain bladder control. (Kegel exercises probably won't help men who are leaking large amounts of urine, but it doesn't hurt for these men to try them.) Start doing them every day after a diagnosis—before cancer treatments begin—to prevent future problems.

What to do: First, identify the pelvic-floor muscles. They're the muscles that you contract to hold urine in the bladder—or to stop the flow of urine in midstream.

Several times a day, squeeze the muscles as hard as you can. Hold for about five seconds, then relax. Repeat this sequence a few times. As the muscles get stronger, try to do 20 or more contractions at a time. Do them a few times a day.

Task Force Recommends Ending the PSA Test

CNN.
American Cancer Society.
US Preventive Services Task Force Web site, *http://www.uspreventiveservicestaskforce.org/*

The US Preventive Services Task Force has recommended that men no longer get screened for prostate cancer by undergoing prostate specific antigen—or PSA—testing, reported CNN recently.

The task force is the same group of independent medical experts that unleashed a storm of controversy in 2009 by stating that there was not enough evidence to recommend that women in their 40s get annual mammograms.

SCREENING TEST GETS A "D"

According to CNN, the task force recommended that the PSA blood test get a "D" rating, which means "there is moderate or high certainty that the service has no net benefit or that the harms outweigh the benefits," according to the group's Web site.

The task force report says that a review of studies indicates that the PSA blood test—which measures the presence of prostate specific antigen, a protein produced by cells of the prostate gland—results in "small or no reduction" in prostate cancer deaths, the news network reported.

The test has been controversial for some time. Many doctors contend that the screen often uncovers tumors that are small and slow growing, and will never cause a man to die. On the other hand, treating the disease can often leave a patient impotent or incontinent.

REACTION FROM CANCER PATIENTS

Some prostate cancer patients were disappointed with the task force's decision.

A spokesman for the Prostate Cancer Foundation, Dan Zenka, described the proposed recommendation as "a tremendous mistake. You're talking to someone whose life was saved by [the PSA test]," CNN reported.

But Kenneth Lin, MD, researcher for the US Department of Health and Human Services and senior author of the paper, said he believes PSA testing does more harm than good, the news network reported.

"Maybe you should get tested if you have this horrible family history where everyone gets prostate cancer before the age of 50. But for most men, testing is harmful," he said.

ABOUT THE US PREVENTIVE SERVICES TASK FORCE

The US Preventive Services Task Force is an independent panel of experts in prevention and evidence-based medicine and consists of primary care doctors, such as internists, pediatricians, family physicians, gynecologists/obstetricians, nurses, and health behavior specialists, according to the organization's Web site.

The task force conducts scientific evidence reviews of a broad range of clinical preventive health care services (such as screening, counseling and preventive medications) and develops recommendations for primary care clinicians and health systems.

BACKGROUND ON PROSTATE CANCER

According to the American Cancer Society, prostate cancer is the most common type of cancer found in American men, other than skin cancer. It's the second leading cause of cancer death in men, behind only lung cancer.

The cancer society estimates that there are approximately 240,890 new cases of prostate cancer diagnosed each year, and about 34,000 men die from the disease annually.

info To learn more, visit the Web site of the National Cancer Institute, *www.cancer. gov/cancertopics/pdq/treatment/prostate/Patient.*

Should You Get A Prostate Cancer Screening?

Sheldon Marks, MD, associate clinical professor of urology at University of Arizona College of Medicine, Tucson, and adjunct assistant professor of urology at Tufts University School of Medicine, Boston. He is author of *Prostate and Cancer: A Family Guide to Diagnosis, Treatment, and Survival* (Da Capo).

An influential government panel recently advised healthy men not to undergo routine screening for prostate cancer. The report has triggered protests from urologists—the doctors who diagnose and treat prostate cancer—who say that the test is very important.

We talked with urologist Sheldon Marks, MD, a noted expert on prostate cancer, about the panel's findings and who should get the prostate-specific antigen (PSA) test...

THE PANEL'S RECOMMENDATION

In October 2011, the United States Preventive Services Task Force concluded that routine PSA screening does not save lives. This conclusion was based on five major clinical studies. The two largest, conducted in the US and Europe, found that the death rates of men who got the test were virtually the same as those who didn't.

The panel also concluded that the PSA test leads to more tests and treatments that needlessly cause pain, impotence and incontinence in many men because most of the cancers that are detected are very slow-growing and unlikely to ever pose a threat.

WHAT MOST PEOPLE DON'T KNOW

What many patients and even doctors don't understand is that the PSA test is not a specific test for cancer. It's a very sensitive test that can detect abnormalities, but it's not designed to identify a particular problem.

It is like an engine warning light in your car. When it flashes, you can't tell if a particular spark plug is bad. It tells you only that something needs to be investigated.

About two-thirds of men with an elevated PSA don't have cancer. They could have an inflamed or infected prostate (prostatitis). They could have a prostate gland that's larger than normal (benign prostatic hyperplasia, or BPH). Also, PSA levels normally increase with age.

There even could be a laboratory error. A doctor should never encourage men to undergo invasive tests or treatments because of a single PSA reading. The test only alerts the doctor to the possibility of disease—and that disease might not be cancer.

BETTER TESTING

Many doctors consider the normal range for PSA to be between zero and 2.5 nanograms per milliliter (ng/mL) of blood. Cancer cells release about 10 times more PSA into the blood than normal prostate cells. This is why an elevated reading is worrisome. But an elevated PSA, taken in isolation, doesn't mean very much. *Next steps…*

•**Repeat the test in six to eight weeks.** Laboratory errors are more common than people realize. A man with an unusually high PSA should have a second test to see if the numbers stay the same.

•**Even if the first test was accurate, the numbers could be transitory.** A high PSA often will return to normal when an underlying condition—infection or inflammation, for example—clears up. I've seen men with a PSA reading as high as 100 that wasn't caused by a cancer.

•**Repeat the test once or twice a year.** If a man tests high on his initial PSA test and it's confirmed with follow-up testing, he may be given the option to get retested in three to six months to a year. If the numbers have dropped, as they often do, nothing more needs to be done. If the PSA still is high, there might be an underlying problem—and cancer is one possibility.

•**Watch for an increase.** A progressive increase of PSA over time, known as velocity, is more worrisome than a single high reading. The larger the jump, the higher the risk for cancer.

•**Schedule a biopsy.** This is the logical next step when a man's PSA continues to rise. The prostate gland is numbed with a local anesthetic. A spring-loaded device extracts a dozen hair-size slivers of tissue from the part of the gland that's most likely to contain cancer cells. The samples then are analyzed in a lab.

•**Biopsies aren't perfect.** They can miss the part of the prostate that contains cancer cells. There also can be uncertainty about the results.

If cancer is present, the pathologist will give it a Gleason score, a measure of the cancer's aggressiveness. Though we have a good idea, it's still not possible to predict with total accuracy how dangerous the cancer is likely to be.

Helpful: The PCA3 urine test. This usually is performed when a man has a negative biopsy but continues to have a high PSA. The PCA3, which identifies genetic markers associated with cancer, can help determine if a man needs a second biopsy.

WHO SHOULD GET TESTED

The task-force recommendations apply only to healthy men. A man with symptoms, such as difficult or painful urination or blood in the urine, must see a doctor and get tested.

I also strongly recommend PSA testing starting at ages 40 to 45 for men with a family history of prostate cancer. They're far more likely to get cancer than men without this history. All African-American men should get tested at ages 40 to 45—they have a higher risk for prostate cancer than Caucasian men.

Men in their mid-70s or older often don't need the PSA test. Even if they develop a cancer—or have harbored cancer cells in the prostate for decades—it's unlikely that the cancer will grow fast enough to cause problems during their expected life span. Virtually all men, if they live long enough, eventually will have cancer cells in the prostate gland. The majority of these cancers are indolent—they grow so slowly that they are unlikely to ever cause disease.

Of course, Americans are living longer than ever, and plenty of 80-year-olds are healthy and active. An older man who thinks that he has a decade (or more) ahead of him should ask his doctor about testing.

BOTTOM LINE

The fact that the PSA test is not perfect does not mean that we should return to the old days of no testing. More than 33,000 American men die each year of prostate cancer. But today, with earlier detection from PSA testing and treatment, about 95% of patients survive for at least 10 years—and many are cured.

The task-force report is a general public-health recommendation that does not agree with those of many prostate cancer experts. The task-force recommendation doesn't exclude men from getting the test—and insurance companies probably will continue to pay for it. Every man should ask his doctor if, or when, he should get tested.

The bottom line is that the PSA remains a valuable and sensitive test that, when interpreted correctly, saves lives and prolongs life span for men with prostate cancer.

■ ■ ■ ■

New Prostate Test Helps Some Men Avoid Biopsy

In a recent study, doctors examined urine samples from 1,312 men (average age 62) who showed elevated levels of prostate-specific antigen, an indicator of increased risk for prostate cancer. A new test was then used to analyze the urine for a fusion of two genes thought to cause prostate cancer.

Result: Biopsy indicated cancer in 69% of those found by the gene fusion test to be at high risk. This new test may allow some men to avoid or delay a painful needle biopsy. The test will likely become widely available within the next year.

Arul Chinnaiyan, MD, director, Michigan Center for Translational Pathology, University of Michigan Medical School, Ann Arbor.

Ginger Slows Tumor Growth by 56%

Geovanni Espinosa, ND, director, Integrative Urology Center, NYU Langone Medical Center, New York City. *www.drgeo.com*

Can ginger really help men with prostate cancer? This time-honored remedy is well known for other, less serious problems—including occasional indigestion, muscle soreness, nausea and even arthritis pain. But if ginger can help men manage, or even someday cure, this dangerous cancer, that puts it on another level entirely.

ANTITUMOR BENEFITS WITHOUT TOXIC EFFECTS

There's no doubt that ginger is a nutritional powerhouse—previous research has shown that many of the phytochemicals that make up ginger are packed with anti-inflammatory, antioxidant and antiproliferative powers. Some have been shown, individually, to reduce the risk of developing cancer, and others have been shown to slow tumor growth if cancer occurs. Researchers at Georgia State University in Atlanta studied what effect whole ginger extract might have on prostate cancer, specifically, because other studies have shown that a high intake of fruits and vegetables (which also are high in phytochemicals) help prevent prostate cancer.

After implanting human prostate cancer in mice, investigators fed half of them whole ginger extract (the human equivalent of about 3.5 ounces of fresh ginger) every day for eight weeks, while the other half, the control group, was fed no ginger. *Researchers found...*

•**In the mice that were fed ginger, there was an inhibition (or slowing) of tumor growth by an average of 56%,** compared with no inhibition of tumor growth in the control group that received no ginger.

•**Among the ginger-fed mice, there were no toxic effects in healthy tissue such as the gut or bone marrow.** This is a promising finding, because if these were humans with prostate cancer and they were given a typical treatment of chemotherapy, there would be a high likelihood of toxic side effects, such as neuropathy, nausea, hair loss, mouth sores, diarrhea and permanent infertility.

These findings appeared in the *British Journal of Nutrition.*

AN ANTICANCER DIET

Geovanni Espinosa, ND, director of clinical trials at the Integrative Urology Center at NYU Langone Medical Center in New York City believes that the Georgia State study provides sufficient information to encourage most prostate cancer patients to include ginger in their diets—so talk to your doctor. And it's easy to do—you can grate it or slice it to mix with vegetables, rice, salad dressings and smoothies. Ginger tea (made from the root) is delicious, and it's easy to brew. Just simmer about and inch or so of ginger slices in water for 10 minutes.

Caution: Dr. Espinosa noted that ginger is not 100% risk-free—for example, in rare cases, high amounts of ginger might worsen a bleeding disorder, reduce blood sugar too much if you're diabetic and interfere with blood pressure drugs and certain heart medications, such as *digoxin* and *digitoxin*. So the possible side effects of extensive treatment with ginger need to be studied in humans.

■ ■ ■ ■

New Drug for Advanced Prostate Cancer

Abiraterone (Zytiga) tablets inhibit the production of testosterone, which fuels the growth of prostate tumors.

Recent study: When combined with the corticosteroid *prednisone*, abiraterone added about four months to the lives of men with advanced prostate cancer, and it helped relieve pain and other disease-related symptoms.

Eleni Efstathiou, MD, PhD, assistant professor of medicine, University of Texas MD Anderson Cancer Center, Houston, and coauthor of a study published in *The New England Journal of Medicine.*

■ ■ ■ ■

Coffee May Fight Lethal Prostate Cancer

In a 14-year study of 47,911 American men (average age 53), those who drank one to three cups of coffee (caffeinated or decaffeinated) per day had a 30% lower risk for aggressive prostate cancer, while six or more cups daily was linked to a 60% lower risk. The reason for this association is still being studied.

Lorelei Mucci, ScD, associate professor of epidemiology, Harvard School of Public Health, Boston.

Men's Breast Cancer Uncommon—But More Deadly

Jon Greif, DO, general surgeon, San Francisco.
Susan K. Boolbol, MD, chief, division of breast surgery, Beth Israel Medical Center, New York City.

Breast cancer in men is much less common than it is in women, but it may be more deadly, recent research suggests.

"Men with breast cancer don't do as well as women with breast cancer, and there are opportunities to improve that," said study author Jon Greif, DO, a breast surgeon in San Francisco. "They are less likely to get the standard treatments that women get."

Although many men may not be aware that they can get breast cancer, nearly 2,200 new cases of male breast cancer were expected in 2012, according to the American Cancer Society. The society estimates 410 men died of breast cancer in 2012 in the United States.

Men should be able to recognize potential symptoms of breast cancer, the American Cancer Society suggests.

Among them: A lump or swelling, dimpling or puckering, a turning inward of the nipple, scaling of the nipple or breast skin, redness of the nipple or skin of the breast, and nipple discharge.

Survival rates for men with breast cancer, overall, are lower than those for women, at least when it is diagnosed in the early stages, Dr. Greif found. The cancers differ in other respects too.

Dr. Greif and his team warn, however, that some of the differences they found may not bear out in clinical practice.

STUDY DETAILS AND LIMITATIONS

Dr. Greif compared about 13,000 men with breast cancer, identified from the National Cancer Data Base, to more than 1.4 million women with breast cancer. The data covered 1998 to 2007.

The investigators evaluated cancer characteristics and survival rates, taking into account age, ethnicity and other factors.

Men with breast cancer were more likely to be black than women with breast cancer (11.7%

versus 9.9%) and less likely to be Hispanic (3.6% versus 4.5%), the researchers found.

In addition, men were older at diagnosis—63, on average, compared with 59 for women.

Men's tumors were larger when diagnosed. Men were also more likely to have later-stage tumors…involvement of lymph nodes…metastasis to other parts of the body and other differences.

Dr. Greif also found that women's overall five-year survival rate was 83%, but men's was 74%. That was looking at all breast cancers, whatever the stage.

When Dr. Greif's team looked at survival stage by stage, women with early stage cancer had better survival rates than men with early stage disease. The gap closed when men and women had more advanced disease.

"Women are encouraged to get breast exams [and] mammograms," Dr. Greif said. That is why their cancers are often diagnosed earlier, when the tumors are smaller, he said.

Men with breast cancer were less likely to get a partial mastectomy and to receive radiation, the study found.

More awareness of male breast cancer is crucial, Dr. Greif emphasized.

A big limitation to the research: The database they drew from keeps track of which breast cancer patients die, but not what they died from. So it is impossible to tell if they died from their cancer or something else, Dr. Greif explained.

EXPERT COMMENTARY

The study is valuable in pointing out gender differences, even with its limitations, said Susan Boolbol, MD, chief of the division of breast surgery at Beth Israel Medical Center in New York City.

"Over the years, it was thought that, stage for stage, women and men had equal outcomes," Dr. Boolbol said. The new research finds otherwise, and includes larger numbers of men with breast cancer than many previous studies did, she noted.

Lack of information on cause of death is a major limitation of the finding, she elaborated. Even so, "this is a very interesting study, and it will open the door to more research being done in male breast cancer."

The study may also raise awareness that men can indeed develop breast cancer, Dr. Boolbol said.

info To learn more about breast cancer in men, visit the Web site of the American Cancer Society at *http://www.cancer.org/cancer/breastcancerinmen/index.*

■ ■ ■ ■

Amino Acid Boosts Libido After Prostate Surgery

Is there a natural treatment to boost libido and erectile function after prostate surgery?

Some degree of erectile dysfunction (ED) does usually occur after most types of prostate surgery. The natural treatment that I recommend most often is the amino acid L-arginine, which is known to dilate blood vessels and improve blood flow. I find that 1,000 mg to 2,000 mg taken three times daily can help ED in most men. The time-released version has the longest-lasting effect. Patients need to take L-arginine daily (not just before having sex). For maximum benefit, it is best to take it between meals. Avoid this supplement if you are prone to herpes outbreaks (L-arginine could cause outbreaks) or if you have a history of a heart attack (since its safety after a heart attack is uncertain).

Mark A. Stengler, NMD, naturopathic medical doctor in private practice, Encinitas, California…adjunct associate clinical professor at the National College of Natural Medicine, Portland, Oregon…author of *The Natural Physician's Healing Therapies* and coauthor of *Prescription for Natural Cures* (both from Bottom Line Books).

FDA Approves New Impotence Drug Stendra

Bruce Kava, MD, acting chairman, urology, University of Miami School of Medicine.
US Food and Drug Administration press release

In April 2012, the US Food and Drug Administration approved Stendra, a new medication for erectile dysfunction. An estimated

30 million American men are affected by erectile dysfunction, according to the FDA.

Stendra (*avanafil*) joins Viagra, Cialis and Levitra, all from a class of drugs known as phosphodiesterase type 5 inhibitors that help boost blood flow to the penis.

According to the FDA, fast-acting Stendra is designed to be taken 30 minutes before sexual activity and at the lowest effective dose.

Stendra's safety and efficacy were established in three double-blind, placebo-controlled clinical studies. A total of 1,267 patients were randomly assigned to take Stendra for up to 12 weeks at doses of 50 milligrams (mg), 100 mg or 200 mg, or a placebo as needed about 30 minutes before sexual activity.

Stendra is marketed by Vivus Inc., based in Mountain View, California.

EXPERT COMMENT

Whether the new drug adds any value to the existing range of impotence medications is unclear, one expert said.

Bruce Kava, MD, acting chairman of urology at the University of Miami School of Medicine, said "the only advantage Stendra may have is a more rapid onset of action over the other drugs. The question is whether there are any advantages to a more rapid onset."

He noted that often patients don't respond to any brand of erectile dysfunction drugs. And there is currently no way of telling who will respond to which drug. "Sometimes it's hit or miss," he explained.

Men will have to try each individual brand to find the one that best suits their lifestyle, Dr. Kava said. For example, for some men Cialis works best because its effects seem to last much longer than that of the other drugs, he said.

The FDA said Stendra's approval means one more option for patients.

"This approval expands the available treatment options to men experiencing erectile dysfunction, and enables patients, in consultation with their doctor, to choose the most appropriate treatment for their needs," Victoria Kusiak, MD, deputy director of the Office of Drug Evaluation III in the FDA's Center for Drug Evaluation and Research, said in a recent FDA news release.

SIDE EFFECTS AND WARNINGS

Stendra comes with the same warnings as its companions in this drug class. It should not be taken by men who take nitrates—drugs used to treat chest pain (angina). This combination can cause a sudden drop in blood pressure, the FDA cautioned.

The agency also warned that these drugs can, in rare cases, cause color vision changes and in a few instances, men have also reported a sudden loss of vision in one or both eyes. Sudden loss or decrease in hearing has also been reported in patients taking these drugs. "Patients who experience a sudden loss of vision or hearing should stop taking PDE5 inhibitors, including Stendra, and call a doctor right away," the FDA said.

The most common side effects reported with Stendra include headache, redness of the face and other areas, nasal congestion, cold-like symptoms and back pain.

Also in rare cases, patients taking these drugs may get an erection lasting four hours or indefinitely. "If this happens, patients should seek immediate medical care," the agency said.

info For more information on erectile dysfunction, visit the site of the US National Library of Medicine at *www.nlm.nih.gov/med lineplus/erectiledysfunction.html*.

■ ■ ■ ■

Testosterone Does Not Help Erectile Dysfunction

Recent research found that replacing testosterone in men who had borderline low levels of the hormone did not improve the men's ability to achieve and maintain erections. Men with ED should discuss treatment options with their physicians.

Lauren W. Roth, MD, obstetrician/gynecologist, University of Colorado, Denver, and coauthor of a study of 167 men age 60 and older, presented at a recent meeting of the American Society for Reproductive Medicine.

Four Ways to Boost Testosterone Production

Jamison Starbuck, ND, naturopathic physician in family practice and a guest lecturer at the University of Montana, both in Missoula. She is past president of the American Association of Naturopathic Physicians and a contributing editor to *The Alternative Advisor: The Complete Guide to Natural Therapies and Alternative Treatments* (Time Life).

These days, a week does not go by without one of my patients—it can be a male or a female—asking me about testosterone supplementation, often after seeing an ad touting its benefits of improved vitality and sexual performance. In some cases, it's a reasonable choice, while in others, it may be safer to use natural approaches.

While most people think of testosterone as being a male hormone, it is essential to male and female health—and in both genders, levels begin to decline with age (as early as age 30 in men and primarily at menopause in women). In both men and women, testosterone helps build muscle and maintain bone density and libido. However, in some very critical areas, the role this hormone plays is unique to each gender. In men, appropriate testosterone levels reduce the risk for heart attack, stroke and type 2 diabetes. Too much testosterone can lead to aggressive behavior and decreased testicle size. Testosterone's effect on a man's risk for prostate cancer is debated—some studies show that high testosterone levels are associated with an increased risk for prostate cancer, while other research disputes this finding. In women, elevated testosterone levels carry an increased risk for such conditions as cardiovascular disease, high blood pressure and insulin resistance.

For these reasons, I often prefer to start with safer and time-tested methods, including herbs, nutrition that helps the body manufacture hormones and exercise, rather than initiating hormone supplementation. *For example…*

•**Zinc helps promote the body's production and utilization of testosterone.** Zinc-rich foods include turkey, Swiss chard, oats, soy, lima beans and pumpkin seeds. In supplement form, zinc picolinate is the most readily absorb-able. To boost testosterone levels, take no more than 60 mg daily.

Caution: Zinc is added to many supplements and nutritional products, so check your formulas for daily totals. Taking too much zinc may increase total cholesterol, lead to a deficiency of copper and cause other ill effects.

•**Damiana is an herb that holistic doctors often use to boost testosterone production.** I typically recommend 20 drops of the tincture twice daily in two ounces of water, taken at least 15 minutes before or after meals.

Caution: Pregnant women should avoid damiana.

•**Vitamins E and B-6.** These basic nutrients are required by the liver for appropriate hormone synthesis. I frequently recommend a simple daily dose of 400 international units of vitamin E and 50 mg of vitamin B-6 for my patients who need to improve their testosterone production.

•**Moderate aerobic exercise helps just about everything, including hormone metabolism.** Get at least two hours weekly of brisk walking or something more strenuous, if you prefer.

If you are experiencing symptoms of low testosterone, such as low libido, and prefer to take testosterone supplements, get accurate testing first. Testosterone can be tested via blood, urine or saliva. Just be sure your doctor has investigated the lab—not all of them provide reliable test results.

■ ■ ■ ■

Depression and ED

Erectile dysfunction (ED) is linked to depression and heart disease. ED and cardiovascular disease share many risk factors, including hypertension and diabetes. ED also is one of the earliest manifestations of a forthcoming cardiovascular event. Men with ED, depression or both should talk to their doctors about being screened for possible heart problems.

Mario Maggi, MD, professor of endocrinology, University of Florence, Italy, and coauthor of a study of 2,303 men, published in *The Journal of Sexual Medicine*.

■ ■ ■ ■

Pain Relievers Are Linked To Erectile Dysfunction

In a recent study, men who regularly used non-steroidal anti-inflammatory drugs (NSAIDs), such as aspirin or *ibuprofen*, were about 40% more likely to have ED than other men. The reason for the link is unknown.

Caution: If you use an NSAID for heart protection or other benefits, do not stop taking it without first consulting your physician.

Steven J. Jacobsen, MD, PhD, director of research at Kaiser Permanente Southern California, Pasadena, and senior author of a study of 80,966 men, published in *Journal of Urology*.

■ ■ ■ ■

Ways to Increase Sperm Count

In a recent finding, men whose anus-to-scrotum (anogenital) distance was shorter than the average of about two inches were 7.3 times more likely to have low sperm counts than men with a longer anus-to-scrotum distance. To increase your sperm count, in addition to consulting with a fertility doctor, avoid stress, quit smoking if you smoke and eat organic food (some pesticides can impact sperm count).

Shanna Swan, PhD, professor, department of preventive medicine, Mount Sinai Medical Center, New York City, and leader of a study of 126 men, published in *Environmental Health Perspectives*.

■ ■ ■ ■

Another Reason for Fertility Problems

Wormlike veins, called *varicoceles*, are caused by misdirected blood flow from the renal vein. They can slow blood flow and cause overheating in a testicle, which can reduce sperm production. Surgery may be necessary.

Also: Men with varicoceles average 11% lower testosterone levels than men who do not have them. The discomfort of varicoceles sometimes can be reduced with *ibuprofen* and by wearing an athletic supporter.

Larry Lipshulz, MD, professor of urology, Baylor College of Medicine, Houston.

You Can Relieve Prostate Pain

Mark A. Stengler, NMD, naturopathic medical doctor in private practice, Encinitas, California...adjunct associate clinical professor at the National College of Natural Medicine, Portland, Oregon...author of *The Natural Physician's Healing Therapies* and coauthor of *Prescription for Natural Cures* (both from Bottom Line Books).

When it comes to men's health, we hear a lot about enlarged prostate and prostate cancer. But there is another prostate ailment that gets much less attention yet affects many men. Prostatitis, a very painful condition, is inflammation of the prostate gland. It can be difficult to diagnose because its symptoms (persistent pain in the pelvis or rectum...discomfort in the abdomen, lower back, penis or testicles...difficult, painful or frequent urination or painful ejaculation) are similar to those of other conditions such as an enlarged prostate or a urinary tract infection.

It is estimated that almost half of all men will be affected by prostatitis at some point in their lives. If the condition lasts for three months or longer, it's considered to be chronic prostatitis.

Mainstream medicine often is unsuccessful in treating chronic prostatitis, leaving men in pain and without hope of feeling better. In my practice, I have had lots of success treating chronic prostatitis as both an inflammatory condition (which it always is) and as a possible fungal infection.

REASONS BEHIND PROSTATITIS

For a long time, it was thought that prostatitis could be caused only by bacterial infection. That view was dispelled when several studies found that the bacteria in the prostates of both healthy men and men with prostatitis were essentially identical. It's now understood that most prostatitis cases are not caused by bacteria. Still, most mainstream physicians routinely prescribe antibiotics for it—a treatment that is appropriate only if your case is one of a very small number actually caused by bacteria.

Although prostate inflammation is not well understood, the inflammation could be the result of inadequate fluid drainage into the prostatic ducts...an abnormal immune response...or a fungal infection.

PROSTATITIS TREATMENT PLAN

If you experience any of the symptoms of prostatitis mentioned above, see your doctor. Your visit should include a rectal exam to check for swelling or tenderness in the prostate...and a laboratory test of prostatic fluid to check for bacterial infection. I also recommend that you have your doctor order a urine culture to test for fungal infection (most medical doctors don't test for this).

In a small number of cases, the lab test does reveal a bacterial infection, and an antibiotic is appropriately prescribed. But if there is no bacterial infection, then I recommend that men with this condition follow an anti-inflammatory, antifungal treatment plan for two months. If symptoms subside but don't disappear, continue for another two months. Even if you don't have a test for fungal infection, I often advise following the antifungal portion of the program (along with the inflammation portion) to see if it helps to relieve symptoms.

FOODS THAT BATTLE PROSTATITIS

•**Anti-inflammatory diet.** Eating a diet of whole foods and cutting out packaged and processed foods go a long way to reducing inflammation in general and prostate inflammation in particular.

Eat: A variety of plant products to maximize your intake of antioxidants, which are natural anti-inflammatories...coldwater fish such as salmon, trout and sardines, which are high in omega-3 fatty acids...and pumpkin seeds, which are high in zinc, a mineral that helps reduce prostate swelling.

Don't eat: Foods that are high in saturated fat, such as red meat and dairy, which can make inflammation worse. Avoid alcohol, caffeine, refined sugar and trans fats, all of which tend to contribute to inflammation.

•**Antifungal diet.** If you already are following the anti-inflammatory diet above, then you have eliminated refined sugar from your diet. (Fungi thrive on sugar!) Also try eliminating all grains (including whole grains and rice) from your diet. Fungi thrive on these foods.

PROSTATE-PROTECTIVE SUPPLEMENTS

The following supplements have targeted benefits for prostate inflammation. They are safe to take together, and there are no side effects. Many men feel much better within two weeks of taking these supplements.

•**Rye pollen extract.** Studies show that rye pollen extract can relieve the pain of chronic prostatitis. In one study published in *British Journal of Urology*, men with chronic prostatitis took three tablets of rye pollen extract daily. After six months, 36% had no more symptoms and 42% reported symptom improvement. Follow label instructions. The pollen component in rye pollen does not contain gluten, but if you have celiac disease or a severe allergy to gluten, look for a certified gluten-free product.

•**Quercetin.** This powerful flavonoid helps reduce prostate inflammation.

Dose: 1,000 milligrams (mg) twice daily.

•**Fish oil.** In addition to eating anti-inflammatory foods, these supplements are a rich source of inflammation-fighting omega-3 fatty acids.

Dose: 2,000 mg daily of combined EPA and DHA.

ANTIFUNGAL SUPPLEMENTS

Many patients benefit from taking one or more antifungal remedies. Several herbs—such as oregano, pau d'arco, garlic and grapefruit seed extract—have potent antifungal properties. They are available in capsule and liquid form. For doses, follow label instructions. Most patients feel better within two to four weeks of taking antifungal supplements.

■ ■ ■ ■

Music Eases Pain and Anxiety During Prostate Biopsy

In a recent study, eighty-eight men (average age 62) undergoing a prostate biopsy were assigned to three groups—one with noise-cancelling headphones...one with headphones that played Bach concertos...and one without headphones. Compared with the other two groups, the men who listened to music reported less pain and had lower diastolic (bottom number) blood pressure, which often rises due to anxiety.

Theory: Music stimulates the frontal cortex of the brain, which modulates perceived pain and anxiety.

If you need a prostate biopsy: Listen to classical music on an iPod or other device during the procedure. Music may also help with other minor procedures.

Matvey Tsivian, MD, postdoctoral associate, division of urology, Duke University Medical Center, Durham, North Carolina.

■ ■ ■ ■

How to Firm Up Man Breasts

Larger-than-normal breasts can be an embarrassment for older men. All men possess breast tissue and some, due to increasing body fat and/or hormones, experience tissue growth in this area. After seeing your doctor to rule out less common causes, such as kidney failure, overactive thyroid or other underlying medical conditions, tackle the excessive fat—the most likely culprit.

Recommended: Most days of the week, perform 30 minutes of calorie-burning interval training, which boosts metabolism for hours.

To interval train: While jogging, spinning or using an elliptical machine, alternate one minute of heavier exertion with two minutes of moderate exertion. Do this for the entire workout. Add push-ups and bench presses (10 repetitions of each, three times a week) to develop chest muscles and fill out your chest area with nonfat tissue. Results may start to appear in four weeks. Meanwhile, try wearing a swim shirt and get back in the pool.

Michele Olson, PhD, professor of physical education and exercise science, Auburn Montgomery University, Alabama.

■ ■ ■ ■

Avoid Belly Fat, Eat More Fiber

Consuming fiber helps to control weight. But now researchers at Wake Forest University School of Medicine in North Carolina have found that fiber can reduce weight accumulation in a specific area of the body—the belly. For every 10-gram increase in daily intake of soluble fiber, the rate of belly fat decreased by 3.7% in adult women. It's not known how soluble fiber, which can be found in apples, oatmeal and legumes, helps to prevent abdominal fat deposits.

Fat deposits in men are different from those in women, but there is no harm in men boosting their fiber consumption.

Mark A. Stengler, NMD, naturopathic medical doctor in private practice, Encinitas, California…adjunct associate clinical professor at the National College of Natural Medicine, Portland, Oregon…author of *The Natural Physician's Healing Therapies* and coauthor of *Prescription for Natural Cures* (both from Bottom Line Books).

■ ■ ■ ■

Wedded Weight

Women tend to gain weight after marriage, while men gain more after a divorce.

Reasons: Married women have less time to stay fit. Divorced men may lose a nutritious diet, which often comes with marriage.

American Sociological Association.

■ ■ ■ ■

Men: Beware of Spine Surgery

Men and obese people are at greater risk for vision loss after spine surgery. Researchers studied 80 postoperative spinal fusion surgery patients (average age 51.6) who suffered vision loss, comparing them with 315 spinal surgery patients who didn't have vision problems.

Result: Two of the strongest risk factors for the vision loss were being male and obesity.

Theory: Men's susceptibility may be due to hormonal or anatomical differences. Obese patients typically have higher venous pressure when lying on their stomachs during a long surgery, which may cause abnormal blood flow in the head, damaging the optic nerve.

Lorri Lee, MD, associate professor of anesthesiology and pain medicine, University of Washington Medical Center, Seattle.

■ ■ ■ ■

Hair-Loss Treatment Can Have Sexual Side Effects

Finasteride, the treatment for male-pattern hair loss sold as Proscar or Propecia, can cause reduced sexual desire, erectile dysfunction, decreased arousal and problems with orgasm. The effects usually reverse when finasteride is no longer taken—but in some cases, they can persist for three months or more.

Michael S. Irwig, MD, assistant professor, department of medicine, The George Washington University, Washington, DC, and coauthor of a study published in *The Journal of Sexual Medicine*.

■ ■ ■ ■

Watch Out, Men!

Skin-prick tests reveal that men who have postorgasmic illness syndrome may be allergic to their own semen. For such men, runny nose, fever and other flulike symptoms may occur within 30 minutes of ejaculating and last up to a week.

Journal of Sexual Medicine

How Safe Is Circumcision?

Harry Fisch, MD, a urologist at New York-Presbyterian Hospital/Weill Medical College of Cornell University, New York City. He is author of *Size Matters: The Hard Facts About Male Sexuality That Every Woman Should Know* (Three Rivers).

Circumcision, of all things, has been in the news of late. The American Academy of Pediatrics announced that the need for circumcision "revision" surgery among infant boys had increased by more than 100% between 2004 and 2009. And a German court recently ruled that circumcising for religious reasons constitutes grievous bodily harm and is a crime, regardless of parental consent.

This latest turn of events contrasts the usual research that confirms the safety and benefits of circumcision.

WHY THE TREND?

Jewish and Muslim males are virtually always circumcised in infancy for religious reasons, but among the rest of Americans, the popularity of the procedure—which involves cutting off the foreskin of the penis—has ebbed and flowed over the years. The proportion of circumcised American male infants rose to about 90% in the 1970s, but since then it has declined to about 55% as of 2010, according to the Centers for Disease Control and Prevention (CDC). Many parents have questioned whether this procedure is necessary, and the American Academy of Pediatrics continues to take a neutral position as to whether or not it is advisable.

Is circumcision more dangerous than we had realized? Are there good reasons to be—or not to be—circumcised?

WHAT THE RESEARCH SAYS

Harry Fisch, MD, a urologist at New York-Presbyterian Hospital/Weill Medical College of Cornell University in New York City explained that like any procedure, circumcision has risks. But, he said, evidence-based research now demonstrates clear and compelling medical benefits of circumcision throughout life—not only for men, but also for the women who are their sexual partners...

• **For men, it decreases the risk of acquiring HIV,** the virus that causes AIDS, by as much as 50%, but it is not clear whether or not it reduces transmission of HIV to a partner.

• **It reduces the risk among men and women of transmitting and acquiring genital herpes** by about 28% and human papillomavirus (HPV), which can lead to cervical cancer in women and penile cancer in men, by 35%.

• **It decreases infant boys' risk of getting urinary tract infections in the first year of life from one in 100 to one in 1,000.** UTIs should be avoided in infancy because in 10% to 30% of cases they scar kidneys for life, and UTIs can lead to major health problems such as hypertension and chronic renal failure.

Dr. Fisch said that it's not entirely clear how circumcision provides all of these health protections, but since the foreskin leaves a warm, moist pouch between the inside of the foreskin and the head of the penis, disease-causing microbes can multiply there. And because the inner surface of the foreskin is especially permeable, said Dr. Fisch, it may facilitate entry of microbes into the male's body.

Removing the foreskin also makes genital hygiene easier and therefore allows men to avoid a wide variety of foreskin-related health problems, such as infections and *phimosis*, a condition that's often triggered by an infection in which the foreskin becomes tightly stretched around the head of the penis and makes retraction impossible. Phimosis may interfere with urination and sexual function, and because it makes genital hygiene even more difficult, it can lead to further infections.

In terms of sexual satisfaction, though, no studies have yet been able to evaluate whether or not being circumcised increases or decreases pleasure for a man or a woman, said Dr. Fisch. He added that they would be difficult to conduct, since pinpointing the exact cause of pleasure isn't easy.

TO SNIP OR NOT TO SNIP?

Experts are looking into the reasons behind the doubling of the need for circumcision revisions among infant boys (it rose up to 119%—from around 2,600 to around 5,600 cases), but, according to Dr. Fisch, it's surprising. Up until now, it has generally been widely accepted that complications from infant circumcision are rare, minor (e.g., bleeding, infection) and easily controlled. He added that a local anesthetic will reduce any associated pain and discomfort and that the penis heals fully in less than 10 days.

According to Dr. Fisch, the most significant health advantages of circumcision do not kick in until many years later when males become sexually active—but he and others in the medical community believe that infant circumcision is a safer and less traumatic procedure than adult circumcision. When you have the procedure done as an adult, it is generally quite painful, often requiring general anesthesia—as opposed to local anesthesia—which makes it a much riskier option. Plus, the healing tends to take longer (four to six weeks).

Parents: It's a tough decision, but it's up to you to decide for yourselves.

■ ■ ■ ■

HPV Affects Half of All Men

Most men don't know that they have the sexually transmitted disease because they usually don't have symptoms and doctors rarely test men for it. While most of the 40 strains of HPV affecting the genital areas aren't harmful,

several strains can lead to a variety of cancers in men and women, as well as genital warts.

Anna Giuliano, PhD, chair of the department of cancer epidemiology at the H. Lee Moffitt Cancer Center & Research Institute, Tampa, and leader of a study of 1,159 men, published in *The Lancet.*

Should You Carry a Condom?

Barbara Bartlik, MD, psychiatrist and sex therapist in private practice and voluntary attending psychiatrist at Montefiore Medical Center, Bronx, New York.

According to a recent study, unprotected sex is not a thing of the past. The Indiana University School of Health, Physical Education, and Recreation conducted a survey of 5,865 individuals (ages 14 to 94) covering condom use in heterosexual sex and found that singles are using condoms only about one-third of the time.

Women tend to be more aware of the dangers of STDs, and according to Barbara Bartlik, MD, psychiatrist at Montefiore Medical Center, Bronx, New York, men are way undereducated on the topic of sexually transmitted infections. The following is a list of infections that can be transmitted by having sex without a condom—all of which are nearly 100% preventable by wearing one.

STD DANGERS FOR MEN

●**Chlamydia.** Testing for chlamydia (usually involving a cervical swab) is a routine part of a gynecological exam, so women are more likely to get tested and treated for chlamydia. But that's not the case for men—if they're not told that they've been exposed, men may go on to infect other partners. Women with chlamydia who don't get treated will often develop *pelvic inflammatory disease* (PID), which can result in scarring in their fallopian tubes that can cause infertility. Men with untreated chlamydia may eventually suffer urinary discomfort (itching, burning, discharge) and scarring of the prostate.

•**Herpes.** A common misperception, even among people who have herpes, is that there's no danger of infection if there are no active sores. That's not so—herpes can be contagious even when the carrier of the virus has no visible sores.

•**Human papillomavirus (HPV).** HPV is among the most dangerous STDs—in fact (depending on the type) one of the deadliest, because it often brings no symptoms and can increase the risk for oral and anal cancer in both genders…cervical cancer in women…and penis cancer in men. According to Dr. Bartlik, HPV infection is so rampant that a person who has had unprotected sex with three or more partners has probably been exposed to it. Six million new genital HPV cases occur each year here in the US.

•**Human immunodeficiency virus (HIV).** Obviously, the stakes are high with HIV. Dr. Bartlik told me that, all other things being equal, in heterosexual sex, women are at higher risk for acquiring HIV than men (because men are more likely to be asymptomatic carriers, and the mucous membrane of the vagina is more vulnerable than the outer skin of the penis). But, she noted, "Even for the man, the risk is not zero."

•**Chronic prostate infections.** Acknowledging that this is anecdotal and not yet confirmed with research, Dr. Bartlik said that she and other doctors are seeing more men with chronic prostate infections—she and her colleagues believe that this may be related to bacterial infections picked up during unprotected sex. "Although I'm speculating, perhaps regular condom use might cut down on some of these bacterial infections as well as on the standard STDs," she said.

SHOULD COMMITTED COUPLES USE CONDOMS?

Dr. Bartlik believes that even couples who are in long-term, committed monogamous relationships ought to still use condoms. "The unexpected happens sometimes," she said, noting that it's not unusual to hear that people who never intended to have encounters or even affairs end up doing so. According to The Kinsey Institute, about 20% to 25% of men and 10% to 15% of women have extramarital sex at least once during their marriages. "Most of the time, these are not discovered," she said. "Often, at the end of the affair, they simply pick up and continue with married life—meaning unprotected sex with their spouse or partner."

Does the idea of using condoms forever make you feel glum? Dr. Bartlik outlined a strategy that allows a committed couple to make a safe segue from using condoms to enjoying the full intimacy of having nothing between you.

Couples making a commitment to a monogamous relationship can agree to get tested to confirm that neither partner is carrying an STD or, if there is evidence of one, to then make a rational decision about whether or not condoms are needed.

See your doctor (individually or together) to discuss the necessary steps, since there are several different types of tests involved, with varying degrees of reliability.

Share and discuss your results. If you both agree that no infidelity will occur—and more importantly, that if it does, you both promise to be honest about it right away—then go ahead and stop using condoms—unless you use them to prevent unwanted pregnancy, of course.

■ ■ ■ ■

Slip into Something Red

Men who wear red appear more powerful to women. Women view powerful men as more attractive and sexually desirable. They also view men in red as wealthier and more likely to climb the social ladder.

Andrew Elliot, PhD, professor of psychology, University of Rochester, New York, and author of the study of 313 people, published in *Journal of Experimental Psychology: General.*

■ ■ ■ ■

If Your Partner Has Breast Cancer…

Men whose partners have breast cancer are at risk for mood disorders serious enough to require hospitalization. The stress of dealing with the partner's disease, and the deprivation of emotional and social support that it brings, makes men more likely to develop major depression, bipolar disease and other serious mood-related conditions.

Self-defense: Men whose partners have breast cancer should be screened for depressive symptoms and treated before any conditions become severe enough to require hospital care.

Christoffer Johansen, MD, PhD, head, department of Psychosocial Cancer Research, Institute of Cancer Epidemiology, Copenhagen, Denmark, and leader of a 13-year study of 20,538 men whose partners were diagnosed with breast cancer, published online in *Cancer*.

■ ■ ■ ■

How Spouses Help Ease Pain

Researchers observed communication patterns between 78 adults with chronic pain and their spouses.

Result: The male patients' pain, marital satisfaction and depression were more affected by their spouse's negative and/or unsupportive behavior than were the female patients'.

Theory: Pain may be disruptive to the husband's traditional role as provider, making men vulnerable to a spouse's negative responses.

If you or your spouse suffers from chronic pain: See a psychologist or social worker who can counsel the couple, not just the pain patient.

Laura Leong, PhD candidate, Wayne State University, Detroit.

Narcissism Especially Bad for Men's Health

Sara Konrath, PhD, assistant research professor, University of Michigan Institute for Social Research, Ann Arbor, Michigan.
Mark Russ, MD, director, psychiatric services, Zucker Hillside Hospital, Glen Oaks, New York.
PLoS ONE

The inflated sense of self-importance common to narcissism can be toxic to relationships, but a recent study suggests the personality trait may also harm men's health.

Researchers from the Universities of Michigan and Virginia determined that men who scored high on two destructive narcissistic traits—entitlement and exploitativeness—had markedly higher levels than others of cortisol, a stress hormone that can lead to high blood pressure and heart problems. While men and women are equally narcissistic, study authors said, the cortisol stress response was not noted in female participants.

"We generally see narcissism as a personality trait that's bad for others but not narcissists. It's bad for people in relationships with them," said study coauthor Sara Konrath, PhD, an assistant research professor at the University of Michigan's Institute for Social Research. "This study was a way of getting under their skin to see if there are physical consequences."

Narcissism levels have increased in both genders in recent years, Dr. Konrath said, perhaps as a byproduct of the so-called "self-esteem movement," which emphasizes praise for children over criticism.

The study was published in the journal *PLoS ONE*.

STUDY DETAILS

Dr. Konrath and her colleagues administered a 40-item questionnaire to 106 college students that measured five components of narcissism, which is also characterized by self-absorption, overestimations of their uniqueness—attractiveness or intelligence, for instance—and a sense of grandiosity. They also measured cortisol levels twice in the students' saliva to assess baseline levels of the hormone, which signals activity in the *hypothalamic-pituitary-adrenal axis* (HPA), the body's key stress response system.

While entitlement and exploitativeness are considered unhealthy narcissistic traits, three of narcissism's five personality components are considered useful or healthy: leadership/authority, superiority/arrogance and self-absorption/self-admiration.

Dr. Konrath noted that narcissists tend to be creative people with low levels of depression, but their fragile views of themselves can lead them to react defensively and resort to aggression when their sense of superiority is threatened.

The authors found elevated levels of cortisol only in the men with unhealthy narcissism, and they speculated that in these men the HPA axis is chronically activated.

While study data didn't explain why only men seem to suffer from a higher stress response to narcissism, Dr. Konrath speculated that societal definitions of masculinity that overlap with the trait—such as arrogance or dominance—may leave men particularly vulnerable physiologically.

"They're at especially high risk because someone who admits they're stressed out is going to get help, but they're not likely to," she said. "There may be a cost to this jerkiness. It's a little sad they're a group that wouldn't get help if they needed it."

EXPERT COMMENTARY

While the study "invites people to look at this issue in a more comprehensive way," it did not prove a cause-and-effect relationship between narcissism and the body's stress response, said Mark Russ, MD, director of psychiatric services at Zucker Hillside Hospital in Glen Oaks, New York.

"People with narcissism may be type-A, very driven, perfectionistic and seek high-stress situations, and the cortisol levels may be measuring that," Dr. Russ said. "There may be an overlap."

Dr. Konrath said future research would focus on the reason women don't respond physiologically to narcissism as men apparently do.

info The US National Institutes of Health's Web site, *www.nlm.nih.gov/medlineplus/ency/article/000934.htm*, has more about the unhealthy aspects of narcissism.

■ ■ ■ ■

Culture Benefits Men's Health

A Norwegian study found that attending cultural events, including religious activities, sporting events and concerts, was associated with health and happiness, especially for men. About 84% of those who attended just one activity in a six-month period said that they were satisfied with their lives.

Mark A. Stengler, NMD, naturopathic medical doctor in private practice, Encinitas, California...adjunct associate clinical professor at the National College of Natural Medicine, Portland, Oregon...author of *The Natural Physician's Healing Therapies* and coauthor of *Prescription for Natural Cures* (both from Bottom Line Books).

Kegel Exercises Are Good For Men Too

Jonathan M.Vapnek, MD, urologist and an associate clinical professor of urology at Mount Sinai School of Medicine in New York City.

Just about every woman who has experienced childbirth or gone through menopause has heard of "Kegels." These simple exercises are widely used to treat and prevent urinary leaks.

What you may not realize: Kegels, named after the American gynecologist Arnold Henry Kegel, are also useful for men—not just for reducing urinary and bowel incontinence but also for easing prostate discomfort and relieving premature ejaculation. *Bonus:* Many men and women report that these exercises enhance sexual pleasure as well.

Good news: You don't have to set aside a specific time to do these exercises. No one can see what you're doing, so you can exercise the muscles almost any time—when you're standing in line, driving your car or watching TV.

But even people who have heard of Kegels—or perhaps tried them—may not be getting all the possible benefits if they're making some common mistakes while performing the exercises.

WHAT GOES WRONG

The goal of Kegel exercises is to strengthen the pelvic floor—a group of muscles that control urination and defecation and help support pelvic organs, such as the bladder (and uterus in women).

In women, pregnancy and vaginal childbirth can stretch and weaken the pelvic floor, leading to urinary incontinence. Women who haven't had children can also suffer from incontinence, in part because age-related declines in estrogen may weaken the urinary sphincter.

In men, urinary incontinence is usually due to prostate enlargement or prostate surgery. Prostate enlargement causes the bladder muscle to become overactive, resulting in urinary incontinence. Prostate surgery can damage the sphincter or nerves that control the sphincter.

HOW TO DO KEGELS PROPERLY

Kegels are simple—they involve contracting and relaxing your pelvic-floor muscles. *Yet many women and men make these mistakes when performing the exercises...*

Mistake 1: Not identifying the pelvic-floor muscles. Some people simply can't "feel" these muscles. When contracting them, there should be no movement of the abdominal muscles and minimal movement of the buttocks. Men can see a "shortening" of the base of the penis, and women should feel a "lifting or narrowing" of the vagina.

Solution: The next time you urinate, try to stop the flow in midstream. If you can do this, you're contracting all of the right muscles. You can also tighten the muscles that prevent you from passing intestinal gas. (Once the proper muscles have been located, do not do Kegels while urinating or defecating.)

If you still can't locate the muscles: A woman can insert a finger into her vagina and tighten the muscles to squeeze her finger. A man can place a finger in his anus. If he is tightening the correct muscles, he will feel a contraction on his finger.

A physical therapist trained in pelvic-floor rehabilitation can also teach you where the muscles are. He/she may use biofeedback, which involves placing electrodes on the abdomen or in the vagina or anus. A machine can then monitor the contraction/relaxation of the appropriate muscles and alert patients when they're doing it right. This procedure is painless.

Mistake 2: Stopping too soon. It's common for women and men to do a few Kegels then stop.

Solution: Make sure you know how to correctly count your repetitions. To begin, squeeze the muscles as hard as you can for three to five seconds. Then relax for five seconds. This is one Kegel. Start with five or 10 repetitions. As your muscles get stronger, you'll easily be able to do 20 in a row and hold each Kegel for about 10 seconds.

Mistake 3: Not doing the exercises often enough. Until you've incorporated Kegels into your daily schedule, it's easy to try the exercises a few times, then forget about them for several days.

Solution: As with any exercise, Kegels are more effective when you do them regularly. To get the most benefit, do 10 or 20 Kegels, relax for a minute, then do 10 or 20 more. Repeat this three times daily. Be patient. It may take six to 12 weeks to see any benefits, but many people report beneficial effects earlier.

For improved sexual function: Men who experience premature ejaculation can learn to delay their orgasms by squeezing the muscles, hard, during masturbation or intercourse. Women can use Kegels to create more friction during intercourse and reach orgasm sooner.

Important: Avoid devices sold online that claim to strengthen pelvic-floor muscles—they aren't necessary and often don't work.

■ ■ ■ ■

Natural Relief for Overactive Bladder

An overactive bladder, which typically refers to a sudden urge to urinate, can lead to urinary incontinence in women and men. In men, overactive bladder is commonly caused by prostate enlargement or a weakened bladder sphincter.

One long-used Native American remedy: Pumpkin seeds to normalize bladder function. Now a Japanese treatment containing pumpkin seeds and soy isoflavone extract has been shown in clinical trials to help urinary incontinence in men and women.

One brand I like: LifeExtension Water-Soluble Pumpkin Seed Extract with Soy Isoflavones (800-544-4440, *www.lef.org*).

Mark A. Stengler, NMD, naturopathic medical doctor in private practice, Encinitas, California...adjunct associate clinical professor at the National College of Natural Medicine, Portland, Oregon...author of *The Natural Physician's Healing Therapies* and coauthor of *Prescription for Natural Cures* (both from Bottom Line Books).

Treatment Options for Prostate Troubles

Peter T. Scardino, MD, chairman of surgery at Memorial Sloan-Kettering Cancer Center in New York City. Dr. Scardino is author of *Dr. Peter Scardino's Prostate Book: The Complete Guide to Overcoming Prostate Cancer, Prostatitis, and BPH* (Avery).

If you're a man over age 50, chances are you spend a fair amount of time running to the bathroom. Prostate enlargement—also known as *benign prostatic hyperplasia* (BPH)—is among the most common problems men face as they age. It affects about 40% of American men in their 50s and 90% of those in their 80s.

Fortunately, BPH is not cancer, nor does it raise cancer risk. But it can cause extremely bothersome symptoms, including frequent and/or urgent urination (which can wake men at night and interfere with sleep)...a weak urine stream...and sometimes urine leakage.

Good news: An increasing number of highly effective treatments now are available for BPH. The question is, which is best for you?

What you need to know...

NONSURGICAL APPROACHES

If you're a man who is concerned about developing BPH, it's wise to focus on your diet. One recent study found diets low in fat and high in vegetables (five-plus servings daily, especially of vitamin C–rich bell peppers, cauliflower, Brussels sprouts and tomato juice) to be associated with lower BPH risk.

Millions of men who have BPH use saw palmetto, an herb, to treat the condition, but research is mixed as to its effectiveness.

When nondrug approaches don't work, medication is usually the next step. Two-thirds of all men treated with medication have shown improvement in BPH symptoms and are able to delay or avoid surgery.

Among the most widely used BPH drugs are *alpha-blockers*, such as *terazosin* (Hytrin) and *tamsulosin* (Flomax), which relax the prostate and bladder-wall muscles to improve urine flow...and *5-alpha reductase inhibitors*, such as *finasteride* (Proscar) and *dutasteride* (Avodart)—these drugs block formation of the hormone *dihydrotestosterone*, which fuels prostate growth.

While both alpha-blockers and 5-alpha reductase inhibitors relieve symptoms, finasteride and dutasteride shrink the prostate and limit growth over time, leading to less risk for sudden blockage or need for surgery. If one drug type does not work well, try using both a 5-alpha reductase inhibitor and an alpha-blocker.

For men who have risk factors for prostate cancer, including a family history of the disease, the 5-alpha reductase inhibitors often are worth considering. These drugs not only treat BPH but also may lessen the risk for a prostate malignancy.

Important: Earlier studies have suggested an increase in aggressive prostate tumors among men who took 5-alpha reductase inhibitors, and subsequent research has failed to fully resolve the issue. Discuss the pros and cons of these drugs with your doctor.

Latest development: Recent research, including a 2010 Mayo Clinic study of more than 1,000 men, has shown that erectile dysfunction (ED) drugs, such as *sildenafil* (Viagra) and *tadalafil* (Cialis), can improve urinary symptoms of BPH.

The *combination* of an ED drug with a standard medication for prostate enlargement might be helpful for men with both erection and prostate problems, but ED drugs should not replace BPH drugs.

DO YOU NEED SURGERY?

Unfortunately, there's no one medication that controls BPH for all men. Surgery can be highly effective, but many men think of it as a last resort, fearing complications such as erection problems and incontinence (though these are rare).

But for some men, there are risks associated with *not* having surgery. For example, when the prostate gland is enlarged, the bladder may never fully empty and urine stagnates. This sets the stage for possible recurrent urinary tract infections and painful bladder stones.

Over time, the pressure of a blocked urinary tract also may damage the kidney and/or the bladder may become irreversibly stretched and unable to function properly. What's more, the larger a man's prostate, the longer, more complicated corrective surgery becomes, increasing the risk for complications.

How can a man tell if he may need surgery for BPH? Surgery is worth considering if symptoms (including slow urinary stream, urinary frequency, difficulty emptying the bladder or waking at night to urinate) persist despite taking medication for at least six months. In other cases, side effects (including dizziness from alpha-blockers and loss of sex drive from 5-alpha reductase inhibitors) keep him from taking medication properly. Surgery is also a reasonable option if a man develops signs of worsening BPH, such as urinary tract infections, bleeding or bladder stones.

Also useful to determine whether BPH requires surgery: No test provides sure answers about when to operate, but a man's responses on the International Prostate Symptom Score (IPSS) questionnaire are the most helpful. It's designed to determine the seriousness of urinary symptoms. Increasing scores over time signal worsening symptoms. Simple office tests (such as flowmetry, which measures the rate at which the bladder empties, and/or ultrasound) are useful indicators but not definitive.

THE LASER REVOLUTION

For men who do require surgery for BPH, the most significant recent change is the increasing use of laser technology, which uses extreme heat to vaporize excess tissue in the prostate.

There are several different types of laser surgery. One of the most effective is performed with a *potassium-titanyl-phosphate* (KTP), or green light, laser.

Clinical trials confirm that results from KTP laser surgery are comparable to those from *transurethral resection of the prostate* (TURP), in which the surgeon manipulates tiny instruments through the penis and urethra to remove excess tissue from the prostate.

Important recent finding: When 120 men with advanced BPH received either KTP laser surgery or TURP, they experienced an equal improvement in symptoms, but recovery was faster after laser, according to a 2010 study reported in the *British Journal of Urology*.

Advantages of KTP: KTP laser causes less bleeding than TURP, and the urinary catheter,

generally necessary after either procedure, can be removed sooner, reducing the risk for infection. While TURP usually requires two to four days in the hospital, with KTP laser, most men can go home after an overnight stay or even the same day.

Possible complications of laser surgery include tissue regrowth, which may necessitate a repeat operation, and/or persistent urinary symptoms, such as urgency and frequency. About 2% to 3% of patients have side effects after TURP or KTP laser.

For some men, including those who take a blood-thinning drug, such as *warfarin* (Coumadin), laser is usually the obvious choice because it causes less blood loss.

However, the risk for problems with laser surgery is greatly increased if the surgeon is not well-qualified. If you choose laser surgery, make sure your surgeon is well-trained and performs the procedure multiple times each year.

Another option: The *holmium* laser. It uses a different energy source than that used for KTP laser to cut prostate overgrowth into fragments that are then ground up with a device and removed—a process that helps reduce the need for retreatment. Holmium laser surgery is effective for prostates of any size, according to a 2010 study reported in the journal *Urology*, and may be a particularly good choice when the prostate is large.

Caution: Unless holmium laser surgery is performed by an extremely skilled surgeon, risk for bleeding or damage to the bladder or rectum is higher than with the KTP laser or TURP. Because this type of surgery is still not widely available in this country, it may be harder to find a well-qualified surgeon. A medical center that is affiliated with an academic institution is generally the best place to find such a surgeon.

■ ■ ■ ■

Medication for Enlarged Prostate Reduces Cancer Risk

Roughly 16% of men will be diagnosed with prostate cancer. Men who take *dutasteride* (Avodart) or *finasteride* (Proscar, Propecia) for benign enlarged prostate are 26% less likely to develop prostate cancer.

But: Men taking either drug who do develop prostate cancer are slightly more likely to have a more dangerous form of the disease.

J. Stephen Jones, MD, FACS, professor and chairman, department of regional urology, and Leonard Horvitz and Samuel H. Miller Distinguished Chair in Urological Oncology Research, Cleveland Clinic.

Cialis Approved to Treat Enlarged Prostate

US Food and Drug Administration news release

The erectile dysfunction drug Cialis (*tadalafil*) has received new approval from the US Food and Drug Administration (FDA) to treat *benign prostatic hyperplasia* (BPH), the medical term for an enlarged prostate.

Symptoms of BPH frequently include difficulty urinating, a sudden urge to urinate, and an increase in having to urinate, notably at night.

The drug was evaluated among men with BPH in three trials. Those who took 5 milligrams (mg) of Cialis once daily showed significant reduction in symptoms of BPH, the FDA said in a news release. The third trial involved men with BPH who also had been diagnosed with erectile dysfunction.

Men who take a class of drugs called nitrates, including nitroglycerin, shouldn't take Cialis in tandem, since the combination could lead to an unsafe drop in blood pressure, the FDA said. The agency made a similar warning about taking Cialis along with alpha-blocker drugs, which typically are prescribed to treat high blood pressure or as well as BPH.

Eight other drugs have been approved to treat symptoms of BPH: Proscar (*finasteride*), Avodart (*dutasteride*), Jalyn (*dutasteride and tamsulosin*), Hytrin (*terazosin*), Cardura (*doxazosin*), Flomax (*tamsulosin*), Uroxatral (*alfuzosin*) and Rapaflo (*silodosin*).

Cialis is produced by Indianapolis-based Eli Lilly and Co.

The US National Library of Medicine has more about tadalfil at the Web site *http://www.nlm.nih.gov/medlineplus/druginfo/meds/a604008.html*.

Natural Remedies

Ordinary Spices With Extraordinary Health Benefits

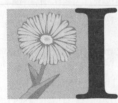

I t's common knowledge that sprinkling cinnamon on your food helps control blood sugar levels, adding cayenne clears the sinuses and using ginger can ease nausea.

What fewer people realize: There are several lesser-known spices that not only give foods wonderful flavors, but also offer significant health benefits.* In some cases, spices can be just as helpful as medication for people with certain conditions—and safer.

Common medical conditions that you can help prevent—or improve—with the use of spices…

*Check with your doctor before using any of the spices mentioned in this article for medicinal purposes. The natural compounds found in spices may interact with some prescription drugs. Pregnant and nursing women should avoid using spices medicinally.

OREGANO FOR ARTHRITIS

Oregano helps alleviate osteoarthritis and other inflammatory conditions, such as rheumatoid arthritis. You might be surprised to learn that this favorite spice of Italian cooking contains natural compounds that have many of the same effects as the powerful anti-inflammatory COX-2 inhibitor drug *celecoxib* (Celebrex).

In addition, oregano contains dozens of other anti-inflammatory compounds that act as muscle relaxants and pain relievers. Unlike celecoxib, which may increase heart attack risk in some people, oregano actually *protects* the heart by helping to prevent blood clots and irregular heart rhythms.

Best uses: Use oregano liberally on salads or on pizzas. Oregano also can be mixed with peppermint and/or spearmint for a hot or iced

James A. Duke, PhD, an economic botanist retired from the USDA, where he developed a database on the health benefits of various plants (*http://www.ars-grin. gov/duke/*). He is author of numerous books including, most recently, *The Green Pharmacy Guide to Healing Foods: Proven Natural Remedies to Treat and Prevent More Than 80 Common Health Concerns* (Rodale).

mixed-herb tea. If you prefer to take an anti-inflammatory supplement, oregano is one of the half dozen spices in a product called Zyflamend (its ingredients also include rosemary and turmeric). The herbs in Zyflamend act synergistically to provide a more powerful effect than each would when used individually. Zyflamend can be purchased in health-food stores and online. Follow label instructions.

CALENDULA
FOR CATARACTS

Calendula, or marigold, contains powerful plant-based carotenoids—particularly *lutein* and *zeaxanthin*—that help protect the eyes. In addition to being powerful antioxidants, these two compounds absorb damaging blue-light wavelengths from the sun. Increased intake of lutein and zeaxanthin has been associated with reduced risk for cataracts.

Best uses: Calendula makes an excellent addition to homemade vegetarian soup. If you prefer to use calendula in supplement form, follow label instructions.

ONION FOR
HIGH BLOOD PRESSURE

Onion contains blood-thinning compounds, all of which have a blood pressure–lowering effect. One of the most potent of these compounds is the flavonoid *quercetin*. Onion also acts as a natural diuretic, which lowers blood pressure by helping the body excrete excess fluids and salt.

Best uses: If possible, use a *full* onion (all types contain some blood pressure–lowering compounds) in onion soup, for example.

Reason: The onion's thin outer skin is the plant's best source of quercetin. Onion powder and cooked onions are not as effective as fresh onion.

Research shows that people who take quercetin as a supplement can lower their blood pressure in less than a month. In a double-blind study, people with hypertension who took 730 mg of quercetin daily for 28 days lowered their systolic (top number) blood pressure by an average of 7 mm HG and diastolic (bottom number) by 5 mm HG.

FENNEL SEED FOR INDIGESTION

Fennel seed is surprisingly effective at relieving indigestion. If I get indigestion, I pick some fennel seeds from the fennel plant in my garden. Fennel is easy to grow, and it keeps coming back year after year. In my experience, it can settle the stomach as well as many over-the-counter products.

Fennel seed relaxes the smooth muscles that line the digestive tract, relieving flatulence, bloating and gas, as well as nausea and vomiting, motion sickness and abdominal pain. If you don't want to grow your own, store-bought fennel seed also works well.

Best uses: Fennel seed can be eaten whole (it tastes and smells similar to anise) or made into a tea by pouring boiling water over it (use one gram to three grams of fennel seed—about one-half to one and one-half teaspoons—per cup). To sweeten the tea, molasses or honey is the best choice.

Caution: Because fennel seed can increase estrogen levels, it should be avoided by women who are pregnant or breast-feeding or who have an estrogen-sensitive medical condition, such as estrogen-responsive breast cancer.

GARLIC FOR THE COMMON COLD

While the research on garlic's positive effect on cardiovascular health is perhaps most widely known, this popular allium also boosts immunity, helping to prevent and treat the common cold.

In one study of nearly 150 people who took a garlic supplement or placebo for 12 weeks during cold season, those taking the garlic had significantly fewer colds (or symptoms that eased more quickly in cold sufferers) than those taking a placebo.

Best uses: To help cure or prevent a cold, add a clove or two of garlic to all soups…sprinkle garlic powder on toast…and/or mix diced raw garlic with olive oil and vinegar.

SAFFRON FOR DEPRESSION

Saffron, a spice derived from a small, blue crocus, acts as a potent antidepressant and has been used for centuries in traditional medicine for this purpose. No one is sure how it works, but its active ingredient, *crocetin*, appears to enhance blood flow to the brain.

Research conducted in Iran has shown that 30 mg per day of saffron powder (about one-tenth of a teaspoon) relieved mild-to-moderate depression as effectively as standard doses of the antidepressant medications *fluoxetine* (Prozac) and *imipramine* (Tofranil).

Best uses: One of the world's most expensive spices, saffron can be used in herbal tea or chicken paella. A five-gram bottle of Exir Pure Saffron Powder is $41 at *www.amazon.com*.

The Wonders of Aloe

Mark A. Stengler, NMD, naturopathic medical doctor in private practice, Encinitas, California…adjunct associate clinical professor at the National College of Natural Medicine, Portland, Oregon…author of *The Natural Physician's Healing Therapies*. (Bottom Line Book).

You may know aloe for its ability to soothe, soften and heal skin. But you might not realize that *Aloe vera*, one of 300 varieties of this plant, is loaded with vitamins, choline, zinc and beta-carotene, giving it potent antiviral and antibacterial properties. It can help a variety of conditions—and researchers are investigating its potential for treating diabetes and cancer.

Aloe can be used topically or internally (juice or capsule form). All forms are available at health-food stores. *How aloe can help you…*

•**Digestive disorders.** Aloe juice has been found to ease stomach ulcers…inflammatory bowel disease…Crohn's disease…and ulcerative colitis. Aloe also can help constipation. But people with these digestive disorders should be cautious when using aloe products that contain aloe latex (from the milky part of the plant) since this component of aloe can be a powerful laxative.

•**Skin conditions.** Aloe cream expedites the healing of cold sores. Because of its anti-inflammatory and emollient properties, it also can ease psoriasis and eczema. Apply an aloe vera cream three times daily.

•**Arthritis.** Taking aloe (either orally or topically) can help joint pain.

How to use aloe: When buying a topical gel, look for a product that contains at least 80% aloe. When drinking aloe juice, start with one teaspoon daily. Add a teaspoon daily to see how well you tolerate it until you reach six teaspoons daily, either on its own or mixed in water or some other juice. Pregnant women and children under age 13 should not use any aloe products orally. Since aloe may lower blood sugar, people with diabetes should speak to their doctors before taking aloe orally.

The Truth About Garlic— Health Claims That You Can Trust…

Ellen Tattelman, MD, director of the faculty development fellowship at the Residency Program in Social Medicine at Montefiore Medical Center in New York City. She is an assistant professor of family and social medicine at Albert Einstein College of Medicine of Yeshiva University, also in New York City.

Garlic is one of the most exhaustively researched herbs—the National Library of Medicine's Web site lists more than 3,700 studies addressing garlic's effect on everything from elevated cholesterol and various types of cancer to fungal infections.

So why is there still so much confusion about the health benefits of garlic?

Even though garlic has been used medicinally by some cultures for thousands of years, much of the contemporary research on garlic is mixed—some studies show that it has positive effects, while others indicate no significant benefits.

Here's what the research shows…

HEART HEALTH

Over the years, scientists have investigated garlic's ability to reduce cholesterol levels and blood pressure and act as an anticlotting agent to prevent blood platelets from being too sticky—a main cause of heart attack.

Key scientific finding: A recent meta-analysis in China looked at 26 randomized, double-blind, placebo-controlled trials—the "gold standard" in scientific research. In that meta-analysis, researchers concluded that garlic reduces total cholesterol by 5.4% and triglyceride levels by 6.5% compared with a placebo. Garlic powder and aged garlic extract were found to be the most effective at lowering total cholesterol, while garlic oil had a greater effect on lowering triglyceride levels.

When it comes to high blood pressure, some credible research shows that garlic can help lower it.

Important scientific findings: Two meta-analyses showed that garlic reduced systolic (top number) blood pressure by 8 mmHg to 16 mmHg and diastolic (bottom number) blood pressure by 7 mmHg to 9 mmHg in people with high blood pressure.

As for garlic's antiplatelet effect—that is, its ability to make blood less sticky and therefore less prone to clotting—a meta-analysis of 10 trials showed a modest, but significant, decrease in platelet clumping with garlic treatment when compared with placebos in most of the studies.

Bottom line: Garlic does help reduce risk for cardiovascular disease, with positive effects on both total cholesterol and blood pressure. It also has enough of an effect on clotting that I recommend patients discontinue garlic supplements seven to 10 days before surgery because it may prolong bleeding.

My advice: If you have a personal or family history of heart disease, ask your doctor about using garlic (in food or supplements) as part of a heart-healthy lifestyle. Be sure to consult your doctor first if you take a blood pressure or statin drug.

CANCER

Large population studies have shown that people who live in countries where a lot of garlic is eaten—as well as onions and chives—are at lower risk for certain cancers.

Key scientific findings: In China, high intake of garlic and other alliums, including onions, was associated with a reduced risk for esophageal and stomach cancers. Specifically, the study found that people who ate alliums at least once a week had lower incidence of both forms of cancer than people who ate these foods less than once a month.

Meanwhile, the European Prospective Investigation into Cancer and Nutrition, which involves 10 different countries, found that higher intakes of garlic and onions lowered the risk for intestinal cancer.

My advice: If you are concerned about cancer—especially if you have a family history or other risk factors for stomach or esophageal cancer—include one to two cloves of garlic in your diet each day.

INFECTIONS

Historically, garlic has received attention as a potent antibacterial agent. In 1858, Louis Pasteur touted garlic as an antibiotic. Garlic was later used in World War I and World War II as an antiseptic to prevent gangrene.

Bottom line: There have been few contemporary studies looking at the use of garlic to treat infections. However, preliminary research suggests that it may reduce the frequency and duration of colds when taken for prevention and may speed the healing of a fungal infection or wart.

My advice: For most people, garlic is worth trying as a preventive/treatment for these infections (see options described below).

SHOULD YOU USE GARLIC?

It's wise to make garlic part of a healthful diet that includes plenty of fruits, vegetables, whole grains and fiber.

Caution: Consuming large quantities of garlic—either in the diet or as a supplement—may cause body odor and/or bad breath. Chewing a sprig of fresh green parsley, mint or cardamom can work as a breath freshener. Hot tea also can help by rinsing away garlic oil still in your mouth. Drinking a glass of milk—full-fat or fat-free—may be effective as well. Garlic, especially on an empty stomach, can cause gastrointestinal upset and flatulence.

Because garlic may also interact with certain prescription drugs, such as *warfarin* (Coumadin), consult your doctor before significantly increasing your intake of the herb if you take any medication or have a chronic medical condition.

Options to consider...

• **Raw garlic.** If you prefer raw garlic, try eating one or two cloves a day. You can chew and swallow it or use it in pesto, guacamole or a salad dressing. Cooked garlic is less powerful medicinally—heat inactivates the enzyme that breaks down alliin, the chemical precursor to allicin.

• **Aged garlic extract (AGE).** If you prefer liquid, AGE is available in this form, which is popular in Europe. Follow label instructions.

• **Powdered garlic supplements.** These are typically sold as capsules or tablets and standardized to contain 1.3% alliin. They usually contain 300 mg.

Typical dose: Two or three capsules or tablets a day.

Find Out What Astaxanthin, The Ocean's Antioxidant, Can Do for You

Mark A. Stengler, NMD, naturopathic medical doctor in private practice, Encinitas, California…adjunct associate clinical professor at the National College of Natural Medicine, Portland, Oregon…author of *The Natural Physician's Healing Therapies* (Bottom Line Books).

Astaxanthin (pronounced as-tuh-ZAN-thin) is a type of red-orange-pink carotenoid that comes from the sea. Carotenoids are pigments that give food their color and have powerful antioxidant properties. Most of us are familiar with beta-carotene, the main carotenoid found in land plants. Well, astaxanthin is the main marine carotenoid. It is found in some types of algae as well as in some fungi and plants—and it gives salmon, shrimp, lobster and crawfish their bright color. You get some astaxanthin when you eat these foods, but most of us don't eat enough of them to benefit.

Astaxanthin is closely related to *lutein*, a carotenoid known to improve eye health, and it has long been used as a supplement to treat aging eyes. But recent studies are finding that this carotenoid provides many other health benefits.

In my own practice, I have found that astaxanthin can especially help patients with diabetes and heart disease. Laboratory studies also show that astaxanthin may fight cancer and enhance cognition, but these findings have not yet been tested in humans. *Here's how astaxanthin can help you…*

HEART DISEASE

Research shows that heart cells have a particular affinity for astaxanthin, which is a potent anti-inflammatory agent. Studies have found that astaxanthin not only reduces inflammation but also lessens oxidative stress. This is particularly important because doctors now believe that coronary artery disease is caused by inflammation in the heart and arteries.

• **LDL cholesterol.** A study published in *Atherosclerosis* found that astaxanthin significantly lowered triglyceride levels and increased HDL (good) cholesterol in adults who were not obese. Astaxanthin also prevents LDL (bad) cholesterol from oxidizing. Oxidized LDL contributes to inflammation and the formation of cholesterol deposits.

• **Diabetes.** High blood glucose levels, which can occur in people with uncontrolled diabetes, increase deposits of fatty materials on the insides of blood vessel walls. This affects blood flow and can result in clogged and rigid blood vessels, increasing the risk for heart attack and stroke. The antioxidant activity of astaxanthin helps keep blood vessels clog-free and flexible by minimizing oxidative damage to the cells that make up blood vessels.

• **Blood flow.** Astaxanthin improves blood *rheology*—the velocity of blood moving through arteries and veins. In a small study of middle-age men, Japanese researchers showed that taking 6 milligrams (mg) of astaxanthin daily for 10 days resulted in smoother, faster blood flow. Improved rheology eases the heart's workload.

• **Heart and brain protection.** Research indicates that astaxanthin can protect the heart and the entire cardiovascular system from ischemic injury. This type of injury occurs when the blood supply to an area of tissue is cut off, such as during a heart attack, stroke or other thrombotic event, including when an *embolus* (a mass of clotted blood) blocks a blood vessel in the heart, brain or veins. Tissue damage occurs when blood supply returns to the area after a period of absence. Reentering blood causes oxidative stress, resulting in inflammation and oxidative damage. This type of injury also occurs during open-heart surgery, when blood flow is stopped and then resumed during the procedure. Similar circulatory damage also may be involved in pressure sores and diabetic foot ulcers. Astaxanthin has not been tested in all of these situations, but it does appear to reduce these types of injuries.

AN IMMUNE BOOSTER

In a Washington State University study, researchers gave college-age women 2 mg or 4 mg of astaxanthin or placebos daily for eight weeks. Astaxanthin increased the immune system's production of natural killer cells, which help us fight infections. The supplements also lowered the women's levels of *C-reactive protein*, a marker of inflammation.

MY RECOMMENDATIONS

To boost immunity and for people with diabetes, I suggest taking 2 mg to 4 mg daily of astaxanthin. For people with coronary artery disease, I recommend taking 8 mg to 16 mg daily (the dose is determined by your weight) as part of a dietary and supplement regimen. You can speak to a holistic doctor about the amount that is right for you. There are no reported side effects. Astaxanthin is safe for everyone but should not be taken by pregnant and lactating women because it has not been studied in these populations. The supplements are derived from algae, so they are even safe for people who are allergic to shellfish (but read your label!).

One brand I like: Source Naturals (800-815-2333, *www.sourcenaturals.com*).

■ **More from Dr. Mark A. Stengler...**

Six Natural Remedies for Warts

My patients always are glad to know that there are natural treatments for unsightly or painful warts—especially because traditional treatments are hard on the body. Conventional wart treatments include applying salicylic acid to the skin (which sloughs off layers of skin and the wart), cryo-surgery (freezing the wart) and standard surgical removal.

Natural solutions take a different approach. They focus on boosting immune function to suppress or eliminate the many viruses that cause warts, including about 70 types of the *human papillomavirus*. First, I have all patients boost their immune systems and fight the virus with the following supplements for two to four weeks—echinacea (300 mg twice daily)...selenium (200 mcg daily)...and a mixed vitamin E supplement that contains tocotrienols and tocopherols (400 IU daily). I also have patients choose either a homeopathic remedy or a topical treatment. If one type of treatment doesn't help them, they can try the other.

●**Homeopathic remedies.** It is important to choose a homeopathic remedy that matches the specific type of wart. The usual dose is two 30C pellets twice daily for two weeks. If the treatment eliminates the wart in that time period, you can stop taking it, although you can resume if the wart starts to return. *Homeopathic remedies to try...*

●***Antimonium crudum*** for hard, flat warts (including plantar warts) on the hands or feet.

●***Causticum*** for large, fleshy and soft warts that bleed easily.

●***Dulcamara*** for large, smooth warts on the back of the hand or the palm.

●***Nitric acid,*** in homeopathic form, is recommended for hard cauliflower-like warts that cluster near the mouth, genital area or anus.

●***Thuja occidentalis*** for groups of large warts that often recur after conventional treatment.

●**Topical antiviral remedies.** Two topical remedies can fight wart-causing viruses. You can try one for two weeks to see if it helps you. If it doesn't, then try the other.

Remedies to use: Thuja oil or garlic oil. Apply one drop of oil directly on the wart twice daily. There is no need to cover the wart.

Surprising Conditions That Chiropractors Can Treat

James N. Dillard, MD, DC, CAc, a pain and integrative medicine specialist in private practice in New York City and East Hampton, New York, *www.drdillard.com*. Dr. Dillard is coauthor of *The Chronic Pain Solution* (Bantam).

If you were asked to name a condition commonly treated by chiropractors, chances are neck and back pain would come to mind. But the list could be much longer.

Even though 11% of Americans seek the services of a chiropractor each year, most people are unaware that chiropractic care—a more than 100-year-old hands-on discipline that focuses primarily on manipulation of the spine—can be used to treat discomfort in many parts of the body.*

To learn more about the surprising conditions that chiropractors can help relieve, we spoke with James N. Dillard, MD, DC, CAc, a medical doctor, chiropractor and acupuncturist who specializes in treating chronic pain. *For example...*

•**Asthma.** The goal of treating people with asthma is to stimulate the rib cage muscles to ease breathing, optimize blood and lymph flow and enhance nervous system activity, all of which help reduce symptoms such as chest tightness and shortness of breath. In treating asthma, chiropractors typically use not only spinal manipulation but also other modalities such as stretching and/or trigger-point massage. Exercise, good eating habits and meditation also may be discussed. Additionally, chiropractic and acupuncture can be an effective combination for asthma.

Scientific evidence: A 2010 study in *The Journal of the Canadian Chiropractic Association,* which compiled data from eight scientific

articles, showed improvements, based on pulmonary function tests, in 5,882 asthma patients who underwent chiropractic care.

•**Carpal tunnel syndrome (CTS).** This condition, which causes shooting pain and numbness in the hand (usually the thumb, index and middle fingers), often occurs in people who have poor posture while performing repetitive tasks, such as working with small hand tools or typing at a keyboard.

Chiropractors can improve CTS by doing stretching and manipulation at the wrist, guiding physical therapy exercises and counseling patients on how they position their hands at the computer or while using hand tools. Wrist splints, worn at night, also may help.

Scientific evidence: Two studies support the use of chiropractic for CTS, including one reporting significant progress in strength, range of motion and pain after several chiropractic sessions. Most improvements were maintained for at least six months.

•**Fibromyalgia.** Characterized by chronic pain and tenderness in joints and muscles, fibromyalgia is a diagnosis of exclusion, meaning other illnesses must first be ruled out, since no laboratory tests can identify it.

Chiropractors can help relieve symptoms by focusing on the tender points—and relaxing these areas as well as the patient's entire frame. They can also apply heat, ice or electrostimulation, which uses electric current to promote muscle contractions, improving blood flow.

A diet that reduces the systemic inflammation that fibromyalgia patients typically have also may be recommended. Such a diet emphasizes fish, fresh vegetables and fruit and discourages fatty meat, fried food and dairy products.

Scientific evidence: A 2009 study of fibromyalgia patients in *The Journal of Alternative and Complementary Medicine* tested the effects of resistance training—including chest presses and leg extensions—combined with chiropractic care. It found that the resistance training's positive impact on patient strength was enhanced by the addition of chiropractic, which improved flexibility, balance and coordination.

In addition to the healing effects of chiropractic's hands-on approach, chiropractors tend to

*Chiropractic care is safe for most people. However, people who have osteoporosis or take blood-thinning medications could be at increased risk for bone fractures and/or internal bleeding, while in extremely rare cases, those with a history of stroke may have an increased risk for a subsequent stroke. If you have these conditions or any other chronic health problem, consult your doctor before seeking chiropractic care.

excel at listening to their patients, which also provides comfort.

•**Headache.** Many of the up to 45 million Americans affected by chronic headache (occurring at least 15 days a month) try one drug after another to find relief. While headache pain obviously manifests in the head, a significant number of headaches are related to the alignment of the cervical spine (neck).

Scientific evidence: Research has found chiropractic care to be especially useful for tension headaches, the most common type experienced by adults in the Western world. Chiropractic may also help with migraines. A study in the *Journal of Manipulative and Physiological Therapeutics* suggested that the combination of spinal manipulation and *amitriptyline* (Elavil), an antidepressant also used for migraine pain, produced stronger results than either alone.

The hand movements chiropractors use to stretch the neck, which often include manual traction to increase space between the vertebrae and/or side-to-side stretches of the neck, may relax the muscle tension at the root of tension headaches in ways that can't necessarily be achieved with drugs.

•**Temporomandibular joint disorder (TMD).** This refers to a variety of conditions marked by intermittent pain in the jaw joints and surrounding tissues, making it difficult to chew or yawn. Many patients have a genuine mechanical malfunction in the jaw, but in my experience, the majority who think they have TMD simply have too much tension in their jaws. They're holding their jaws too tightly and/or grind their teeth at night.

Chiropractic, which may involve manually stretching the jaw and the surrounding muscles, can be enormously helpful for jaw pain. Spinal adjustments to the upper neck and jaw can properly realign the joints, and exercise and lifestyle changes can prevent a relapse. Mouth guards also can be used by people who grind their teeth at night.

Scientific evidence: Research published in 2003 in the *Journal of Manipulative and Physiological Therapeutics* tracked nine TMD patients who suffered pain while opening their mouths. After eight weeks of chiropractic therapy, all

of the patients were able to open their mouths more widely and with less pain.

To find a chiropractor near you: Consult the American Chiropractic Association, 703-276-8800, *www.acatoday.org.*

Acupuncture Can Help You Get Pregnant

Lisa Lilienfield, MD, family practice and pain management specialist, Kaplan Center for Integrative Medicine, McLean, Virginia, and clinical assistant professor, community and family medicine, Georgetown University, Washington, DC.

Jamie Grifo, MD, director, division of reproductive endocrinology, New York University (NYU) Langone Medical Center, and director, NYU Fertility Center, New York City.
*Journal of Endocrinological Investigation
Acupuncture in Medicine*

When a couple is trying to have a baby and can't, it can be emotionally and financially draining. But help may be available in an unexpected form: acupuncture.

Medical experts believe that this ancient therapy from China, which involves placing numerous thin needles at certain points in the body, can help improve fertility in both men and women.

"Acupuncture has been around for almost 3,000 years. It's safe and there are rarely any side effects," explained Lisa Lilienfield, MD, a family practice and pain management specialist at the Kaplan Center for Integrative Medicine in McLean, Virginia. "It may not be the only thing that is done in isolation to treat infertility, but it helps get the body primed and maximizes the potential effects of fertility treatments," she added.

Jamie Grifo, MD, director of the NYU Fertility Center and director of the division of reproductive endocrinology at the NYU Langone Medical Center in New York City, said, "it's not a panacea, but acupuncture does help some patients have better success."

"It's one non-traditional modality to help manage the stress of infertility, and it does improve pregnancy rates and quality of life in some people," he said.

BACKGROUND

Studies that have been done on acupuncture and fertility have had mixed results, with some showing benefits and others showing none. Dr. Grifo said the differing results might have something to do with the design of the studies. Two areas that appear to be more consistently helped by acupuncture treatments are in vitro fertilization (IVF) and women who are infertile due to polycystic ovary syndrome (PCOS). IVF is a procedure that manually combines an egg and sperm in a laboratory dish. If fertilization occurs, the embryo is then transferred into a woman's uterus. PCOS, a condition in which a hormone imbalance occurs, affects a woman's menstrual period, making it difficult to become pregnant.

THE STUDIES

Two studies—one published in *Acupuncture in Medicine* and the other in the *Journal of Endocrinological Investigation*—found a benefit when acupuncture was used on the day an embryo was transferred into a woman's uterus.

The study from the *Journal of Endocrinological Investigation* also found that women with PCOS and infertile men could also benefit from acupuncture.

HOW ACUPUNCTURE BOOSTS FERTILITY

In addition to relieving stress, Dr. Lilienfield said that acupuncture can help increase a woman's fertility by improving blood flow to the ovaries and uterus. This improved blood flow can help thicken the lining of the uterus, increasing the chances of conception.

It may also help correct problems with the body's neuroendocrine system. Acupuncture can help activate the brain to release hormones that will stimulate the ovaries, adrenal glands and other organs that are involved in reproduction, according to Dr. Lilienfield. Acupuncture's effect on the neuroendocrine system may also help infertile men by stimulating sperm production, she said.

ACUPUNCTURE TREATMENT

The actual acupuncture treatment session involves placing very thin needles at specific points in the body. In Chinese medicine, these points are believed to be areas where a person's "qi" (pronounced chee), or life force, is blocked, according to the US National Center for Complementary and Alternative Medicine. In Western medicine, it's believed that the needle placement may release the body's natural painkillers.

Acupuncture is commonly used to treat pain, such as back pain, headache and menstrual cramps, according to the center.

WHEN TO GET HELP FOR INFERTILITY

In general, someone younger than 35 is often advised to try to get pregnant for about a year before seeking treatment for infertility. "But, if you're anxious to get going, six months is a reasonable time to wait," Dr. Lilienfield said. And women older than 35 probably shouldn't wait more than six months, she added.

Dr. Grifo said he doesn't favor waiting that long to seek treatment. "If you are trying to get pregnant and struggling with it, you don't need to wait a year," he said. "And, if you're over 35, don't wait six months if it's causing you distress."

info For more on acupuncture, visit the US National Center for Complementary and Alternative Medicine Web site, *http://nccam.nih. gov/health/acupuncture*.

Acupuncture Safe For Children

Sunita Vohra, MD, professor, department of pediatrics, and director, CARE program, University of Alberta, Canada.

Raymond Pitetti, MD, associate medical director, emergency department, Children's Hospital of Pittsburgh.

Jeannie Kang, president, American Association of Acupuncture and Oriental Medicine.
Pediatrics

When done by well-trained professionals, acupuncture can be a safe treatment for children, recent research suggests.

In an analysis of 37 studies or case reports, Canadian researchers found that in over 1,400 children treated with acupuncture, just 168 experienced a mild adverse reaction, such as crying or pain. The investigators found 25 reports of serious adverse events.

"In trained hands, acupuncture seems safe in children," said the study's senior author, Sunita Vohra, MD, a professor in the department of pediatrics at the University of Alberta in Canada.

Results of the study are published in *Pediatrics*.

ABOUT ACUPUNCTURE

Acupuncture is a treatment that is said to have originated in China thousands of years ago. In Eastern medicine, acupuncture is believed to open the channels where a person's *qi* (pronounced chee), or life force, is blocked. In Western medicine, it's more commonly believed that acupuncture works by stimulating the release of the body's natural painkillers, according to the US National Center for Complementary and Alternative Medicine.

Stimulation of certain areas to release the blocked qi (called acupoints) can be done through the insertion of very thin needles or with heat, pressure or a laser, according to the study authors.

Acupuncture is used for a variety of problems, such as pain, nausea, vomiting, anxiety and muscle spasm, according to Dr. Vohra and Raymond Pitetti, MD, the associate medical director of the emergency department at Children's Hospital of Pittsburgh. Jeannie Kang, president of the American Association of Acupuncture and Oriental Medicine, added that acupuncture is also used for sprains, allergies, asthma, and menstrual cramps and irregularities.

In the United States, recent estimates suggest that as many as three million people have tried acupuncture therapy.

STUDY ON CHILDREN AND ACUPUNCTURE

Because acupuncture is growing in popularity, and no specific studies have been conducted on the safety of acupuncture in children, Dr. Vohra and her colleagues wanted to assess the available evidence to determine whether or not acupuncture is a safe treatment for children.

The researchers reviewed all of the available literature on acupuncture in children. They found 37 studies and case reports that met their inclusion criteria.

The rate of adverse events was significantly lower in children than what has been reported in adults, the results showed.

The current analysis found a mild adverse event rate of nearly 12% in children. Mild events included bleeding, pain, crying, bruising and worsening of symptoms.

Serious events occurred in 25 children. Twelve children had thumb deformities, and five experienced infections after acupuncture. There were also isolated heart problems, lung problems, bleeding issues, nerve impairment, intestinal obstruction, hospitalization and a reversible coma.

Many of the serious adverse events were believed to be the result of substandard practices, said Dr. Vohra.

EXPERT ADVICE

All three experts recommended making sure your child's acupuncturist is well trained. In Canada, acupuncture is regulated in a standard fashion and acupuncturists have to have specific training. In the United States, requirements vary by state, although most require that acupuncturists be licensed, according to Kang. Dr. Vohra and Kang both recommended contacting national acupuncture associations for a practitioner recommendation. Practitioners certified by national organizations will likely have more training.

Kang said that there are some acupuncturists who specialize in acupuncture on children, but that most practitioners will have had some pediatric experience. She said that it's uncommon to do needle insertions on children younger than 11 years old. Instead, she said, acupuncture practitioners will usually use something that "looks like a spiky rolling pin" to put pressure on acupoints.

Dr. Pitetti said he didn't know if there were specific areas of the body where acupuncture absolutely shouldn't be used, but "into the neck, into the brain would make me more concerned. Also, when you start to go near major organs, like the heart, or right around the spinal cord, that would make me nervous."

But, he said, "This study should give parents a little reassurance that it's probably a safe procedure, but it should also make them take a hard look at who's doing the acupuncture to make sure that they're reputable and skilled."

And, he added, it would be very helpful for parents if pediatricians were more aware of complementary medicine therapies, as well as the practitioners in the local area.

info Learn more about what to look for in an acupuncture practitioner from the National Certification Commission for Acupuncture and Oriental Medicine, *www.nccaom.org/consumers/frequently-asked-questions-consumer.*

How to (Finally) Get Rid Of That Lingering Cough

Mark A. Stengler, NMD, naturopathic medical doctor in private practice, Encinitas, California…adjunct associate clinical professor at the National College of Natural Medicine, Portland, Oregon…author of *The Natural Physician's Healing Therapies* and coauthor of *Prescription for Natural Cures* (both from Bottom Line Books).

Your cold disappeared weeks ago—but you're still coughing. This cough usually isn't due to the infection itself but to its inflammatory aftereffects. Postnasal drip is your body's attempt to clear out your respiratory tract through a "productive cough." Or a virus can leave your bronchial tubes sensitive and irritated by airborne substances. A "dry cough" (no mucus is produced) is your body's attempt to get rid of these irritants.

It may take one to three weeks to get rid of a lingering cough. If your cough doesn't ease up within three weeks, see your doctor. Tea and honey always help, but so can the remedies below, which are safe for everyone except as noted. You can try one remedy at a time, but I find that using all of them in combination works best. These natural options work as well as, or better than, over-the-counter cough formulas and have a better safety record. Children also can take these remedies—in doses that are one-quarter to one-half that of adults, based on their weight.

For a cough with mucus or a dry cough…

- **N-acetylcysteine (NAC).** This amino acid derivative thins mucus so that your body can expel it more easily.

Dose: 1,000 milligrams (mg), twice daily.

- **Cherry bark extract.** An extract from black cherry tree bark (*Prunus serotina*), this expectorant loosens phlegm so that it can be expelled.

Dose: 500 mg in capsule form or 1 milliliter (ml) of herbal tincture, three or four times daily. It should not be used by women who are pregnant.

- **Licorice root extract.** This herb has a soothing effect on the respiratory tract and also is a cough suppressant.

Dose: 500 mg in capsule form or 1 ml of herbal tincture, three or four times daily.

For a dry cough…

In addition to the remedies above, I often recommend…

- **Marshmallow root extract.** This herb, derived from the marshmallow plant, reduces inflammation in the respiratory tract.

Dose: 500 mg in capsule form or 1 ml of herbal tincture, three or four times daily.

Flaxseed May Protect You from Radiation Exposure

Keith Cengel, MD, PhD, researcher, assistant professor of radiation oncology, Perelman School of Medicine, The University of Pennsylvania, Philadelphia.

Melpo Christofidou-Solomidou, PhD, professor of medicine, research associate, Perelman School of Medicine, The University of Pennsylvania, Philadelphia.

It's too bad that our risk for radiation poisoning didn't end along with the Cold War. Today, we have nuclear terrorist attacks and power plant leaks to worry about. And if you aren't concerned about those, there's always the possibility of needing radiation therapy for cancer. So it's on multiple levels that a recent study is intriguing: A common food may protect us against radiation—and that food is flaxseed.

The study, done on mice at the Perelman School of Medicine at The University of Pennsylvania in Philadelphia, revealed that a fairly small daily serving of flaxseed (the human equivalent of four tablespoons) is protective against radiation. To find out more, we spoke with researchers Keith Cengel, MD, PhD, assistant professor of radiation oncology at the university, and Melpo Christofidou-Solomidou, PhD, research associate and professor of medicine at the university. Their findings were published in the June 24, 2011, issue of *BMC Cancer*.

DIETS STOP DAMAGE

The researchers said that groups of mice were fed two very similar but not identical diets—the sole difference was that some mice ate no flaxseed and others ate 10% flaxseed. The mice were exposed to a large dose of radiation. Certain groups were given these diets three weeks before the radiation exposure, while others were fed these diets immediately after or two, four or six weeks after the radiation exposure.

Four months after the mice received radiation, the researchers examined their survival rates. They found that 70% to 88% of the mice who ate the flaxseed diet (either before or after radiation exposure) were alive, versus just 40% of the mice who didn't eat any flaxseed. Not only did the mice who ate the flaxseed live longer, but they also had fewer side effects from the radiation—they lost less weight, had less indication of inflammation and had fewer lung problems, such as fibrosis.

SEEDS OF HOPE

The researchers think that it's reasonable to theorize that this protective effect of flaxseed might benefit radiation-treated cancer patients and possibly even victims of a nuclear power plant leak or a "dirty bomb." Even astronauts—who are exposed to radiation during space flight—and frequent fliers might benefit from flaxseed. It might also be useful for the "worried well"—those who fear that they've been exposed to radiation but show no symptoms or those who fear that they might be exposed in the future.

How does flaxseed work to stem radiation damage? The mice in the study received a single radiation dose that is equivalent to getting about 135,000 chest X-rays (the same amount that a cancer patient might get over an entire course of radiation treatment lasting perhaps many months). The researchers aren't completely certain of the mechanism of protection, but they think that the flaxseed may have somehow prevented the DNA damage that typically occurs among normal, noncancerous cells immediately after radiation exposure. If this holds true among humans, then it might mean that eating flaxseed would help the radiation destroy malignant cancer cells without harming so many normal cells—that's an important benefit, since damage to normal cells is one of the major drawbacks of radiation therapy.

But it's important to realize that the results of the mice studies are preliminary, and Drs. Cengel and Christofidou-Solomidou hope that they can be replicated (without the unneeded radiation, of course) in studies of humans. If flaxseed pans out to be a good source of radiation protection among humans, imagine how cheap and easy it would be to hand out small packets of flaxseed to cancer patients or even to everyday healthy citizens if there is concern about a potential nuclear event or a radiation accident, such as the one that happened this past spring in Japan. The daily dose of flaxseed might be just a few tablespoons—for such a huge return.

Meet the Mushroom That Heals Bronchitis, Altitude Sickness and More

Mark A. Stengler, NMD, naturopathic medical doctor in private practice, Encinitas, California…adjunct associate clinical professor at the National College of Natural Medicine, Portland, Oregon…author of *The Natural Physician's Healing Therapies* and coauthor of *Prescription for Natural Cures* (both from Bottom Line Books).

You may be surprised to find that sometimes a remedy is very effective at treating several seemingly unrelated conditions. That's the case with the mushroom reishi (*Ganoderma lucidum*) that grows wild in

China and Japan. Reishi is well-known in the East for its potent and wide-ranging medicinal properties, but most people in the West have never heard of it. Used in traditional Chinese medicine for more than 4,000 years, reishi promotes longevity. Research has shown that it can stimulate the immune system…support liver function…improve circulation…reduce inflammation…and lower blood sugar and cholesterol. *I recommend it for the following conditions…*

•**Chronic bronchitis.** Studies have shown that reishi helps ease chronic bronchitis symptoms. It inhibits the release of histamine, a compound that causes swelling and inflammation.

•**Altitude sickness.** Because of its ability to thin blood, reishi can help prevent symptoms of altitude sickness, such as nausea, dizziness and light-headedness. It is most effective if taken daily, starting two weeks before needed (whether you are traveling to a high-altitude location or mountain climbing) and then throughout the trip.

•**Liver problems.** Studies show that reishi can help support liver function, especially in people with hepatitis B.

Dosage: Reishi is available in multiple forms, though I generally recommend it in capsule form. For all of the medical conditions described above, you can take two to five 400-milligram (mg) to 500-mg capsules twice daily of a reishi mushroom extract standardized to at least 10% polysaccharides.

Brand to try: Nature's Way Standardized Reishi (800-962-8873, *www.naturesway.com,* for a store locator).

Side effects: Very rarely, reishi initially causes digestive upset. Reduce the dose, and the upset should go away. Then gradually increase the dose. Because reishi has blood-thinning effects, check with your doctor if you take a blood thinner, such as *warfarin* (Coumadin). If you have diabetes, talk to your doctor about reishi because it lowers blood sugar and you might need a lower dose of your diabetes medication.

▪ ▪ ▪ ▪

White Willow Bark Fights Osteoarthritis

It contains salicin, a pain reliever similar to the analgesic in aspirin. White willow bark takes longer to start working than aspirin, but its effects generally last longer.

Usual dose: A standardized willow bark extract containing 100 milligrams of salicin (in capsule or tablet form) two or three times a day.

Caution: Avoid willow bark if you have ulcers or stomach problems or are allergic to aspirin.

Laurie Steelsmith, ND, naturopathic physician and acupuncturist based in Honolulu and author of *Natural Choices for Women's Health* (Three Rivers). *www.drsteelsmith.com*

Natural Remedies for Your Eyes Only

Jeffrey R. Anshel, OD, an optometrist and founder of Corporate Vision Consulting, Carlsbad, California. He is president and founding director of the Ocular Nutrition Society and author of *Smart Medicine for Your Eyes: A Guide to Natural, Effective and Safe Relief of Common Eye Problems* (Square One). *www.cvconsulting.com*

Much of the eye discomfort we suffer from every day can be treated naturally at home.

Best overall remedy: Eat fish high in omega-3 fatty acids, such as salmon, anchovies, mackerel and herring. People who eat fish regularly produce less *arachidonic acid*, a substance that can lead to chronic inflammation and eye damage. Aim for two to three fish meals a week. If you are not a fish lover, take a fish oil supplement.

Here, common eye problems—and the best home treatments…

"COMPUTER EYE"

The average American spends up to seven hours each day looking at digital images on computers, TVs, etc.

Result: Eyes that are irritated and dry.

Studies show that we blink at only about one-third of the normal rate when using a computer or watching TV. This causes eye dryness and an increase in muscle tension. Prolonged sitting also reduces respiration and oxygen saturation in eye tissues.

Natural care: Practice the "three B's." Blink more often…take deep breaths every minute or two to relax your eyes and your body…and take a break every 20 minutes. Look away from the TV or computer screen, and focus on various objects at varying distances for about 20 seconds—preferably while standing—to get your eyes moving more fluidly.

DRY-EYE SYNDROME

Dry-eye syndrome usually is due to a decline in the quality and quantity of tear film, the oily liquid that coats the eyes when you blink.

Natural care: Practice the "three B's" described earlier.

Also helpful: An oral supplement called BioTears, which improves the quality of the tear film. It contains a blend of omega-3 and omega-6 fatty acids and other natural ingredients, such as vitamin E and curcumin. The use of preservative-free eyedrops, such as Tears Naturale Forte, also can help.

Important: Don't smoke. Cigarette smoke is a leading cause of dry-eye syndrome.

BLOODSHOT EYES

Redness typically occurs when blood vessels in the clear covering of the *sclera*, the white part of the eyes, dilate.

Main cause: Irritation from allergies, dust and/or excessive sunlight.

Natural care: Take 250 milligrams (mg) of vitamin C, four times daily. It strengthens blood vessels and helps with the formation and maintenance of collagen in the cornea, the transparent dome that covers the iris and pupil.

I also advise patients to take a B-complex supplement. B-vitamin deficiencies have been linked to bloodshot eyes.

Important: Do not use over-the-counter eye whiteners, such as Visine. These products reduce redness by temporarily shrinking blood vessels. The next day, most patients experience a "rebound phenomenon," in which the blood vessels dilate even more.

FLOATERS

These are the squiggles, dots, strands and other shapes that drift in and out of your field of vision. They're the remnants of old, broken-down blood vessels that float in the vitreous, the transparent gel of the eye. Floaters also can occur when protein fibers in the gel clump together.

Floaters tend to get worse with age—not because they increase in number, but because the vitreous becomes more fluid and less gel-like. This allows the floaters to move more freely.

Natural care: An antioxidant-rich diet that includes fruits, vegetables (especially leafy greens) and whole grains. The antioxidants in these foods make the vitreous less watery.

Important: See an eye doctor if you notice a sudden increase in floaters or if floaters are accompanied by flashes of light. These additional symptoms could indicate inflammation of the retina or a retinal detachment.

BLEPHARITIS

This is an inflammation of the small glands and/or eyelash follicles on the surface of the eyelids. In addition to eyelid swelling, some patients may develop small sores. Also, some eyelashes may fall out.

Blepharitis that is accompanied by sores usually is caused by a bacterial infection. Other cases are caused by *seborrheic dermatitis*, a form of dandruff that also may affect the eyelids and eyebrows, along with the ears and the area around the nose and lips. Environmental irritants, such as allergens and smog, also can cause it.

Natural care: For blepharitis, apply a warm, moist washcloth to the eye. Keep it in place until it cools. Continue using compresses three or four times a day until the inflammation is gone. Heat and moisture increase circulation and the flow of nutrients to the eye. They also flush away inflammatory chemicals.

Also helpful: Use green or black tea to moisten the washcloth. The polyphenols in teas shrink swollen tissues and reduce inflammation.

If the condition doesn't improve in two to three days, see your doctor. Bacterial blepharitis can be treated with an over-the-counter antibiotic ointment such as Neosporin.

STYE

Caused by a bacterial infection in one of the tiny glands on the edges of the eyelids, a stye is a small pimple that can be painful as well as unsightly. Styes almost always clear up on their own within a week. Those that last longer (or that hurt a lot) may need to be drained by a doctor who also may prescribe antibiotics.

Natural care: Steam. Boil some water, and pour it into a cup. Close the affected eye, and bring it close to the cup to let the steam rise toward the stye. Be careful not to burn yourself. Repeat three or four times a day. Or you can apply warm, wet washcloths. These help bring the stye to a head.

Caution: Do not squeeze the stye or "pop" the head. It can spread bacteria to the eye.

There are over-the-counter remedies that can help, such as Similasan. Avoid any that contain mercuric oxide, which can irritate the eye.

CORNEAL ABRASIONS

A scratch on the cornea—usually caused by dust or other debris—can make the eye feel "scratchy." Patients often have the sensation that something is stuck under the eyelid even when the debris is gone.

Most corneal abrasions heal within a few days. To relieve the pain, you can take aspirin (not acetaminophen, which does not help with inflammation). See your doctor if the discomfort is severe or doesn't get better within 24 to 48 hours.

Natural care: Any sterile saline solution can help, and sleeping does, too. Also, keep the area around the lids clean to reduce the chance of bacteria getting into the eye.

PTERYGIUM

This is a triangular-shaped growth that forms on the white of the eye—it usually is flat and yellowish with blood vessels going through it. People who spend a lot of time in the sun, such as farmers or surfers, tend to get it. Other risk factors include dust and living in a hot, dry climate. A pterygium (the "p" is silent) doesn't need to be removed unless it spreads onto the cornea and interferes with vision.

Natural care: Try to stay inside when the wind is blowing. Avoid smoky environments.

Reducing environmental irritants can slow or stop further growth.

Also important: Always wear a brimmed hat when you're out on sunny days. Also, wear sunglasses that block 100% of UV radiation—close-fitting wraparound styles are best.

Chinese Herbal Remedies You Can Make Yourself

Daisy Dong, LAc, OMD, licensed herbalist and professor at Southwest Acupuncture College in Boulder and a senior acupuncturist at The Center for Integrative Medicine at University of Colorado Hospital in Aurora.

Traditional Chinese Medicine (TCM) offers natural topical remedies that can soothe joint pain, sprains and minor burns and promote healing. Some TCM herbal remedies are simple enough for you to make and use at home (though for any serious injury or significant ongoing pain, you should see a health-care professional first).

The recipes below were provided by Daisy Dong, LAc, OMD, a licensed herbalist and professor at Southwest Acupuncture College. Ingredients for these remedies are available at many herbal stores and Asian markets as well as online. (Dr. Dong recommended Spring Wind Dispensary, *www.springwinddispensary.com*, 866-731-4372.) Ask for the herbs by their Chinese names and/or their Latin or common names. Herbs often are measured in grams, so you may want to invest in a small kitchen scale...or, in most cases, you can use the teaspoon, tablespoon and cup measurements that are provided by the dispensary.

Important: These are topical remedies, meant to be applied directly to the affected area. Do not ingest them! Used as directed, they have no side effects.

FOR ACHY JOINTS: HONG HUA LINIMENT

This remedy invigorates blood flow to reduce blood stasis (stagnation) in the joint...lessens swelling...and eases aching pain.

Note: The preparation must soak for a week before it is ready to use, so make a batch to keep it on hand, ready for when you need it. *Ingredients…*

50 g (10 tsp.) dried, raw *hong hua* (also called carthamus)

300 ml (1¼ cups) of 70% isopropyl rubbing alcohol

To prepare: Place the hong hua into a container that has a tight-fitting lid and pour the alcohol over the herb. Cover and refrigerate for one week. Strain the liquid through cheesecloth, removing and discarding all solid remnants of the herb. Store the liquid liniment, tightly covered, in the refrigerator for up to three months.

To use: Up to four times per day as needed, soak a cotton ball or gauze pad in the liniment, then rub on the aching joint. Avoid getting the liniment on your clothing as it may stain.

FOR SPRAINS: HUANG LIAN SALVE

This remedy reduces blood stasis…combats inflammation…and alleviates pain. All herbs for this salve should be purchased in powdered (granule) form. For maximum effect, the salve should be prepared fresh each day, Dr. Dong recommended, but the dry ingredients can be combined ahead of time and stored for easy future use. *Ingredients…*

30 g (6 tsp.) *huang lian* (coptis root)

12 g (2½ tsp.) *yan hu suo* (corydalis rhizome)

12 g (2½ tsp.) *hong teng* (sargentodoxa vine)

10 g (2 tsp.) *bai zhu* (atractylodes rhizome)

10 g (2 tsp.) *qiang huo* (notopterygium root)

10 g (2 tsp.) *du huo* (pubescent angelica root)

10 g (2 tsp.) *mu xiang* (saussurea)

3 g (⅔ tsp.) *xue jie* (dragon's blood)

Fresh egg whites

To prepare: In a container, combine all herbs (not the egg whites) and mix together thoroughly. Cover and store this powdered mixture in a dry place until ready to use. When the remedy is needed, combine 6 g (1¼ tsp) of the mixed powder with one fresh egg white and stir to form a pasty salve.

To use: Rub the salve on the affected area, cover with gauze and leave on for one to two hours. Apply once daily until pain is gone. Avoid applying to skin that is broken or cut.

FOR MINOR BURNS: DANG GUI SALVE

Applied to small burns that are reddened or blistered, this salve helps eliminate toxins…invigorates blood flow…and moistens skin to promote tissue healing and regrowth. *Ingredients…*

30 g raw, sliced *dang gui* (Chinese angelica root)

120 g (8 Tbsp.) sesame oil

30 g (2 Tbsp.) beeswax

To prepare: In a frying pan, fry the raw, sliced dang gui with the sesame oil for several minutes until the herb turns blackish and the oil changes color. Remove from heat. With a slotted spoon, remove and discard the dang gui. Add the beeswax to the hot oil and stir quickly until completely mixed. Pour the mixture into an oven-safe container and place in a 200°F oven for about one hour, stirring mixture two or three times as it bakes. Toward the end of the baking time, check the consistency by placing a small amount of the mixture on a metal spoon and putting it in the freezer for one minute—ideally, it should be soft and pasty (no longer watery but not yet hard) when mixture is the proper consistency. Remove the mixture from the oven and stir again to mix well. Let cool, then transfer to a glass or metal container. Cover and store in the refrigerator for up to nine months.

To use: Spread 1 Tbsp. of salve on a gauze pad and apply to the burned area, changing the dressing once or twice daily, Dr. Dong recommended. Repeat applications until the burned tissue heals.

■ ■ ■ ■

Flaxseed Oil Helps Ease Dry Eye

Patients with dry eye who took 9,000 milligrams (mg) orally of flaxseed oil every day for three months had less dryness, irritation and eye fatigue.

To use flaxseed oil for dry eye: Start with 1,000 mg three times a day for two weeks, then gradually increase the dosage to 3,000 mg three times a day.

Jack Greiner, DO, PhD, clinical instructor in ophthalmology at Harvard Medical School, Boston, and leader of a study presented at a recent meeting of the American Academy of Ophthalmology.

The Spice That Fights Food Poisoning

Fernanda Domingues, PhD, lead researcher, associate professor of microbiology and toxicology, University of Beira Interior, Portugal.

Here's good news for those of us who lean toward the natural way of doing things: A recent in vitro study has found that the oil from ordinary coriander seeds is effective at killing bacteria that can cause food poisoning and other illnesses. With listeria still in the headlines, this is big news.

PUNGENT FLAVOR, RICH HISTORY

If "cilantro" comes to mind when you hear "coriander," it's because the pungent cilantro used in Mexican and Mediterranean cooking is the leaf of the same coriander plant. Coriander has been associated with good digestion for thousands of years, with evidence of its use dating as far back as 5,000 BC. It is mentioned in Sanskrit texts, ancient Egyptian papyri, the Old Testament and the writings of Greek physician Hippocrates. The Roman armies brought coriander to Europe, where it was used to preserve meats, and the Chinese believed that coriander counteracted food poisoning—in addition to serving as an aphrodisiac and bestowing immortality!

Coriander oil, which is what was used for this new research, is "steam-distilled" (a process that uses low heat, so the oil's components won't degrade) from the seeds of the coriander plant (*Coriandrum sativum L.*). The resulting liquid is what's called "coriander essential oil," meaning its distinct properties reflect the essence of the plant.

THE 21ST-CENTURY TAKE

A research group at the University of Beira Interior in Portugal tested the antimicrobial properties of coriander oil against 12 bacteria strains, including some of the bad guys whose names you'll recognize—*E. coli*, *Salmonella* and *B. cereus* (all bacteria that can cause foodborne illnesses), MRSA (methicillin-resistant Staphylococcus aureus—which can cause virulent infections throughout the body) and *E. faecalis* (which can cause urinary tract infections, meningitis and other health problems).

Though they had reason to believe coriander oil would be effective, the researchers were surprised at just how well it worked—10 of the 12 strains of bacteria were killed with a relatively mild concentration of coriander oil (1.6%). In the two strains that were not effectively killed—B. cereus and E. faecalis—the coriander oil still reduced their growth significantly.

WHAT WILL THE FUTURE HOLD?

After all these centuries of use in traditional medicine for treating nausea, pain and fungal infections, coriander has some distinctly modern applications as well. According to Fernanda Domingues, PhD, associate professor of microbiology and toxicology, the food industry may be able to use coriander oil to protect against foodborne diseases and bacterial spoilage—and also as a safe ingredient in antibacterial food packaging that might improve the shelf life of fresh foods. It shows promise in medicine as well, specifically as a potential treatment for drug-resistant infections and a variety of hospital-acquired infections.

There is a rub, however—though the Food and Drug Administration has given coriander oil "generally-regarded-as-safe" (GRAS) status and considers it a recognized flavoring, not much is known about its toxicity in humans. So Dr. Domingues doesn't advise people to inhale coriander oil or to take it orally…for now…until more research provides additional information. "Coriander oil might someday become a natural alternative to common antibiotics," she said. That's something to look forward to—and in the meantime, it is, of course, fine to use coriander seeds (whole or ground) in your cooking.

Castor Oil—The "New" Wonder Cure

Andrew L. Rubman, ND, founder and director, Southbury Clinic for Traditional Medicines, Southbury, Connecticut. *www.southburyclinic.com*

Castor oil, which looks and smells like gooey glycerin, is an oily extract that comes from the *Ricinus communis* plant native to India and Africa. In days of yore, parents

routinely dosed girls and boys with a teaspoon or two in order to prevent constipation. It also was thought to cure headaches. Today, internal use is considered unwise because of its strong, often irritating laxative effect...but external application of a castor oil "pack"—meaning a cloth soaked in the oil—can help in all sorts of ways.

THE WONDER CURE?

According to Andrew L. Rubman, ND, castor oil packs mold comfortably to the body...stay warm much longer than hot water...and deeply and gently stimulate circulation, removing inflammation from underlying organs and tissues (e.g., the liver, intestines, tendons, ligaments). You can buy castor oil packs inexpensively at most drugstores, or you can make your own (see below).

Dr. Rubman describes his favorite uses for castor oil...

•**Soothing arthritis pain.** To relieve that ache in your knee or hip, apply a castor oil pack that is roughly the same temperature as a hot bath (105°F). Put the pack directly on the area that hurts, cover with a plastic wrap of some sort (a ziplock bag is a good choice) and then cover that with a hot water bottle or electric heating pad to maintain the temperature. Leave it in place for about 20 to 30 minutes. Repeat every few hours or so. For long-standing conditions, it may be more practical to do this once a day and leave the pack in place for the better part of an hour, Dr. Rubman said.

•**Reducing swelling and inflammation.** A castor oil pack is helpful in soothing a muscle strain or a bruise.

•**Relieving congestion.** If you have a nagging cold, cough or bronchitis, place the castor oil pack on your chest for quick relief.

•**Making a boil disappear.** Before you schedule an appointment to have your doctor lance a boil, try using a castor oil pack, which will encourage the boil to open and drain. For this purpose, make a smaller pack...make it a bit hotter...and use for shorter periods of time, Dr. Rubman suggests.

If you'd like to make your own castor oil pack, buy castor oil (available at pharmacies) and follow these simple instructions from Dr. Rubman...

•**Pour enough castor oil to cover the cloth you are going to use (such as a clean washcloth) into a pan,** ovenproof or microwavable bowl and heat on the stove, in the oven or microwave to hot bathwater temperature (about 105°F). Take care to not leave it in too long or it will get too hot and you may get burned when you remove it.

•**Soak the cloth in the warm castor oil until it is saturated.**

•**Wipe excess oil off the cloth (so it's not dripping) and place the cloth on the affected area of your body...**cover the cloth with a sheet of plastic wrap...and cover that with a heating pad or hot water bottle to keep it warm. As explained above, leave on for 20 to 30 minutes twice a day—or, for chronic conditions, up to an hour, once a day. Rest during this time.

•**When you are finished using the pack, wring as much oil as you can out of the cloth and cover it in plastic,** such as by placing it into a resealable plastic bag, until its next use.

CASTOR OIL PACKS—MAKING THEM LAST

Between uses, store castor oil packs in the refrigerator. When reusing, refresh the packs with additional oil as needed. Dispose of them after about 10 (commercial packs) to 20 (homemade ones) applications. The homemade packs tend to retain the embedded oil longer, Dr. Rubman said, adding they should be discarded when they no longer feel sticky.

Hot tip: Dr. Rubman says that you can intensify the effectiveness of a castor oil pack by sprinkling a teaspoon of cayenne (hot pepper) powder onto the pack (after you've heated it) on the same side you apply to your skin. He explained that the capsaicin in the hot pepper is a pain reliever that increases the stimulating effect on circulation. (Wash your hands with soap and water afterward—you don't want to get this stuff in your eyes or, frankly, on any other sensitive place, such as on mucous membranes!)

Dr. Rubman had another bit of practical advice—he said that castor oil has a tacky, glue-like texture and that handling it can be a messy business. So make sure when you are using the pack that plastic covers it completely—to avoid staining clothing, bedding or upholstery with castor oil.

Pain Relief

A Pain-Free Life— Without Drugs

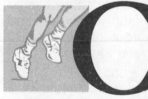

Chronic pain from an injury, arthritis or nerve damage can be so uncomfortable that the sufferer will do almost anything to relieve it—including regularly using over-the-counter (OTC) painkillers that can cause stomach upset, internal bleeding and even death...and/or prescription narcotics that can lead to addiction and cognitive impairment.

But chronic pain sufferers often do not need these drugs...or can take them far less often. Newest thinking on when—and when not—to take drugs for pain...

DRUG OR NO DRUG?

If you have occasional short-term pain, it is OK to take a nonsteroidal anti-inflammatory drug (NSAID), such as aspirin or *ibuprofen* (Motrin).

But chronic pain, defined as pain that lasts more than six months, is a different story. This type of pain affects about 116 million-plus Americans each year—more than cancer, heart disease and diabetes combined.

Shocking fact: Each year, about two million Americans suffer NSAID-related gastritis, ulcers and other types of gastrointestinal irritation—and about 16,000 die from internal bleeding associated with OTC and/or prescription NSAID use.

Among the millions of people who treat chronic pain with prescription narcotics, such as *oxycodone* combined with *acetaminophen* (Percocet) and *oxycodone* (OxyContin), about 3% will progress to abuse or addiction and about 12% will suffer cognitive and/or behavioral side effects.

SAFER WAYS TO MANAGE PAIN

More and more scientific evidence now shows that various nondrug approaches can be highly effective in fighting chronic pain.

Vijay Vad, MD, a sports medicine physician and researcher specializing in minimally invasive arthritis therapies at the Hospital for Special Surgery in New York City. Dr. Vad is the author of *Stop Pain: Inflammation Relief for an Active Life* (Hay House). *www.vijayvad.com*

People who are overweight can help curb their pain by losing weight (which reduces the mechanical stress placed on the body). Recent research has also uncovered that fatty tissue actually secretes inflammatory compounds that increase pain and pain-sensitivity. *Other non-drug approaches to relieve chronic pain...**

1. Exercise the right amount. A recent study found that the majority of back patients who performed stretching and strengthening exercises for 15 minutes, three days a week—with a day off in between to allow muscles to recover—had a 50% reduction in pain. The patients were allowed to use the painkiller *hydrocodone* with acetaminophen, but only as needed. In those who used medication but didn't exercise, pain was reduced by only 33%.

Why does exercise help? For one thing, it increases blood flow to injured tissues. This promotes a flow of nutrients that accelerates healing and reduces pain. Exercise also increases the body's production of endorphins, neurotransmitters that have effects that are similar to morphine and other narcotic painkillers.

Important: Exercise must be tailored to each individual to help strengthen specific parts of the body and avoid additional injury. Walking and swimming are good choices for most patients because they put little stress on muscles and joints. Consult with your doctor or a physical therapist.

2. Supplement with vitamin D. Low vitamin D levels have been linked to chronic pain—in part because the vitamin curbs inflammation. You can potentially get enough vitamin D from sun exposure, but up to one-third of Americans are deficient. Most people can get adequate vitamin D by spending 10 to 15 minutes in the sun without sunscreen twice a week. Sunscreen should be used at other times.

In people who suffer more pain in the winter, it may have less to do with cold temperatures than with the lack of sunshine and vitamin D production. Because food generally does not provide significant levels of the vitamin, I suggest taking a vitamin D supplement.

*The nondrug approaches described in this article can be used at the same time, but it's helpful to initially use them one at a time for one to two weeks each so you can determine which approach works best for you.

Typical dose: 1,000 IU to 2,500 IU daily. To determine the best dose for you, get an annual blood test to check your vitamin D level.

3. Take ginger or turmeric daily. Both are potent anti-inflammatories that reduce pain as effectively as ibuprofen and other NSAIDs. They do this by blocking the enzyme COX-2, which causes inflammation. Unlike NSAIDs, ginger and turmeric do not block the COX-1 enzyme—a lack of COX-1 is what leads to gastric bleeding.

Scientific evidence: A yearlong study published in the journal *Osteoarthritis and Cartilage* found that participants with osteoarthritis of the knee who took ginger supplements had significant relief from knee pain. Other studies have found that turmeric also can reduce pain from knee osteoarthritis.

Typical dose: Follow label instructions. Ginger and turmeric supplements are available at most health-food stores.

Caution: Ginger and turmeric have mild blood-thinning effects. If you take *warfarin* (Coumadin) or another blood-thinning medication, or medications to lower blood sugar or blood pressure, check with your doctor before using ginger or turmeric supplements.

4. Use fish oil. It's well-established that omega-3 fatty acids in fish can help reduce cardiovascular disease, arthritis and other conditions. That's because omega-3s are among the most potent anti-inflammatory agents found in nature.

Scientific evidence: A study at the University of Pittsburgh School of Medicine found that 59% of patients with neck or back pain who were given omega-3s experienced enough pain reduction that they were able to stop using NSAIDs.

Typical dose: 2,000 mg daily.

Caution: Fish oil can have a mild blood-thinning effect, so consult your doctor before taking it.

5. Take care of your mental health. Patients with chronic pain tend to experience higher-than-normal levels of stress, fatigue and depression—all of which, in turn, increase pain in most patients.

If you're depressed—symptoms include changes in sleep habits, difficulty concentrating, unexplained changes in appetite and/or a loss of interest in things that you used to enjoy—see a therapist. About 20% to 25% of patients with both chronic pain and depression will experience a significant reduction in pain just from treating the depression.

6. Increase REM sleep. Patients who don't get enough rapid eye movement (REM) sleep tend to be more sensitive to pain. Researchers speculate that decreased amounts of this deep sleep boost levels of amino acids, such as glutamate, which increase pain signal transmission.

My advice: To promote restful sleep, spend a few minutes doing deep-breathing exercises just before you go to bed. Breathing slowly and deeply stimulates the lower lobes of the lungs and activates the part of the nervous system that reduces stress as well as pain.

FOR ACUTE PAIN

Acute pain should be promptly treated with lifestyle measures as well as prescription or OTC painkillers. Pain that is reduced or eliminated within six to eight weeks is less likely to become a lifelong problem than pain that isn't treated quickly.

Important: If you're suffering from acute or chronic pain but don't know the cause, see your doctor.

You May Not Need a Knee Replacement

David C. Wang, DO, osteopathic physician at The Kaplan Center for Integrative Medicine in McLean, Virginia. A former instructor at Harvard Medical School, he is a nationally recognized expert in treating musculoskeletal pain.

If physical therapy, pain medications and commonly used injections of cortisone or *hyaluronic acid* (Synvisc) no longer relieve your knee pain, don't assume that you need surgery.

Knee replacement is widely known to significantly reduce pain, but 15% of knee-replacement patients still have severe pain several years later. In some cases, scar tissue from the surgery can irritate the surrounding knee structure, which leads to lasting pain.

What's more, the recovery period after knee replacement can be very difficult for some people—for example, it usually takes four to six weeks after the operation before you can drive again, go shopping and do most of your everyday activities. And some knee-replacement patients can never again participate in high-impact sports, such as tennis, jogging or downhill skiing.

Fortunately, there are some highly effective nonsurgical alternatives to knee replacement.

LESS INVASIVE THAN SURGERY

The procedures that show promise for long-term relief are less painful and have a quicker recovery time than knee-replacement surgery. *Nonsurgical approaches…**

•**Platelet-rich plasma (PRP) therapy.** This is rapidly emerging as one of the most popular remedies for knee pain. It's been successfully used by professional athletes, including the golfer Tiger Woods, to improve healing after a knee injury.

How it's done: A small amount of blood is withdrawn from the patient. The blood is then spun in a centrifuge to concentrate platelets, which are then injected back into the knee to stimulate healing. Injections given in the open space inside a joint are only slightly painful…those given directly into a ligament or tendon typically require a local anesthetic to reduce discomfort. The procedure takes about an hour. Moderate to significant soreness lasts a few days.

How it works: Platelets are small cells in blood that initiate clotting. More importantly, they produce growth factors that stimulate, and accelerate, the body's natural healing process. An injection of PRP stimulates the movement of collagen-producing cells to the injured area. The body uses collagen to repair cartilage and other tissues.

My clinical experience: I've found that about 90% of my patients given PRP treatment for knee osteoarthritis report at least a 50% reduction in knee pain after two to four injections given at four- to eight-week intervals. PRP

*To find a physician with expertise in evaluating and treating musculoskeletal disorders, click on "Find a Doctor" at the Web site of the American Association of Orthopaedic Medicine (*www.aaomed.org*).

can heal damaged cartilage, but it won't stop the progression of osteoarthritis. Many patients need a booster shot every couple of years.

Best candidates: PRP can potentially be helpful for anyone with mild-to-severe arthritis who wants to avoid knee-replacement surgery, but seems to work best in younger patients with less severe arthritis.

Typical cost: Each injection ranges from $500 to $1,000. Most patients need at least two injections. PRP usually is not covered by insurance. Risks are minimal but include infection and injury to surrounding tissue.

•**Prolotherapy.** Using sugar (dextrose) injections to treat knee pain sounds like a scam. But this approach, known as prolotherapy, has been extensively researched.

Scientific evidence: In a recent study of arthritis patients published in *Alternative Therapies in Health and Medicine,* patients who received dextrose injections had a 44% decrease in pain, 63% decrease in swelling and 85% fewer episodes of knee buckling after one year.

How it's done: Dextrose solution is injected into the painful area. A topical anesthetic can be used to reduce discomfort from the injections. Most patients get several injections during each session. It takes about 15 minutes. Prolotherapy injections are given every three to six weeks. It usually takes one to three months to notice results, which can last for several years.

How it works: The sugar solution stimulates production of collagen fibers, the body's natural healing response. Sometimes other solutions are used, including sodium morrhuate or phenol.

Best candidates: Most effective for patients with mild-to-moderate knee pain from arthritis or ligament and tendon injury.

Typical cost: $150 to $500 per session. The average patient needs five to seven sessions. It probably won't be covered by insurance. Prolotherapy has a small risk for infection, temporary or permanent nerve irritation or injury, or allergic reaction.

•**Stem cell therapy.** Stem cells are undifferentiated cells that have the ability to turn into specialized cells in different parts of the body. They also have the unique ability to repair damaged tissue by dividing and multiplying almost indefinitely. Stem cell therapy is often used to repair damaged cartilage.

How it's done: Stem cells are "harvested" from the patient, often from fatty tissue or from bone marrow. The cells are spun in a centrifuge to separate stem cells and get a high concentration of them. Patients are given a local anesthetic to reduce discomfort, then the cells are injected into the injured/painful area.

How it works: When stem cells are injected into specific parts of the knee, they transform themselves into chondrocytes, or cells that build cartilage. They can also be transformed into cells known as *fibroblasts* (for soft-tissue repair) or *osteoblasts* (for building bone).

Unlike PRP and prolotherapy, which mobilize the body's repair mechanisms, stem cell therapy directly repairs damaged areas. I've seen arthritis patients with severe bone damage, who I thought would require joint-replacement surgery, improve dramatically enough from this therapy to not need surgery.

Best candidates: People with severe osteoarthritis who didn't get significant pain relief from PRP or prolotherapy.

Typical cost: About $2,000 to $3,000 per treatment. One treatment might be enough—patients with more severe joint damage may need more. The therapy is not covered by insurance.

New Help for Plantar Fasciitis

Raymond R. Monto, MD, orthopedic surgeon, Nantucket Cottage Hospital, Nantucket, Massachusetts.

Howard Luks, MD, chief, sports medicine, Westchester Medical Center and New York Medical College, Hawthorne, New York.

For people struggling with plantar fasciitis—a painful and sometimes disabling foot condition—a small, preliminary study suggests that a new type of therapy is more effective than standard cortisone injections in restoring mobility.

So-called "platelet-rich plasma" therapy is injected directly into the foot. It harnesses two main ingredients found in blood—plasma and platelets—to promote inflammation, connective-tissue growth and vascular healing. This contrasts with cortisone injections, which are designed to reduce inflammation.

"The focus here is on very difficult patients for whom well-recognized nonsurgical and surgical approaches are not effective," said study author Raymond R. Monto, MD, an orthopedic surgeon with Nantucket Cottage Hospital in Nantucket, Massachusetts. "Because while 90% of patients usually get better with standard treatment, about 10% don't.

"For these patients cortisone shots just don't help," Dr. Monto added. "The initial benefit degrades very quickly, and eventually by six months, and certainly by one year out—you are back where you started.

"But among these sorts of patients I was very encouraged by the results with [platelet-rich plasma therapy]," Dr. Monto continued. "For most, after just one shot, we saw dramatic improvements. We're talking about the restoration of well over 90% of normal function lasting at least a year after treatment."

ABOUT PLANTAR FASCIITIS

According to the American Academy of Podiatric Sports Medicine, plantar fasciitis is the most common musculoskeletal problem in the United States, typically prompted by aerobic injury or poor shoe support.

The painful condition arises from inflammation of the connective tissue running from the heel to the ball of the foot, tissue known as plantar fascia, which in turn places heavy stress on the bottom of the foot. Commonly, the condition will begin when a person feels a sharp pain in their heel as they step down after being at rest.

Standard treatment can involve a mix of nonsteroidal anti-inflammatory drugs, stretching exercises, steroid injections, rest, orthotics, improved arch support, shockwave therapy and, in some cases, surgery.

STUDY DETAILS

The new study focused on 36 patients (16 men and 20 women), ages 21 to 74, struggling with a severe and chronic form of plantar fasciitis. None had experienced any relief following standard nonsurgical treatments.

The participants were divided into two groups. One received an ultrasound-guided injection of *methylprednisolone* (a steroid) at the injury site, while the other was treated with platelet-rich plasma.

While the steroid group showed notable improvement within the three months following treatment, foot function started to decline by the sixth month and continued on a downward trend through to the one-year mark.

The platelet-rich plasma group experienced better initial improvement and maintained increased function throughout the following year.

"Pretty much, if the patient treated with [platelet-rich plasma therapy] saw function go up by the four-week mark, then that function was maintained," Dr. Monto said.

"But, of course, one study doesn't change patterns of treatment," he noted. "So this should be viewed as a beginning point that raises awareness of the potential of [platelet-rich plasma therapy] for this type of treatment, and hopefully initiates more research."

Dr. Monto presented his findings at a meeting of the American Academy of Orthopaedic Surgeons in San Francisco.

EXPERT COMMENTARY

Howard Luks, MD, chief of sports medicine at Westchester Medical Center and New York Medical College, both in Hawthorne, New York, described the platelet-rich plasma therapy exploration as "worthwhile," but added that questions remain.

"The reason there has been such an interest in [platelet-rich plasma therapy] is because cortisone is degenerative," he said. "It doesn't heal tissue. It actually can damage tissue with repeated injections. So we never, as orthopedists, really had a regenerative injection option available to us."

However, platelet-rich plasma therapy "is somewhat of a controversial subject, because at this point not all [platelet-rich plasma therapy] is equal," Dr. Luks added. "Different manufacturers take a different level of the blood. Some take the white cells, some don't; some exclude platelets, some don't. So the orthopedics community at large is still sort of saying that before we adopt this widely, let's figure out exactly what we're doing and what's the best preparation. And those studies are now under way."

Unlike cortisone treatments, platelet-rich plasma therapy is not covered by insurance. Dr. Luks said that, in his experience, costs for the new treatment can range anywhere from $270 an injection to as much as $3,000.

Self-Help for Painful Heels

Jim Johnson, PT, is a physical therapist and clinical instructor at Emory University Hospital in Atlanta. He is the author of 11 books, including *The 5-Minute Plantar Fasciitis Solution and Treat Your Own Knee Arthritis* (both from Dog Ear Publishers). *www.bodymending.com*

If you have heel pain, your podiatrist or physical therapist can confirm a plantar fasciitis diagnosis. Often the condition eventually goes away on its own, according to physical therapist Jim Johnson, PT, a clinical instructor at Emory University Hospital, but since this can take months, you'll want to know what you can do to alleviate pain and hasten healing. *What helps…*

•**Stretch the plantar fascia.** Do this before getting out of bed and twice more during the day, continuing until symptoms are gone. Sit on the edge of your bed or in a chair and rest the ankle of the affected foot on the opposite knee. With either hand, grasp the base of the toes and gently pull the toes back toward the shin until you feel a stretch through the sole. Hold for 10 seconds…rest…repeat 10 times. For detailed instructions and illustrations, see Johnson's book, *The 5-Minute Plantar Fasciitis Solution.*

•**Stretch your calves.** Increasing calf muscle flexibility helps support the plantar fascia.

Four times daily: Stand on the bottom step of a stairway, facing the stairs and holding the railing. Place the ball of each foot on the edge of the step so your heels hang off. Keeping knees straight, slowly lower your heels until you feel a mild stretch in your calves. Hold for 20 seconds…rest…repeat three more times.

•**Use shoe inserts that support the arch and cushion the heel.** These change the way your feet sit in shoes, reducing stress on the feet as you stand or walk. The inserts sold at drugstores for about $15 to $20 generally work as well as more expensive custom-made inserts, Johnson noted. Put inserts in both shoes even if only one heel hurts and use them daily for eight to 12 weeks.

•**Wear a night splint.** Tissues in the sole tend to constrict and tighten at night, which is why plantar fasciitis patients often experience pain upon arising in the morning. The night splint, which looks like a big plastic boot, prevents constriction by keeping the ankle and foot at a 90° angle overnight, Johnson explained. Unless you have pain in both feet, it's OK to wear just one splint. Use it nightly for 12 weeks. Night splints start at about $40 and are sold at medical-supply stores and online (for instance, check *www.footsmart.com/c-night-splints-20.aspx*).

Johnson advised that surgery on the plantar fascia be considered only as a last resort. And even then, beware—surgery can cause the arch to drop and compromise foot stability and there is no conclusive evidence that it helps. A better medical treatment option to try is *extracorporeal shockwave therapy,* in which a machine sends ultrasonic waves through the sole, causing micro-injuries that are thought to increase the flow of blood and healing nutrients to the tissues. Fortunately, though, for most patients the aforementioned self-help techniques are enough to make heel pain a thing of the past.

Pain in Your Big Toe? You May Have Gout

Robert T. Keenan, MD, MPH, rheumatologist and assistant professor of medicine in the division of rheumatology at Duke University School of Medicine and medical director of the Infusion Center at Duke University Medical Center, both in Durham, North Carolina.

Approximately six million Americans suffer from gout, the most common form of inflammatory arthritis. Although gout is most often associated with pain, it is now thought that the condition also increases risk for hypertension and cardiovascular disease.

WHAT IS GOUT?

Gout occurs when uric acid, a by-product of metabolism, is produced in excessive amounts or when it is not excreted efficiently by the kidneys. A buildup of uric acid causes the formation of urate crystals in the fluid that lubricates joints. These crystals can trigger an immune response that causes inflammation and excruciating pain.

AGONIZING ATTACKS

Gout often strikes at the base of the big toe, causing pain that increases for eight to 12 hours and subsides within three to 10 days without treatment. Other joints can also be affected. The attacks are intermittent and unpredictable. They may occur every few weeks or months, once or twice a year or every few years. But without treatment, the attacks generally increase in duration as well as frequency.

The risks: Untreated gout can cause permanent joint damage. Some patients progress from *recurrent gout* to *tophaceous gout*, a severe form in which lumps of urate crystals form in and around joints or even under the skin. Gout increases the risk for kidney stones, and patients who don't achieve good control of their elevated uric acid levels are more likely to develop cardiovascular disease than those without gout.

EASY TO DIAGNOSE

Patients who are suspected of having gout are usually advised to have a blood test to measure uric acid. However, some asymptomatic patients have high levels of uric acid, while those in the midst of an attack may have apparently normal levels (3 mg/dL to 7 mg/dL). Typically, the uric acid level peaks around two weeks after an acute attack.

Joint aspiration is the best test for gout, especially in its early stages. Your doctor will insert a needle into the inflamed joint (lidocaine and numbing sprays minimize the pain of the needle) and withdraw fluid, which is then examined under a microscope. The presence of urate crystals means that you have gout, regardless of the uric acid concentrations in your blood.

Ultrasound is now used by some doctors to diagnose gout. It's painless and completely noninvasive. It's good for detecting gout (which may not be evident with a physical exam), but harder to diagnose in the early stages without joint aspiration.

BEST TREATMENTS

Treating gout is a two-step process. Depending on the severity of the attack, various medications can be used to reduce pain and inflammation.

Examples: Nonsteroidal anti-inflammatory drugs, such as *ibuprofen* (Motrin)…*colchicine* (Colcrys), the oldest medication used for treating gout…and corticosteroids, which serve as fast-acting anti-inflammatories.

To reduce uric acid, medications such as the following are taken one to two weeks *after* a gout attack (using these drugs during a gout attack can worsen symptoms)…

• *Febuxostat* (Uloric) is the first new oral drug for gout in 40 years. Taken daily, it can reduce uric acid to an optimal level within a few weeks. Most people with gout need to continue taking this drug indefinitely, but in rare cases it can be discontinued after about a year without subsequent flare-ups.

• *Allopurinol* (Zyloprim, Aloprim), like febuxostat, reduces uric acid concentrations. It's much less expensive than febuxostat ($40 versus $185 for 30 tablets), and it works well for most patients. It usually takes at least six to eight weeks to see a reduction in uric acid levels and may take subsequent dose increases to reduce uric acid to an appropriate level. An older gout drug, allopurinol is more likely to cause kidney problems than febuxostat.

• *Probenecid* (Benemid, Probalan) increases the excretion of uric acid by the kidneys. Most patients who take it can achieve reductions in uric acid levels within two weeks. Potential side effects include kidney stones, gastrointestinal upset and rash. Probenecid can't be taken by patients with kidney disease.

• *Pegloticase* (Krystexxa) has just been approved by the FDA for the treatment of *refractory gout*, which can't be managed with other approaches. It's given by intravenous infusion once every two weeks. Side effects may include nausea, confusion and vomiting.

Natural Gout Remedies

Mark A. Stengler, NMD, naturopathic medical doctor in private practice, Encinitas, California...adjunct associate clinical professor at the National College of Natural Medicine, Portland, Oregon...author of *The Natural Physicians Healing Therapies* and coauthor of *Prescription for Natural Cures* (both from Bottom Line Books).

Gout sounds like an old person's or an old-fashioned disease. But it is neither. This painful form of arthritis is very much with us today—and it affects adults of every age.

An attack of gout comes on quickly—it commonly affects the joint at the base of the big toe or other joints, such as the ankle, thumb, wrist, elbow or knee. Inflammation leaves the joint red, swollen and so tender that it hurts to have clothes or bedsheets touch it.

Good news: Gout can be treated very effectively with a natural approach that features detoxification...nutritional supplements...and diet changes. *Here's what you need to know...*

WHY IT OCCURS

Gout results from elevated blood levels of uric acid, a waste by-product created when your body breaks down *purines*, compounds found in foods such as organ meats, anchovies, asparagus, mushrooms and beer. Gout traditionally was associated with the consumption of fatty foods and alcohol, which is why it was once known as a rich man's disease. Today, we know that gout is not always related to diet. With this condition, the kidneys are unable to filter high levels of uric acid out of the blood. Over time, excess uric acid forms crystals that accumulate in joint tissue, leading to attacks of joint pain. Men are more likely than women to get gout. Women are more susceptible after menopause.

Insulin resistance, obesity, fungal overgrowth and hypothyroidism all have been linked to gout. Taking niacin for heart disease can exacerbate gout. Regular use of aspirin (any dose) and some blood pressure medications (thiazide diuretics) can cause gout.

Gout medications lower blood levels of uric acid, but these medications all have side effects, ranging from nausea and skin rash to disruptions in liver enzymes and blood-cell production. Fortunately, gout can be treated very effectively without these harsh drugs.

TREATING AN ACUTE GOUT ATTACK

I recommend starting the following regimen at the first sign of joint pain caused by gout.

Do first: The first two on the list below, then the others. These remedies, which all are available at health-food stores, are safe to take together. There are no side effects except as noted.

•**Juice detoxification.** In an acute gout attack, it's essential to quickly eliminate uric acid from your body. You can do this with a three-day juice fast, which flushes excess purines from the body. I usually recommend drinking eight to 10 cups of juice daily, mainly from vegetables.

Good choices: Green drinks, such as those made from wheatgrass, chlorella and spirulina... pure water...and herbal teas.

Another good choice: Unsweetened cherry juice. Just a few tablespoons give you the beneficial *anthocyanins* that can decrease blood uric acid levels. Dilute the juice with as much water as you like. Don't fast for more than three days. Prolonged periods without food can raise uric acid levels. (Most middle-aged people with gout have no trouble going without solid food for a few days, but it is wise to consult your doctor before fasting.)

•**Celery seed extract.** This anti-inflammatory herb (not to be confused with the spice celery seed, which is much less concentrated) can ease joint pain. Celery seed extract contains compounds that inhibit the enzymes that produce uric acid. The extract comes in tablet and capsule form.

Dose: 400 mg to 500 mg three times daily during an acute attack. Do not use this herb if you have kidney disease (because of its diuretic effect) or if you are pregnant.

Other helpful remedies to take during an attack of gout...

•**Homeopathic *colchicum*.** This remedy can relieve acute gout attacks in which pain worsens with movement.

Dose: During waking hours, take a 30C-potency pellet every two hours for no more than two days.

•**Nettle root** (also known as stinging nettle root). This herb, available in liquid or capsules, neutralizes uric acid.

Dose: 250 mg of concentrated root extract three times daily during an attack.

LONG-TERM GOUT PROTECTION

When gout symptoms have eased, I have my patients implement the following preventive regimen...

Supplements...

•**Celery seed extract.** I recommend taking this important antigout supplement at a reduced dose of 400 mg to 500 mg only once daily.

•**Fish oil.** Omega-3 fatty acids can help prevent gout-related joint inflammation.

Dose: 2,000 mg of combined EPA and DHA daily.

•**Vitamin C.** Studies have shown that vitamin C can reduce the risk for gout.

Dose: 500 mg daily.

•**Antigout diet.** You will want to avoid foods that increase uric acid production, including those with refined flour or sugar, and those containing saturated, hydrogenated and partially hydrogenated fats. Concentrate on consuming moderate amounts of protein (such as cold-water fish and soy products) and plenty of plant foods. And high-fiber foods, such as whole grains and nuts, can help your body eliminate uric acid. Drink eight to 10 eight-ounce glasses of water throughout the day to keep uric acid flushed from your body.

•**Antifungal diet.** Fungal overgrowth in the digestive tract may increase uric acid. You may want to try an antifungal diet, which involves eliminating sugar, grains and yeast products and taking antifungal herbs.

Science Shows How Massage Eases Sore Muscles

Buck Institute for Research on Aging, news release

Having a massage after strenuous exercise not only feels good, it reduces inflammation in muscles at the cellular level, researchers have found.

Massage also appears to promote the growth of new mitochondria in skeletal muscle. Mitochondria are cells' energy-producing "powerhouses," explained the researchers at the Buck Institute for Research on Aging and McMaster University in Hamilton, Ontario.

STUDY DETAILS

For the study, the investigators analyzed muscle biopsies from the quadriceps of 11 men before and after they exercised to exhaustion on stationary bicycles. After the workout, one of each participant's legs was massaged. Biopsies from both legs were taken after the 10 minutes of massage, and 2.5 hours after the end of the workout.

The researchers found that massage reduced the activity of inflammation-inducing proteins called *cytokines* in muscle cells and promoted the growth of new mitochondria.

The study was published in an online edition of the journal *Science Translational Medicine*.

IMPLICATIONS

Many people find that having a massage after exercise reduces muscle pain. This pain reduction may involve the same mechanisms as those targeted by common anti-inflammatory drugs, explained Simon Melov, PhD, an associate professor at the Buck Institute.

"There's general agreement that massage feels good; now we have a scientific basis for the experience," said Dr. Melov.

The findings provide validation for massage, which is growing in popularity, said lead author Mark Tarnopolsky, MD, PhD, of the pediatrics and medicine department at McMaster University.

WHO CAN BENEFIT FROM MASSAGE

"The potential benefits of massage could be useful to a broad spectrum of individuals including the elderly, those suffering from musculoskeletal injuries, and patients with chronic inflammatory disease," Dr. Tarnopolsky said. "This study provides evidence that manipulative therapies, such as massage, may be justifiable in medical practice."

info The US National Center for Complementary and Alternative Medicine has more about massage therapy at *http://nccam.nih.gov/health/massage*.

Natural Painkiller Works Better Than Morphine

Andrew L. Rubman, ND, founder and director, Southbury Clinic for Traditional Medicines, Southbury, Connecticut. *www.southburyclinic.com*

Scientists may have come up with a lead on a new painkiller—a compound derived from an Asian tree bark that appears to alleviate serious pain without causing addiction or serious side effects...which often occur with opium-based painkillers (such as morphine, hydrocodone and oxycodone).

CAN A STICK DO THE TRICK?

At The Scripps Research Institute in Florida, researchers have undertaken a study of *Tabernaemontana divaricata*, also known as crepe jasmine, a tropical flowering plant that has long been used in traditional medicine in China, India and Thailand. Natural practitioners in these countries prescribe various parts of the plant (from flowers to leaves, roots and bark) to heal wounds, fight toothaches and treat skin diseases, fever, pain, scabies and dysentery, notes Andrew L. Rubman, ND. When it comes to pain, it turns out that one of the most promising elements in crepe jasmine is *conolidine*, an extremely rare constituent of the stem bark of Malayan *T. divaricata*.

In the Scripps laboratory, researchers looked for a way to get sufficient quantities of this hard-to-obtain substance and for the first time created a synthetic conolidine compound. Once they accomplished this feat, they tested its effectiveness on mice. *In various pain models (the researchers used acid to cause pain and inflammation on the paws of the mice), investigators found that the newly synthesized compound...*

• **Was present in high concentrations for up to four hours after administration and passed readily through the blood-brain barrier.** This is important as many areas in the brain are involved in the perception of pain.

• **Effectively relieved acute inflammatory pain in mice.** Scientists measured this by observing such things as how often mice attended to and licked injured paws.

• **Did not show harmful side effects.** Mice demonstrate certain characteristic movements when exposed to morphine—for instance, they become disoriented and walk in circular patterns—which did not happen after conolidine injections.

These findings were published in *Nature Chemistry*.

Researchers are not sure exactly how conolidine relieves pain. It does not bind to opiate receptors in the body and thus is not an opiate like morphine. But it certainly appears to be effective. Much more study is needed, but this may finally turn out to be the alternative to opiates we've been hoping for. Its broad and effective usage over time in India, Thailand and China is yet another reason for hope.

DMSO—Rub On Quick Pain Relief

Mark A. Stengler, NMD, naturopathic medical doctor in private practice, Encinitas, California...adjunct associate clinical professor at the National College of Natural Medicine, Portland, Oregon...author of *The Natural Physician's Healing Therapies* and coauthor of *Prescription for Natural Cures* (both from Bottom Line Books).

When I am helping patients achieve immediate pain relief for burns, sprains, back pain or arthritis, I often turn to *dimethyl sulfoxide* (DMSO), a remarkable topical alternative medication for pain that has its own remarkable history. *Find out how it can help you...*

THE POWER OF DMSO

DMSO works in several ways. First, as a topical compound, it has analgesic properties and reduces pain quickly—which is why it is great for rubbing on sore muscles and joints. Laboratory studies suggest that it decreases pain by blocking peripheral nerve C fibers. DMSO reduces inflammation by acting as an antioxidant—and so it neutralizes some of the free radicals that promote inflammation. Some evidence suggests that it also can ease swelling, further helping with aches and pains.

Second, DMSO is rich in sulfur—and sulfur is found in every cell and is essential for life. From what we know about DMSO, some of its sulfur is used to create new cells involved in the healing process and in the production of gluta-thione, the body's most powerful antioxidant.

Third, DMSO dissolves and transports other substances through the skin, which makes it a great carrier and helper in getting other substances into sore or damaged tissues. I have often mixed DMSO with pharmaceutical anti-inflammatory and pain medications, such as *ketoprofen* (Actron) or *gabapentin* (Neurotin), so that people can use these combinations topically without damaging the heart and digestive tract. The best way to mix DMSO with drugs is to have a holistic doctor write a prescription for you and to have it made at a compounding pharmacy.

Used in this way, DMSO can provide real relief of symptoms for many conditions, including back pain, severe arthritis of the hands, shingles, severe nerve pain and many other localized problems. It also has been found to promote the healing of leg and foot ulcers and to speed up healing after surgery.

Where to get DMSO: You can buy DMSO for basic pain relief at health-food stores and online at such Web sites as *www.herbalremedies.com* and Jacob Lab, the Web site of Dr. Stanley Jacob, who helped discover DMSO. (*www.jacoblab. com*). It generally comes in two concentrations, with either 70% or 90% DMSO. Most people find pain relief with the 70% solution. At Jacob Lab, the 70% solution costs $28 for four ounces. This may seem expensive compared with many conventional pain relievers such as NSAIDs, but it works so effectively, has no side effects and is often needed only short-term, so my patients don't mind spending the extra money.

How to use DMSO: Make sure your hands are clean before applying DMSO, especially since it is efficient at transferring substances through the skin. For acute injuries, apply up to four times daily. For chronic conditions, apply twice daily. It can be used for a few days, a few weeks or indefinitely, depending on the condition. Apply a small amount to the painful area and rub it in. Wash your hands after applying DMSO so that excess is not absorbed by your skin.

Within minutes of applying DMSO, many people experience a taste of sulfur or garlic in their mouths that can last for several hours. In general, this is not a big problem. People who are allergic to sulfites can use DMSO. (There is no such thing as an allergy to sulfur.)

The Right Way to Relieve Muscle Aches

Ice the muscles for at least 10 minutes immediately after you are done exercising. Later, apply heat, either with a heating pad or by taking a warm bath—but not until 24 hours later, because heat can increase inflammation if applied too soon. Do 20 to 30 minutes of low-impact exercise, such as walking, to enhance the blood flow to the area and facilitate healing. Do some gentle stretching, holding each stretch for about 30 seconds at a time. Use a nonsteroidal anti-inflammatory drug (NSAID), such as aspirin, ibuprofen or naproxen, sparingly, because it actually slows the body's muscle-repair process.

Allan Goldfarb, PhD, professor, department of kinesiology, School of Health and Human Performance, University of North Carolina at Greensboro.

Experts Offer Tips to Avoid "iPain"

IOS Press, news release

If working with your iPad or other tablet computer gives you shoulder or neck pain, there are ways around it, a new study suggests.

Researchers from Harvard School of Public Health, Microsoft Corp. and Brigham and Women's Hospital say this type of pain can be avoided if people do not use the tablet while it's resting in their laps, and by using cases that offer higher viewing angles.

TABLETS LINKED TO NECK AND SHOULDER PAIN

"Compared to typical desktop computing scenarios, the use of media tablet computers is associated with high head and neck flexion [flexed] postures, and there may be more of a concern for the development of neck and shoulder discomfort," said lead investigator Jack Dennerlein, PhD, senior lecturer on ergonomics and safety in the Department of Environmental Health, Harvard School of Public Health.

THE STUDY

For the study, Dr. Dennerlein's team asked 15 experienced tablet users to complete certain tasks, such as surfing the Internet, reading, playing games, watching movies and emailing, with two types of tablet devices—an Apple iPad2 and a Motorola Xoom.

All the tablets had a proprietary case that allowed it to be tilted up for use at a low or high angle. (The Apple Smart Cover offers tilt angles of 15° and 73°, and the Motorola Portfolio Case enables tilt angles of 45° and 63°.)

The participants positioned their tablets in various ways, such as in their lap and on a table at various angles, to test how the configurations affected their neck and shoulders.

The researchers found that the iPad2 case design forced participants' head and neck into more flexed postures. For both tablet devices, head and neck flexion angles were greater than those associated with desktop or notebook computers.

BEST TABLET POSITIONING

When used on a table at their highest angle, however, users' postures become more neutral. The study's authors concluded when using tablets, people should place the devices on a table at a steep angle—not in their lap—to avoid looking down.

However, there was a caveat: The researchers noted that this position may not be ideal if users perform a task that requires input with their hands. They believe more studies are needed to determine how tablet positioning could affect arms and wrists.

"Our results will be useful for updating ergonomic computing standards and guidelines for tablet computers. These are urgently needed as companies and health care providers weigh options to implement wide-scale adoption of tablet computers for business operations," concluded Dr. Dennerlein.

The findings appear in the journal *Work: A Journal of Prevention, Assessment, and Rehabilitation.*

Two of the study's authors are employees of Microsoft, a partial funding source for the study. These researchers did not contribute to the analysis and interpretation of the results.

info For more information on shoulder pain, visit the Web site of the US National Institutes of Health, *www.nlm.nih.gov/medline plus/ency/article/003171.htm.*

Landmark Study Reveals Exercises That Ease Neck Pain

Gert Bronfort, DC, PhD, vice president of research at Northwestern Health Sciences University in Bloomington, Minnesota. Dr. Bronfort is coauthor, with Roni Evans, DC, of the neck pain study in *Annals of Internal Medicine.* Dr. Evans also contributed to this article.

If you suffer from neck pain, chances are you've tried heating pads, painkillers and perhaps even repeated visits to a physical therapist, osteopath or chiropractor.

But new research shows that simple neck exercises can relieve neck pain.

Important new research: In a landmark study published earlier this year in *Annals of Internal Medicine*, researchers followed 272 people suffering from neck pain of less than three months' duration with no specific known cause. One group received pain medication and muscle relaxants for 12 weeks…another had 12 weeks of spinal manipulation sessions…and a third group did 12 weeks of special daily neck exercises.

Findings: Spinal manipulation was more effective than medication at improving neck pain by the end of 12 weeks of treatment and one year later—and participants who did home neck exercises experienced improvement in their pain similar to that achieved with spinal manipulation.

WHY THESE EXERCISES WORK

Various factors contribute to neck pain, including chronic strain on the joints and ligaments due to poor posture, minor trauma and excessive work in front of a computer.

The neck exercises used in the neck pain study described above were adapted from a program developed by New Zealand physical therapist Robin McKenzie. The "McKenzie Method" brings the neck into normal alignment by reinforcing its natural curves and rebalancing supporting muscles. Through numerous gentle repetitions, these exercises help you develop a healthier posture, eliminating stress on the neck's joints and ligaments.

HOME EXERCISE PROGRAM

If you suffer from neck pain or stiffness, the following sequence of exercises should be performed six to eight times throughout the day (a total of about 30 to 40 minutes daily).*

Keep doing the routine as long as your neck pain continues to improve. Once you reach a plateau, do the exercises just once a day to maintain a healthy neck and prevent a recurrence.

All of the exercises should be done while sitting on a straight-backed chair or stool, except for the two lying-down versions. As you hold each position, take one full, deep breath—inhaling, then exhaling and relaxing.

Exercise 1: Head retraction. While sitting in a relaxed position and looking straight ahead, slowly move your head backward as far as you can. Next, tuck in your chin as much as possible toward your throat while continuing to look straight ahead. Hold this position for three seconds, then return to starting position. Repeat 10 times.

If this exercise is too difficult: While lying on your back on a bed (without a pillow), tuck

---

*Check with your doctor before trying these exercises. If your neck pain worsens as a result of the exercises, stop them and see your doctor for advice.

---

in your chin toward your throat. Hold this position as you push your head backward into the bed for three seconds. Repeat 10 times.

Exercise 2: Head retraction with extension. Tuck in your chin and pull your head backward, as in Exercise #1. While keeping your head pulled back, lift your chin up and tilt your head back as far as you can. Hold this position for three seconds as you rotate your head a half inch to the right and then a half inch to the left. Return to the starting position. Repeat the sequence 10 times.

If this exercise is too difficult: While lying on your back on your bed with your head, neck and the tops of your shoulders extending off the bed, support your head with one hand. Next, tilt your head backward as far as you can. Hold this position for three seconds as you rotate your head a half inch to the right and then a half inch to the left. Return to the starting position. Repeat the sequence 10 times.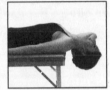

Exercise 3: Head retraction with side bending. Tuck in your chin and pull your head backward, as in Exercise #1. While continuing to look straight ahead, put your right hand on your head and 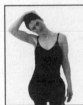 gently tilt your head so that your right ear moves as far as possible toward your right shoulder. Hold this position for three seconds, then return to the starting position. Repeat five times on each side.

Exercise 4: Head retraction with rotation. Tuck in your chin and pull your head backward, as in Exercise #1. While maintaining this posture, turn your head to the right as far as you can and hold this position for three seconds, 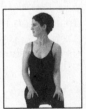 then return to the starting position. Repeat five times on each side.

Exercise 5: Head flexion. Relax completely, then let your head fall forward so that your chin drops to your chest.

Put your hands behind your head, then let your arms relax so your elbows point downward and the weight of your arms gently pulls your chin even closer to your chest. Hold this position for three seconds, then return to the starting position. Repeat five times. After completing Exercise #5, do 10 additional repetitions of Exercise #2.

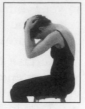

Exercise 6: Scapular retraction. This exercise strengthens the shoulders' scapular muscles, which help support the base of the neck. Hold your arms at your sides with your elbows bent at 90° angles. While maintaining this position and continuing to look straight ahead, pull your elbows back behind you until you feel a squeezing between your shoulder blades. Hold for three seconds, then return to the starting position. Repeat five times.

Exercise photos: Courtesy of Spinal Publications New Zealand Ltd.

■ ■ ■ ■

Help for Arthritic Hand Pain

In a recent study, half of 162 people with osteoarthritis in the hands took 800 mg of chondroitin sulfate daily for six months, and the rest took a placebo. Both groups took an average of two 500-mg *acetaminophen* (Tylenol) tablets each week.

Result: Those who took chondroitin had 44% less pain and morning joint stiffness, compared with 33% in those taking a placebo.

Caution: Be sure to consult your doctor if you take blood-thinning medication—chondroitin can interact with these drugs.

Cem Gabay, MD, professor of medicine and head, division of rheumatology, University Hospitals of Geneva, Switzerland.

■ ■ ■ ■

Spice Eases Arthritis

Frankincense is a traditional arthritis treatment that blocks the production of inflammatory molecules and helps protect joint cartilage.

Cardiff University

■ ■ ■ ■

New Treatment for Severe Migraines

An implanted device called Genesis uses mild electrical impulses to stimulate the occipital nerves, just beneath the skin at the back of the head, and block pain transmission in the brain stem. Genesis already is in use in the US for chronic back pain and is approved for migraine treatment in Europe. Some US doctors prescribe it for migraine on an off-label basis.

Stephen D. Silberstein, MD, is professor of neurology and director of Jefferson Headache Center, Thomas Jefferson University, Philadelphia, and past president of the American Headache Society.

■ ■ ■ ■

Drug-Free Headache Fix

Here's a drug-free solution for headache pain—a headband with reusable cool/heat packs. The packs, when cooled, gently constrict blood vessels in the forehead, and when heated, relax tense muscles, depending on which works best for you. Developed by a neurologist, the wrap was the subject of a study in *Archives of Family Medicine* that showed it helped relieve headaches in 87% of patients. Adjustable and insulated headband, one size fits all.

Hammacher Schlemmer, 800-321-1484, *www.hammacher.com.*

■ ■ ■ ■

Don't Look Away— Face Your Pain

Did you know that looking at a body part that hurts reduces the pain? People who had a heat probe placed on their hand felt less pain when they looked at their hand than when they looked at a wooden object.

Flavia Mancini, PhD, research assistant, Institute of Cognitive Neuroscience, University College London, and leader of a study published in *Psychological Science.*

Slow Rheumatoid Arthritis with Early Detection

Beth L. Jonas, MD, assistant professor of medicine and rheumatology and director of the Rheumatology Fellowship Program at the University of North Carolina Thurston Arthritis Research Center in Chapel Hill.

Unfortunately, many individuals with rheumatoid arthritis (RA) postpone seeking medical care...and once they do, doctors may not accurately diagnose the disease or may fail to refer patients to rheumatologists, the specialists best equipped to treat RA. In a recent study in *Arthritis & Rheumatism*, 69% of RA patients did not see a rheumatologist within the crucial first 12 weeks when the disease's progression can be limited—and the delay contributed to a 30% faster rate of joint destruction and an 87% lower likelihood of remission, compared with patients who saw a specialist promptly.

"Permanent joint damage can occur at a very early stage of the disease. Medication can slow and sometimes prevent joint destruction—but once damage is done, we can't reverse it," said Beth L. Jonas, MD, director of the Rheumatology Fellowship Program at the University of North Carolina Thurston Arthritis Research Center.

New concern: Some research links the high levels of inflammation associated with RA to cardiovascular disease, Dr. Jonas said.

What about people who have already missed that window of opportunity for early treatment? Avoiding further delay is vital because the new medications still can help somewhat...whereas RA sufferers left untreated face a significantly increased risk of becoming disabled.

SPOTTING THE SIGNS

With RA, the immune system attacks the synovial membranes that line the joints. This lining becomes inflamed and thickened...fluid builds up...ligaments and tendons weaken and stretch out...cartilage is destroyed...and bone is damaged. Over time, patients develop crippling chronic pain and joint deformity.

Women are two to three times more likely than men to get RA. The disease can arise at any time but usually appears in midlife. While genetics may play some role, most RA patients have no close relatives with the disease—so we all should be on the lookout for RA. *See your doctor without delay if you experience any of the following...*

•**Pain, tenderness and/or stiffness in any of the small joints**—fingers, wrists, toes, ankles—usually occurring symmetrically on both sides of the body. (As RA progresses, the neck, shoulders, elbows, hips and/or knees also may be affected.)

•**Morning stiffness that lasts for more than 30 minutes.**

•**Redness, swelling and/or sensations of heat at the joints.**

•**Numbness, tingling or burning sensations in the hands or feet.**

Confirming an RA diagnosis can be tricky because the symptoms mimic those of lupus, Lyme disease and other forms of arthritis. Diagnosis is based on a physical exam...blood tests for antibodies (including *rheumatoid factor* and *anti-cyclic citrullinated peptide*) plus various markers of inflammation and imaging tests (ultrasound, MRI, X-ray).

So if your doctor suspects RA, ask to be referred to a rheumatologist or get a referral through the American College of Rheumatology (visit *www.rheumatology.org* and click on "Find a member").

■ ■ ■ ■

Better Posture Eases Pain

People feel more powerful, in control and able to tolerate pain when they stand tall. Better posture may increase levels of testosterone, which improves pain tolerance and decreases stress hormones.

Vanessa Bohns, PhD, assistant professor, department of management sciences, University of Waterloo, Ontario, Canada, and Scott Wiltermuth, PhD, assistant professor of management and organization, USC Marshall School of Business, Los Angeles, and leaders of a study of 129 people, published in *Journal of Experimental Social Psychology*.

■ ■ ■ ■

Three Most Overused Back Pain Tests

The American College of Physicians' new guidelines state that X-rays, CT scans and MRI scans ordered for back pain are frequently not needed and that routine imaging does not improve outcomes…is costly…needlessly exposes patients to radiation (except with MRI)…and often uncovers abnormalities that may be treated unnecessarily. Back pain often vanishes after a month—with exercise and staying active.

Roger Chou, MD, general internist, Oregon Health & Science University, Portland.

You May Have a Broken Back and Not Know It…

David Borenstein, MD, clinical professor of medicine at George Washington University Medical Center in Washington, DC. He maintains a private practice at Arthritis and Rheumatism Associates and is author of *Back in Control!* (M. Evans).

Don't assume that an aching back means just a pulled muscle. It's among the most common symptoms of vertebral fractures, small cracks in the vertebrae of the spine.

About 25% of postmenopausal women in the US eventually will develop a vertebral fracture. Men over age 60 are prone to them, too. Up to two-thirds of these fractures never are diagnosed because the pain is so minor that patients don't bother to tell their doctors—or, as is often the case, because there's no pain at all.

The risk: Hairline cracks in the vertebrae eventually can cause the bone to crumble and collapse, a condition known as a *vertebral compression fracture.* When you see someone with a hunched-over posture, the so-called dowager's hump, you'll know that he/she has a compression fracture. These fractures also can cause patients to lose inches in height over the years.

Studies have shown that patients with compression fractures face a 23% higher risk for death than those with stronger bones. Difficulty breathing and pneumonia also can occur in severe cases because the stooped-over posture often interferes with normal lung function.

BONE LOSS

Unless you've had a severe injury (from a car accident, for example), vertebral fractures usually are due to *osteoporosis*, the leading cause of bone loss. They also can be caused by *osteopenia*, less severe bone weakening that can start decades before the development of full-fledged osteoporosis. People who have one fracture are at greater risk of developing another.

For women, the main cause of bone loss is the postmenopausal decline of estrogen. In the first five years after menopause, women can lose up to 25% of their bone density.

Men have thicker bones to begin with, and they lose bone more slowly, but they're not immune to fractures. About 25% of men develop osteoporosis by age 70. By the time they reach 75 to 80, they're just as likely as women to have severe bone weakening.

The only way to know that you have osteoporosis is to get a bone-density test. The most accurate test is a dual-energy X-ray absorptiometry (DXA). The test is painless, takes about 10 minutes and exposes patients to less radiation than a chest X-ray.

Cost: $150 to $200. The test usually is covered by insurance. Newer DXA machines also are able to scan the spine to detect spinal fractures. This test is referred to as a *vertebral fracture assessment* (VFA).

You might see kiosks at pharmacies and malls that offer a heel sonogram. It's a fast, inexpensive test that measures bone density in the heel. It can indicate which patients might have low bone density. However, the test is not as accurate as DXA. I don't recommend it.

Every woman should get a DXA test around the time of menopause. Men should have the test if they have a family history of osteoporosis…if they're taking steroids (which can cause bone loss) for another condition…or if they have low testosterone, which also leads to bone weakness.

PREVENTING FRACTURES

Early diagnosis of osteoporosis and then adopting bone-building strategies can protect the spine. Patients with low bone density who don't improve with lifestyle measures may need to take bisphosphonates (such as Fosamax) or other medications. Drug therapy can improve bone density by at least 4% a year and reduce the risk for future fractures by 30% to 40%. The general recommendation for bisphosphonates is to take them for five years because long-term bisphosphonate therapy has been linked to a rare type of thigh fracture.

Here, important lifestyle steps…

•**Get more calcium.** It improves the body's ability to develop new bone. Women need 1,200 milligrams (mg) daily until menopause and 1,500 mg afterward. Men should get 1,000 mg until age 65 and 1,500 mg thereafter.

Dairy foods and fortified juices and cereals are the best dietary sources of calcium. (One cup of milk or fortified juice has about 300 mg of calcium.)

Supplements can help if you don't eat a lot of high-calcium foods. Both forms of supplements—calcium citrate and calcium carbonate—are effective.

Helpful: Take calcium supplements with meals. The stomach's acidic environment during digestion improves calcium absorption.

•**Supplement with vitamin D.** A majority of Americans are low in this nutrient, which is needed for calcium absorption. The recommended daily amount is 600 international units (IU) for those ages 51 to 70 and 800 IU after that. However, higher amounts—usually between 1,000 IU and 2,000 IU daily—often are recommended, particularly for those who have dark skin and/or those who don't get a lot of sun exposure.

•**Eat leafy green vegetables, such as spinach and kale.** These are high in vitamin K, which helps calcium in the blood enter the bones. The Harvard Nurses' Health Study found that women who ate at least one daily serving of leafy green vegetables were 50% less likely to suffer a hip fracture than those who ate less. It's not known whether these foods protect the vertebrae, but increasing vitamin K intake as part of a healthy diet is probably helpful.

•**Walk for 30 minutes four times a week.** Walking and other types of weight-bearing exercise (in which the muscles and joints work against gravity) significantly increase bone density. People who exercise regularly throughout their lives put more bone "in the bank" to protect against future fractures.

Riding a bicycle (including a stationary bike) has similar effects. The spine benefits from any exercise that requires you to be upright. This includes jogging, aerobics, yoga and jumping.

•**Swim for pain relief.** Swimming isn't a weight-bearing exercise, so it won't increase spinal strength—but it's very useful for strengthening the muscles that surround the spine and helping to prevent pain and stiffness.

•**Strengthen abdominal muscles.** Strengthening the muscles that surround the spine and abdomen (the so-called "core muscles") can help reduce back pain if you have a fracture. Also by improving muscular support around the spine, strong core muscles may help protect the back from future injuries.

Try this: Lie on your back with your knees bent and your feet flat on the floor. Tighten the abdominal muscles while gently pressing your lower back toward the floor. Hold the tension for five to 10 seconds, relax, then repeat the movement 10 times. Do this daily.

You also can do crunches to strengthen the core muscles in the abdomen and lower back. Crunches are safe for most patients, but they do put pressure on the spine—talk to your doctor before doing them if you have significant bone loss and/or fractures.

To do them: Lie on your back with your knees slightly bent…cross your arms over your chest…and gently raise your shoulders a few inches off the floor. Hold the stretch for a second, then relax. Repeat 10 times. Do this daily.

•**Use heat and/or cold for pain.** To relieve pain initially, apply an ice pack to your lower back. Keep it there for about 10 minutes. Do this several times during the first 48 hours.

After that, heat reduces muscle spasms and can minimize back pain. It also increases circulation, which flushes pain-causing chemicals from the injured area. Apply a hot water bottle or heating pad to your lower back for 10 to 20 minutes several times daily.

■ ■ ■ ■

Treat Cuts with Water

Treat cuts with water, not hydrogen peroxide. Hydrogen peroxide can damage healthy tissue. (The same is true of alcohol and iodine.) Rinsing with water first, then cleaning the surrounding area with mild soap and water is sufficient for most cuts.

Richard O'Brien, MD, attending emergency physician, Moses Taylor Hospital, and associate professor of emergency medicine at The Commonwealth Medical College of Pennsylvania, both in Scranton.

Should You Ease the Pain of a Shot...or Not?

Sergei Frenzel ND, MD, founder of Integrative Natural Health, Stamford and Southington, Connecticut. www. integrativenaturalhealth.com

If your arm feels sore after getting a flu shot or other vaccination, is it OK to take an over-the-counter pain reliever to minimize the discomfort?

Not really—and here's why. The purpose of vaccination is to create an immune reaction...and that includes inflammation. Pain is a natural consequence of inflammation. If you try to reduce the pain and inflammation, whether with a pain-relieving drug or with ice, it may decrease the effectiveness of the vaccination, research suggests. For instance, in a study published in *The Lancet*, babies who received *acetaminophen* (Tylenol) after their injections produced significantly fewer antibodies against the diseases for which they had been vaccinated than babies who were not given the pain reliever. It makes sense that this same effect might apply to adults.

Think of it this way—pain actually is a good sign that your body is reacting to the vaccine the way you want it to. The discomfort should go away within about 10 hours. If it has been more

than a day and your arm is still very sore, alert the doctor who prescribed the injection. You may need to be evaluated to make sure there are no other forces at play.

Sjögren's Syndrome: The Mysterious Disease Takes the Spotlight

Alan Baer, MD, associate professor of medicine and clinical director, Johns Hopkins University Rheumatology Practice, Good Samaritan Hospital, founder and director of the Johns Hopkins Jerome L. Greene Sjögren's Syndrome Center, Baltimore.

When tennis superstar Venus Williams recently announced that she had been diagnosed with Sjögren's syndrome, the tennis world issued a collective gasp. It was followed by the question: What on Earth is Sjögren's syndrome? Venus had been plagued by, as she put it, an "energy-sucking" disease for some time. She suffered from so much fatigue and joint pain that it was sometimes hard for her to even lift her racket. Fans were incredulous. Venus appeared to be in such good shape and, in fact, had won her first match at the 2011 US Open. But then she withdrew from the competition suddenly. Many were bitterly disappointed and suggested that this was just an excuse for her to drop out of the tournament.

The idea that Sjögren's patients are "faking it" is nothing new. This misconception is due to two major factors—the disease is difficult to diagnose, and patients, like Venus, often appear to be perfectly healthy. But this serious autoimmune disease is hardly the product of hypochondriacs.

FOUR MILLION AMERICANS HAVE THIS DISEASE

Sjögren's syndrome is a chronic inflammatory disorder in which disease-fighting white blood cells mistakenly attack the body's own moisture-producing glands, causing symptoms such as dry eyes and dry mouth. The disease can strike children and older adults, but typically, patients develop it between the ages of 40 and the mid-50s. (Venus, who is only in her early thirties, got it very young.) Up to four million Americans have Sjögren's (90% of them are female), and unfortunately there is no cure. However, it can be managed.

MYSTERY DISEASE

Alan Baer, MD, director of the Johns Hopkins Jerome L. Greene Sjögren's Syndrome Center, explained that Sjögren's can present many challenges…

•**It's tough to diagnose.** On average, it takes six and a half years for doctors to put the puzzle pieces together.

•**Symptoms seem unrelated.** When the body's immune system attacks the moisture-producing glands, it causes complications all over the body. The eyes and mouth become dry—without the benefit of cleansing saliva teeth develop cavities…and fatigue and joint pain may develop. In women, there may be a lack of vaginal lubrication, which leads to increased risk for infection and pain during intercourse.

•**It's dangerous.** The longer a person goes without getting a diagnosis, the higher the health risks. If the disease advances undetected, it can set off a widespread inflammatory reaction that can harm the lungs, kidney, liver, pancreas and blood vessels as well as the gastrointestinal and central nervous systems. Up to 30% of Sjögren's patients suffer organ damage, and about 5% develop lymphoma (lymph node cancer).

TOP TREATMENTS

Patients can choose from a variety of over-the-counter preparations that are generally very helpful for symptom relief, says Dr. Baer. Lubricants help with vaginal dryness. For dry eyes, there are drops and ointments…and for dry mouth there are sprays, gums, gels, lozenges, mouthwashes and toothpastes.

More powerful prescription drugs can also help dry eyes and mouth. The drug *hydroxy-chloroquine* (Plaquenil), originally developed to treat malaria, is useful in Sjögren's to relieve fatigue and joint pain. To quiet an overactive immune system, patients can take *methotrex-ate* (brand names Rheumatrex or Trexall)—it is used in high doses as chemotherapy, and now it's also used in low doses to treat autoimmune disorders. Methotrexate can be well-tolerated but can also cause some nasty side effects, including mouth sores, stomach upset, skin rash, hair loss and liver toxicity.

One bright spot: Research on drugs for autoimmune diseases is extremely active, and as general awareness of Sjögren's increases, patients are not likely to be left behind.

STEPS FOR QUALITY OF LIFE

Sjögren's can be mild, moderate or severe. Severe cases can cause renal failure, disability due to peripheral neuropathy, impaired vision, hepatitis or pneumonitis. But Dr. Baer says that most cases are mild. To help maintain quality of life, exercise of any kind is important for physical and psychological reasons. An anti-inflammatory diet built on healthy foods is essential—eat plenty of vegetables, fruits, fish and other proteins, and limit processed foods and refined grains. Dr. Baer says that fish oil supplements and flaxseed oil may help the problem of dry eyes. To maintain a good level of energy, patients need plenty of sleep. They also need to avoid triggers such as extreme heat, fumes, cigarette smoke, dust and winds—all of which can aggravate symptoms.

Quality of life also has much to do with finding doctors who are well-versed in Sjögren's. Rheumatologists are the primary doctors who handle it, but the nature of the disease also requires the involvement of ophthalmologists, otolaryngologists, dentists, neurologists and for women, gynecologists. Ideally, a patient will be treated at a Sjögren syndrome center, such as the one at Johns Hopkins, but these centers are relatively rare. More typically, doctors treat Sjögren's within rheumatology centers, where expertise on autoimmune diseases is available. Once a patient has been diagnosed, his/her primary care doctor will locate an appropriate place for treatment. For an impressive amount of information about the disease and tips for living well with it, go to the Sjögren's Syndrome Foundation Web site, *www.Sjogrens.org.*

■ ■ ■ ■

Shine Helps Fibromyalgia

SHINE stands for Sleep, Hormones, Infections, Nutritional supplements and Exercise—and this approach has led to improvements in 91% of fibromyalgia patients. Patients should get eight to nine hours of sleep a night…be tested for hormone deficiency and treated if necessary…get treated for any symptoms of infections…have nutritional supplementation, such as B-12 and magnesium…and exercise as much as possible.

Also effective: Taking 5,000 milligrams of *ribose* (Corvalen), a nonprescription medical food, twice a day increased energy by an average of 61%.

Jacob Teitelbaum, MD, medical director at Fibromyalgia & Fatigue Centers, Addison, Texas. *www.endfatigue.com*

■ ■ ■ ■

How to Avoid Injury When Doing Yard Work

Before performing any outdoor chores, do a few stretching exercises to warm up your muscles. Also, be sure to avoid muscle strain by taking a break every 20 minutes or so—switch activities or rest briefly.

Proper body mechanics help prevent muscle soreness as well. Switch sides every few minutes when raking, hoeing or digging, even though it may feel awkward on the side that you don't usually use. Stand close to the area where you are working to avoid reaching, which strains back muscles. Don't overload the shovel when digging, and bend your knees so leg and buttock muscles do the heavy lifting—not your back.

A garden stool with wheels, raised garden beds and a riding mower will ease the strain on your back. If you prefer a walk-behind mower, get one that is self-propelled and avoid back-and-forth motions that can hurt your back—push it, don't pull it. Use both hands to carry heavy bags of mulch or potting soil. Be sure to use a shoulder strap with a weed trimmer.

Jay M. Lipoff, DC, chiropractor in private practice in California, Maryland, and author of *Back at Your Best: Balancing the Demands of Life with the Needs of Your Body* (Back at Your Best).

Women's Health

Estrogen and HRT— What You Need to Know

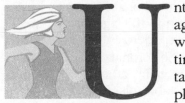 **U**ntil about 10 years ago, menopausal women were routinely advised to take hormone replacement therapy (HRT), including estrogen, to prevent heart disease, strengthen bones and improve mental and emotional health.

Then women began avoiding HRT when an important study announced in 2002 that it increased the risk for heart disease, stroke, pulmonary embolism and breast cancer.

Latest development: A new analysis of data from the same study indicates that for the estimated one-third of women over age 50 who have had a hysterectomy, using estrogen alone actually reduces breast cancer risk, while among the younger study participants, risk for heart disease was reduced. The new findings were reported in

The Journal of the American Medical Association (see also page 35).

John E. Morley, MD, a leading gerontologist who also specializes in the study of hormones, answers questions concerning the latest findings...

•**Why has hormone replacement therapy for menopausal women become so controversial?** A decade ago, more than one-third of postmenopausal American women were taking estrogen, alone or with other hormones, to help fight hot flashes, vaginal dryness and other menopausal symptoms.

HRT was assumed to be both effective and safe—but this assumption had never been tested in a large-scale clinical trial.

In 1991, the National Institutes of Health launched the Women's Health Initiative study to investigate the long-term health effects of

John E. Morley, MD, a gerontologist and endocrinologist who is the Dammert Professor of Gerontology and director of the division of geriatric medicine at Saint Louis University School of Medicine. Dr. Morley is also director of geriatric research at the St. Louis VA Medical Center and coauthor, with Sheri R. Colberg, PhD, of *The Science of Staying Young* (McGraw-Hill).

HRT. The study, which included more than 160,000 women, was stopped early when investigators concluded that study participants on HRT with estrogen and the hormone *progestin* had a higher risk for stroke, breast cancer and other health problems than participants taking placebos.

Reports of the study had an immediate effect—the number of prescriptions for HRT decreased by 50% almost overnight. Today, millions of menopausal women refuse any form of HRT, even though this decision greatly increases their risk of getting osteoporosis.

•**Based on the original findings, aren't women correct in refusing HRT?** In the original study, for every 100,000 women treated with estrogen and progestin, we would expect to see about seven additional cases of heart disease and about eight additional cases of cancer. It's a concern, but the risk for a particular woman is, on average, small.

Remember, these complications occurred only in women taking the two hormones.

•**Why is the new analysis important?** The conclusions are different from the earlier ones, but only because the analysis looked at a different group of women—those who had previously had a hysterectomy (which surgically induces menopause with removal of the uterus) and were taking only estrogen (or a placebo), rather than the estrogen-progestin combination.

The results were striking. Women taking estrogen alone had a 23% lower risk of developing breast cancer than those in the placebo group. We don't know why estrogen was protective in this group.

No one is recommending that women take estrogen solely for breast cancer prevention. However, this finding should be reassuring to the women who have had hysterectomies and are using estrogen therapy for relief from hot flashes or other menopausal symptoms.

•**Why were postmenopausal women historically instructed to take progestin if it's dangerous?** Supplemental estrogen increases the risk for endometrial cancer. The addition of progestin mitigates that risk. It's not a perfect solution because progestin/estrogen has been linked to a slight increase in breast cancer. In the past, many doctors routinely prescribed the two hormones together. This was not the right approach for all women.

A woman who has had a hysterectomy obviously can't get endometrial cancer because she doesn't have a uterus. In these women, as the new analysis has shown, taking estrogen without progestin actually reduces breast cancer risk.

Important: Some types of breast cancer proliferate in the presence of estrogen. Women who have had estrogen-dependent cancers, or have a high risk of getting them due to such factors as obesity, also need to be cautious about estrogen-only therapy.

Women who still have their uteruses and are suffering from severe menopausal discomfort will be advised to continue using the combination treatment at the lowest possible dose and for the shortest period of time—say, for three to five years.

•**Does estrogen help or hurt the heart?** While the original study found an increase in heart problems in women using a combination of estrogen and progestin, the new analysis found that the increase applied to only the older women who had had hysterectomies and took estrogen alone.

The researchers estimate that for every 10,000 women age 70 or older who are taking estrogen, there would be 16 additional heart attacks. It's possible that women in this age group already have advanced atherosclerosis.

Estrogen causes the coronary arteries to relax excessively. With existing atherosclerosis, this could dislodge unstable plaques (deposits) in the arteries and trigger a heart attack.

For younger women (generally age 59 or younger), the situation was the opposite. The analysis found that participants who had undergone a hysterectomy and started taking estrogen in their 50s had nearly 50% fewer heart attacks compared with those taking placebos.

My advice: It's clear from this study that older women who have had a hysterectomy probably should not start taking estrogen—the risks are likely to outweigh the benefits. Younger women without uteruses, on the other hand, can clearly benefit.

•**How young should a woman be to consider HRT?** A woman without a uterus who is age 59 or younger and is experiencing moderate-to-severe menopausal symptoms or has a high risk of developing osteoporosis—due, for example, to low body weight—could benefit from estrogen.

We advise women who do use HRT to not exceed 10 years of use. The risks rise with longer use, with the highest risk for those who take it for 15 years or longer.

•**Are bioidentical forms of estrogen safer than prescription versions?** This topic is controversial. One criticism of the Women's Health Initiative study is that the participants were given prescription Prempro or Premarin, conjugated estrogens made from mare's urine. However, study skeptics argue that *estradiol*, a so-called bioidentical hormone that's touted as being more similar to the estrogen produced by a woman's ovaries, is a safer choice.

Bioidentical forms of estrogen are typically synthesized from soy or yams, foods that contain estrogen-like compounds. Despite the fact that many women use bioidentical hormones, there's no clear evidence, in my opinion, that they're safer or more effective than traditional hormone therapy. Estrogen (traditional or bioidentical) in nonpill forms, such as creams or patches, may have fewer side effects because they are metabolized differently than the oral form. Ask your doctor for advice.

Women in my practice who have added soy and yams to their diets weren't able to get enough of the hormonelike substances from these foods to significantly improve menopausal symptoms.

How Caffeine Alters Women's Estrogen Levels

Enrique Schisterman, PhD, Division of Epidemiology, Statistics and Prevention Research at the Eunice Kennedy Shriver US National Institute of Child Health and Human Development.
American Journal of Clinical Nutrition

Caffeine changes women's estrogen levels and has different effects in Asian and Caucasian women, a recent study reveals.

Estrogen is the reproductive hormone produced primarily by the ovaries.

STUDY DETAILS

More than 250 women, ages 18 to 44, took part in the BioCycle Study between 2005 and 2007. On average, they consumed 90 milligrams of caffeine a day, about the equivalent of one cup of caffeinated coffee.

The caffeine consumed by the women in the study came from any of these sources: Coffee, black tea, green tea and caffeinated soda. The findings differed slightly when the researchers considered the source of caffeine individually.

HIGHER LEVELS FOR ASIAN COFFEE DRINKERS

Asian women who consumed an average of 200 milligrams or more of caffeine a day (equivalent to about two cups of coffee) had elevated estrogen levels compared with women who consumed less. But Caucasian women who consumed the same amount of caffeine had slightly lower estrogen levels than women who consumed less.

African American women who consumed 200 or more milligrams of caffeine daily had elevated estrogen levels, but this finding was not statistically significant, said researchers at the US National Institutes of Health.

Consuming 200 milligrams of caffeine from coffee mirrored the overall findings. But consumption of more than one cup each day of caffeinated soda or green tea was associated with higher estrogen levels in all three groups of women.

The study was published online in the *American Journal of Clinical Nutrition*.

POSSIBLE LONG-TERM EFFECTS

The caffeine-related changes in estrogen levels did not appear to affect women's ovulation, said the researchers, who followed the women for up to two menstrual cycles.

"The results indicate that caffeine consumption among women of child-bearing age influences estrogen levels," said study coauthor Enrique Schisterman, PhD, Division of Epidemiology, Statistics and Prevention Research at the

Eunice Kennedy Shriver US National Institute of Child Health and Human Development, the NIH institute where some of the research was conducted.

"Short term, these variations in estrogen levels among different groups do not appear to have any pronounced effects. We know that variations in estrogen level are associated with such disorders as endometriosis, osteoporosis, and endometrial, breast and ovarian cancers. Because long-term caffeine consumption has the potential to influence estrogen levels over a long period of time, it makes sense to take caffeine consumption into account when designing studies to understand these disorders," Schisterman said.

About 89% of US women ages 18 to 34 consume the caffeine equivalent of 1.5 to two cups of coffee a day, according to the authors.

info For more information of caffeine and health, visit the Web site of the US National Library of Medicine, *http://www.nlm.nih.gov/medlineplus/caffeine.html*.

■ ■ ■ ■

Hysterectomy Linked to Heart Disease

Hysterectomy is linked to cardiovascular disease.

Recent finding: Women who have hysterectomies before age 50 are nearly 20% more likely to develop coronary artery disease or heart failure or have strokes than women who have not had hysterectomies.

Possible reason: Removal of the uterus disrupts blood flow to the ovaries, decreasing heart-protective estrogen. No link has been found between hysterectomy and heart disease in women over age 50.

Daniel Altman, MD, PhD, associate professor of medical epidemiology and statistics, Karolinska Institute, Stockholm, Sweden, and senior author of a study of 824,484 women, published in *European Heart Journal*.

■ ■ ■ ■

Calcium Supplements May Increase Heart Risk

Recent finding: People who take 1,000 milligrams of calcium per day have a 25% higher risk for heart attack and 15% higher risk for stroke than people who do not take the supplements.

Possible connection: The supplements may increase the blood calcium level rapidly, contributing to arterial disease.

Best: Get calcium naturally from food.

Ian Reid, MD, is professor of medicine and endocrinology at University of Auckland, New Zealand, and senior author of a study published in *British Medical Journal*.

The Artery-Clearing Procedure That's Safest For Women

Virginia J. Howard, PhD, is an associate professor of epidemiology at the University of Alabama at Birmingham School of Public Health, and lead author of a study of 2,502 people.

It's scary to be told that your carotid arteries—the big blood vessels in your neck that supply oxygenated blood to the brain—are dangerously clogged with plaque, leaving you at increased risk for stroke. People with this condition, called carotid artery stenosis, often undergo one of two different surgical procedures…and in men, both surgeries appear to have similar benefits and risks.

But: Among women, one of the procedures seems to be significantly riskier than the other, according to a new study published in *The Lancet Neurology*.

Researchers recruited more than 2,500 patients from 117 centers in the US and Canada. The two procedures being compared were the traditional *carotid endarterectomy*, in which a surgeon makes an incision to open the carotid artery, removes the plaque and then stitches up the artery...and the *newer carotid artery stenting*, a less invasive procedure in which a stent (mesh tube) is inserted into the carotid via a catheter and left in place to keep the artery open.

Results: Compared with women who underwent endarterectomy, women who received stents were more than twice as likely to have a stroke within 30 days after their surgery.

Bottom line: If your doctor recommends carotid artery stenting rather than endarterectomy, be sure to discuss the gender-based differences in stroke risk found in this study.

Can Early Menopause Hurt Your Heart?

Melissa Wellons, MD, is an assistant professor in the division of reproductive endocrinology and infertility at the University of Alabama at Birmingham.

Some women experience menopause quite early in life—even in their early or mid-40s. If this describes you or someone you're close to, you'll be especially interested in learning the results of a recent study on early menopause and the risk for heart disease. It's important stuff—if you fall into a particular category, it's not an overstatement to say that it could even be life-saving.

What the study showed: Women who reached menopause before age 46 were at double the risk for heart disease or stroke later in life, compared with women whose menopause came later.

That's a startlingly high increase in risk—enough so that women who had early menopause should take extra precautions to protect their health. The study's lead researcher, Melissa Wellons, MD, an assistant professor in the division of reproductive endocrinology and infertility at the University of Alabama at Birmingham (UAB), said that her goal with this research was to help women at high risk make decisions about how to protect themselves from heart disease. It's a big group, she noted, since 5% to 10% of women experience menopause before age 46.

The UAB research team studied more than 2,500 women, 28% of whom had experienced early menopause either naturally or because their ovaries had been surgically removed. The reason for the apparent link between early menopause and cardiovascular disease isn't entirely clear, but the researchers have several theories—the most obvious relating to the postmenopausal loss of hormones produced by the ovaries. Another theory, said Dr. Wellons, is that some lifestyle-based cardiovascular disease risk factors may be more common in women with early menopause. "For example, these women are more likely to be smokers, a factor that may have contributed to their early loss of ovarian function," she explained.

HOW TO STAY YOUNG AT HEART

While menopause isn't something women get to schedule, there are other risk factors that can be controlled, both before and after menopause—most importantly lifestyle. "There's no doubt that losing weight and exercising will reduce your cardiovascular risk no matter what your ovary status is," said Dr. Wellons. She also noted that a woman who is lean, nonsmoking and exercising at early menopause is at significantly lower risk for future heart disease than a woman who is overweight, smokes and doesn't exercise, regardless of her age at menopause.

"The study findings should give an extra nudge to women with increased heart disease risk to work on things they can control to reduce that risk," Dr. Wellons said. "If you smoke, stop. Exercise, eat a healthy diet and control your weight. Pay attention to cholesterol and blood pressure levels and get those treated, if necessary."

According to Andrew L. Rubman, ND, medical director of the Southbury Clinic for Traditional Medicines in Southbury, Connecticut, certain nutritional supplements also have been shown to protect cardiovascular health. Ask your doctor about taking 200 mg to 300 mg of magnesium daily (as long as you don't have kidney problems)...and 3,000 mg a day of fish oil (as long as you are not on a blood thinner).

Ob/Gyn Visit a Good Time to Screen for Heart Disease

American College of Cardiology, news release

The annual visit to the gynecologist provides an opportune time for heart disease screening, a new study suggests. Heart disease is a leading cause of death among women in the United States.

Researchers from Mount Sinai Medical Center in New York City found that heart screenings performed during visits to obstetrician/gynecologists could help identify women with undetected risk factors for the condition. In addition, the screenings could significantly increase awareness among women about heart disease prevention and treatment, the researchers added.

"There is a real disparity in the medical community where we tend to think heart disease is a disease of men, and historically we have not done a very good job of screening women for cardiovascular risk factors," said the study's principal investigator, Roxana Mehran, MD, director of interventional cardiovascular research and clinical trials at Mount Sinai Medical Center.

"It often doesn't occur to women that they could have a heart problem until their symptoms are very advanced, so we have to think differently and be creative about how we identify, educate and treat women at risk," Dr. Mehran explained.

SCREENING PROGRAM REVEALS RISK FACTORS

In conducting the study, the researchers asked 10 ob/gyn clinics to put a screening program in place to identify women with symptoms or risk factors for heart disease. Over the course of two years, more than 2,200 women completed a one-page survey on traditional and gestational heart disease.

The program revealed that 69% of the middle-aged women screened had heart disease risk factors. Meanwhile, 42% also had symptoms of the condition. The investigators also found that 18% of the women screened considered their ob/gyn to be their primary health care provider.

Among the women in the study, a significant number either had never been checked or were unsure if they had been checked for high blood pressure (21%), high cholesterol (38%) or high blood sugar (19%). Following the screenings, 25% of the women were referred to a primary care physician or another specialist for further treatment for heart disease.

"We found a real lack of awareness among many of these women that they had risk factors, including diabetes, high blood pressure and high cholesterol. Ob/gyn practices have an incredible opportunity to make an impact on heart disease in women by screening, educating and directing women to the right providers, so we hope to see continued research in this area," Dr. Mehran said.

The study authors noted that more research involving a larger group of women is needed to determine if screenings at ob/gyn clinics improve outcomes among women with heart disease.

info The US National Library of Medicine has more information about heart disease in women at their Web site *www.nlm.nih.gov/med lineplus/heartdiseaseinwomen.html.*

Are You Done with Those "Yearly" Exams?

Diane M. Harper, MD, MPH, is vice-chair for research and a professor in the departments of community and family medicine, obstetrics and gynecology, and biomedical and health informatics at the University of Missouri–Kansas City School of Medicine.

According to current cervical cancer screening recommendations from the American College of Obstetricians and Gynecologists (ACOG) for women age 30 and older, if a woman's last three consecutive Paps were negative (meaning that her cervix showed no abnormal cells or potentially cancerous changes) or if her HPV tests did not detect any of the *human papillomavirus* types that can cause cervical cancer, she can wait three years before seeing her gynecologist again for additional cervical cancer screening.

It could be argued that most women age 30 and older do not need to have both an HPV test and a Pap—and in fact, the HPV test may one day replace the Pap as the initial screening for cervical cancer. But for the time being, either the Pap alone or both the HPV test and Pap are recommended by ACOG.

From the patient's point of view, an HPV test is performed just like a Pap and both can easily be done at the same time. A gynecologist sweeps the cervix with a soft brush to collect the cells that are shedding from the cervix, then places the sample in a vial of liquid and sends it to a lab. For the Pap, the cells suspended in the liquid are examined under a microscope to analyze their shape. For the HPV test, DNA from the cells is separated from that same liquid sample and tested for the presence of the 14 high-risk types of HPV associated with cervical cancer. Insurance typically covers the Pap and may cover the HPV test.

Important: If you use your gynecologist as your primary care provider, as some women do, you will still need to see him or her annually or as often as the doctor recommends for your regular checkup, even if you don't get a Pap or HPV test at those visits.

Chinese Remedy for Menstrual Cramps

Xiaoli Chen, OMD, LAc, is an associate professor of classical Chinese medicine at National College of Natural Medicine and a private practitioner, both in Portland, Oregon. She also is the author of three books on Chinese medicine.

Moxibustion is a safe remedy for menstrual cramps, if used correctly. This traditional Chinese technique uses moxa-wool made from the dried leaves of the mugwort plant. In addition to relieving menstrual cramps and regulating menstruation, it can reduce pain from injuries, such as sprains, and ease muscle spasms or weakness associated with chronic fatigue. A study in the *Journal of the American Medical Association* showed that moxibustion also could help "turn" unborn babies who were in breech position prior to delivery.

The moxa-wool is rolled up in special paper to create a moxa stick that resembles a cigar. One end is lit and then the smoldering tip is held an inch away from the painful area or associated acupuncture points, without touching the skin, for five to 10 minutes. According to Chinese medicine traditions, when moxa is burned, its unique vapors enter the body via the skin and acupuncture points, opening the meridians (energy pathways). This regulates blood and *qi* (the body's life energy), expels cold and dampness, warms the uterus and increases circulation specifically to the pelvic area. Also, the warmth of the smoldering moxa relieves stagnation or cold in the blood and improves the flow of qi.

For maximum effectiveness and safety, you should see a licensed acupuncturist, who will direct the moxa stick at specific acupuncture points, depending on the diagnosis. Thereafter, you can do moxibustion on yourself as needed by pointing the moxa stick at the exact area of pain—though you should stop immediately if the skin turns pink or feels very hot.

Moxibustion is not recommended for anyone who is overheated or running a fever. Moxa sticks are sold at Chinese medicine stores and on *www.amazon.com* starting at about $7 for a box of 50.

The Smokers Most Likely To Have Hot Flashes

Journal of Clinical Endocrinology and Metabolism, news release

Women smokers with certain gene variants are at increased risk for menopausal hot flashes compared with smokers without these genetic differences, a new study says.

An analysis of data from nearly 300 late reproductive–age women who were followed for 11 years showed that smokers with specific variations (*single nucleotide polymorphisms*) in genes that affect metabolism are more likely to have hot flashes than smokers without these gene variants.

"Our report demonstrates the impact of smoking on hot flashes as a function of variants in genes involved in sex steroid metabolism in late reproductive–age women, and suggests that certain smokers have increased susceptibility to hot flashes based on their genetic background," said lead author Samantha Butts, MD, Perelman School of Medicine at the University of Pennsylvania in Philadelphia.

"Women who smoke and carry a particular gene variant may benefit from aggressive targeted approaches to smoking cessation, especially if they know that smoking is a significant contributor to their menopausal symptoms," she added.

The study appeared in the *Journal of Clinical Endocrinology and Metabolism.*

Previous research has shown that smoking is linked with earlier onset of menopause, increased risk of hot flashes and heightened risk of postmenopausal osteoporosis.

"The toxins in cigarette smoke that are believed to be associated with hot flashes are also present in many forms in the environment, which means even non-smokers who have certain [single nucleotide polymorphisms] could be at risk for symptoms," Dr. Butts said.

info The US Department of Health and Human Services Office on Women's Health offers advice for dealing with hot flashes and other menopause symptoms.

■ ■ ■ ■

Wrinkles Can Predict Women's Bone Fracture Risk

We usually think of wrinkles as a sign of aging, but researchers at Yale School of Medicine believe that the severity of wrinkles also may indicate bone mineral density levels in menopausal women.

Reason: Bones and skin share common proteins. The researchers found that the worse the wrinkles (severity and distribution throughout

the body), the greater the risk for low bone density and bone fracture risk. If wrinkles are an indicator of bone health, they may tell you that your bone density needs to be checked.

L. Pal, et al., "Skin Wrinkling and Rigidity Are Predictive of Bone Mineral Density in Early Postmenopausal Women" presented at the Endocrine Society Meeting (June 2011).

■ ■ ■ ■

Tomato Juice Boosts Bone Health

Tomatoes contain the antioxidant lycopene, which reduces harmful oxidative stress that causes the body to resorb bone and damage cells responsible for bone formation.

Recent finding: Postmenopausal women who got at least 30 milligrams daily of lycopene through tomato juice or supplements showed improved bone health.

Leticia Rao, PhD, director, Calcium Research Laboratory, St. Michael's Hospital, and associate (adjunct) professor of medicine, University of Toronto, Canada, and leader of a study of 60 postmenopausal women, published in *Osteoporosis International.*

Take the Online Osteoporosis Risk Test Now

Bruce Ettinger, MD, is an emeritus clinical professor of medicine at the University of California Medical Center, San Francisco, and an adjunct investigator in the Division of Research at Kaiser Permanente Medical Care Program for Northern California.

Women are at significantly higher risk than men for osteoporosis, the disease that weakens bones and leads to fractures. Risk increases with age. Previous USPSTF guidelines, set in 2002, recommended bone density testing to screen all women age 65 and older (that part has not changed), plus women ages 60 to 64 who were at increased risk for osteoporotic fractures. Those guidelines were recently revised to more specifically define the level of risk that merits bone density testing for the 60-to-64 age group and to address the needs of younger women by utilizing a new online fracture risk assessment tool called FRAX.

Bruce Ettinger, MD, an emeritus clinical professor of medicine at the University of California Medical Center, San Francisco, and osteoporosis expert whose input helped set the new guidelines, explained that FRAX prompts you to input your status with regard to various risk factors. These include age…height and weight…ethnicity (since genetic influences put Caucasians at higher risk than Asians, Blacks or Hispanics)…alcohol and tobacco use…diseases or drugs that can affect bones…and personal and family history of fractures. Then the Web-based program instantly calculates your 10-year probability of experiencing a fracture due to osteoporosis.

To use FRAX: Visit *www.shef.ac.uk/FRAX/ index.jsp,* enter the pertinent information and answer simple yes/no questions. The FRAX calculator gives you two percentages. The main number to consider is your risk of having a fracture at any of the four major osteoporotic fracture sites—hip, spine, wrist or upper arm/ shoulder—within the next 10 years. Once this risk reaches 9.3%, which is the risk level of a healthy 65-year-old white woman, bone density screening is recommended. (The other percentage given is your 10-year risk of fracturing a hip specifically. Hip fractures are singled out because they are the most serious of the osteoporotic fractures—but since these are rare before age 70 to 75, for younger women it is more useful to consider the combined risk at all four major sites.)

A fair number of women in their 50s do have a FRAX score higher than that of the hypothetical 65-year-old. Dr. Ettinger explained, "If you are 55 and you smoke, are thin and have a parent who had a hip fracture, then you're more like a typical 65-year-old in terms of osteoporosis risk."

Bottom line: If your major fracture site FRAX score is…

• **Below 9.3%**—continue to follow your doctor's recommendations on diet, exercise and lifestyle habits that protect bones…and complete the FRAX questionnaire again in three to five years. Fracture risk typically doubles every seven to eight years, Dr. Ettinger said, so you can estimate when in the future your score might cross the threshold for bone density testing.

• **9.3% or higher**—the recommendation is for your doctor to order a dual-energy X-ray absorptiometry (DEXA) test to measure your bone density. Those results can be entered into the FRAX calculator to further refine your risk level. If your bone density is right at the expected level for your age, your FRAX score won't change much. But if your bone density is much lower than expected, this new factor could easily double your risk, Dr. Ettinger said. Your doctor will take this into account in determining the next appropriate step in your care.

Is the Pill Still Right for You?

Richard P. Dickey, MD, PhD, is a clinical professor and chief of reproductive endocrinology and infertility in the department of obstetrics and gynecology at Louisiana State University Medical School in New Orleans. He also is the founder of the Fertility Institute, which has three clinics in Louisiana, and author of *Managing Contraceptive Pill/Drug Patients* (EMIS). *www.fertilityinstitute.com*

If you are heading toward menopause, you are due to discuss the Pill with your gynecologist, according to Richard P. Dickey, MD, PhD, chief of reproductive endocrinology and infertility in the department of obstetrics and gynecology at Louisiana State University Medical School.

Reason: Recent research provides surprising revelations about the benefits and risks of oral contraceptives. So if you are not taking "the Pill" now and thought that you were too old, you might want to reconsider. If you are on it, you need to make sure that it is still safe, given your lifestyle and medical history…and also make sure that the type you are taking has minimal side effects for you.

To minimize the risk for an unintended pregnancy, you should continue to use birth control until one full year has passed without a menstrual period. And despite what many women think, oral contraceptives do not delay the onset of menopause.

Here's what you need to know now about oral contraceptives…

The Pill recently celebrated its 50th birthday (like many of its users), and it is taking middle age quite well despite earlier fears that it might be detrimental to users' long-term health.

Evidence: A recent study in *BMJ* (*British Medical Journal*), which involved more than 46,000 women who were observed for up to 39 years, found a significantly lower rate of death from any cause among women who had used the Pill, compared with women who had never used it. Also, a study published in *Contraception* found that oral contraceptives strongly protected against death from uterine cancer and ovarian cancer. Surprisingly, many of these protective effects persisted for years after users stopped taking the Pill—which means that oral contraception often is a particularly good choice for women with a family history of uterine or ovarian cancer, Dr. Dickey said.

Good news for the perimenopausal: Combination estrogen/progestin oral contraceptives (the most common type) alleviate many annoying menopausal symptoms, including hot flashes, night sweats and vaginal dryness…and also may help midlife women maintain muscle tone in the pelvic floor, which is important for preventing incontinence.

Bonus: Oral contraceptives (particularly the low-dose type) often lighten perimenopausal menstrual periods or make them stop altogether.

All birth control pills are not created equal—different brands have different ratios of estrogen to progestin—so if one brand causes side effects for you, talk to your doctor about other options. For instance, Dr. Dickey said, developing migraines might mean that your pill has too much estrogen…developing depression, fatigue or increased appetite might suggest too much progestin.

Some studies indicate that being overweight interferes with the contraceptive effects of the Pill. To reduce pregnancy risk, overweight women may be advised against using a low-dose formulation and also should be careful to take their pills exactly as prescribed, Dr. Dickey suggested.

Important: Many drugs and supplements (including acetaminophen, antibiotics and St. John's wort) can interact with progestin, reducing the Pill's effectiveness. Be sure to tell your doctor about any medications or supplements you take.

Who should not use the Pill: If you are over age 35 and a smoker, oral contraception is not an option for you—there is a clear link between Pill users who smoke and an increased risk for breast cancer, cardiovascular disease and potentially life-threatening blood clots.

Also: Oral contraceptives containing estrogen are not appropriate for women with a history of heart disease, uncontrolled hypertension, blood clots or estrogen-dependent cancer. It is not that the Pill is believed to cause those conditions, Dr. Dickey said, but rather that it can exacerbate existing conditions. Some women with such conditions can take a progestin-only oral contraceptive, however, so discuss this possibility with your doctor.

■ ■ ■ ■

Depression Raises Stroke Risk 29%

Depressed women have a 29% greater stroke risk than women who are not depressed.

Possible reason: Depression is linked to increased inflammation, which raises stroke risk.

Also: People with depression may not exercise regularly, use prescribed medications consistently or take other steps that help prevent strokes. The study looked only at women, but the findings likely apply to men as well.

Kathryn Rexrode, MD, is associate professor of medicine at Harvard Medical School and associate physician at Brigham and Women's Hospital, both in Boston. She is senior author of a study of 80,574 women, published in *Stroke*.

■ ■ ■ ■

Coffee Lowers Depression Risk In Women

Recent research found that women who drank two to three cups of caffeinated coffee per day had a 15% lower risk of becoming depressed over a 10-year period than those who drank one cup or less per week. Those drinking four cups a day were at 20% lower risk. But further research is needed. It is too soon to recommend that women drink coffee to prevent depression.

Michel Lucas, PhD, RD, is an epidemiologist and nutritionist and a postdoctoral fellow in the department of nutrition at Harvard School of Public Health, Boston, and lead author of an analysis of data on more than 50,000 women, published in *Archives of Internal Medicine.*

The Link Between Depression and Celiac Disease

Joshua M. Smyth, PhD, professor of biobehavioral health and medicine, Penn State University.
Chronic Illness, news release

New research shows that women with celiac disease face a higher risk for also suffering from depression and so-called "disordered eating," regardless of whether they stick to a gluten-free diet.

"We found that most [study] participants frequently adhered to a gluten-free diet, and this greater compliance with diet was related to increased vitality, lower stress, decreased depressive symptoms and greater overall emotional health," said study coauthor Joshua M. Smyth, PhD, a professor of biobehavioral health and medicine at Penn State University.

"However, even those people who were managing their illness reported higher rates of stress, depression and a range of issues clustered around body image, weight and shape when compared to the general population," he added.

The study results appeared in the journal *Chronic Illness.*

BACKGROUND

Celiac patients are often plagued by abdominal pain, lack of appetite, constipation, nausea, vomiting and diarrhea, stemming from an inability to process foods containing gluten such as wheat, barley and rye.

At least one in every 1,750 Americans is forced to make dietary adjustments to the disease by avoiding such foods, according to the release.

STUDY DETAILS

To gauge how adherence to such eating routines might affect other health issues, the research team conducted a poll of 177 women who were diagnosed with celiac disease.

Patients responded to questions regarding how well they stuck to their gluten-free diets, physical symptoms, physical functioning, stress levels and management, signs of clinical depression and their thoughts and actions reflecting upon their sense of body image and eating habits. The study authors compared their answers with prior research that looked into the same issues among non-celiac patients.

While concluding that celiac patients are more liable to develop depression and eating issues regardless of diet, the team noted that it still remains unclear which comes first: Do people with celiac disease start with depression that leads to eating issues or does the onset of disordered eating lead to depression?

"In the future, we plan to investigate the temporal sequence of these symptoms," Smyth said.

info For more on celiac disease, visit the Web site of the Celiac Disease Foundation, *www. celiac.org.*

What You Don't Know About Hair Loss

Carolyn Goh, MD, director of the inpatient dermatology service at the Ronald Reagan Medical Center at the University of California, Los Angeles (UCLA). Dr. Goh directs the Clinic for Hair and Scalp Disorders, also at UCLA.

The term "hair loss" often conjures up images of older, balding men. But women make up at least 40% of American hair loss sufferers.

What causes this problem in women? A combination of fluctuating hormone levels, drug side effects, stress, aging and general health issues are often to blame.

My story: My interest in hair loss stems, in part, from my own experience. After developing an incurable type of hair loss myself, I have dedicated myself to finding the most effective treatments possible for women.

WHAT'S NORMAL?

It's normal for a woman to lose, on average, 50 to 100 strands of hair a day. However, if you notice any increase in hair loss that persists for more than a month, it's time to visit your primary care doctor.

Blood tests will be given to check your iron stores and thyroid hormone levels (anemia and hypothyroidism or hyperthyroidism can trigger hair loss). If blood tests do not indicate an underlying medical condition, your doctor can refer you to a dermatologist.

TYPES OF HAIR LOSS

Common types of hair loss in women include...

•**Telogen effluvium (TE).** At any given time, about 90% of the hairs on your head are in a growing phase. The rest of the hairs are in the "telogen," or resting, phase—and that's when they shed.

Sometimes, though, a stressful event (for example, the death of a loved one, a divorce, surgery or crash diet) causes more hairs to enter the resting phase. This rarely leads to true baldness but sometimes results in up to three times more shedding than usual.

This type of hair loss—which, at its peak, can cause you to lose handfuls of hair or, in less severe forms, clog the shower drain—typically occurs within a few weeks of the stressful event. In some cases, however, there can be a delay of up to three months.

Medication, such as blood pressure drugs (especially beta-blockers), cholesterol-lowering drugs and antidepressants, can cause TE. Over-the-counter products, including diet pills and excess vitamin A or zinc supplements, are also common culprits.

Diagnosis: TE is diagnosed with a "hair pull." When performing this test, I give a gentle, yet firm, tug to about 40 of a patient's hairs. In women with healthy scalps, no hairs—or just one or two—come out. In women with TE, I might get six or seven.

Treatment: If there is an ongoing underlying medical condition, such as anemia or a thyroid problem, correcting it usually stops the

hair loss. If medication is the cause, the dosage may be reduced or another drug may be substituted. If no underlying medical cause exists and it's just stress, TE usually resolves on its own within six months. Getting support after a stressful event that triggered hair loss can sometimes help, too.

In the meantime, topical *minoxidil* 2% (Rogaine), applied twice a day, helps keep hair in the growing phase. Side effects may include an itchy rash on the scalp. Since most cases of TE are temporary, minoxidil can usually be stopped within a year. If excessive shedding lasts longer than six months, then long-term use may be necessary.

•**Androgenetic alopecia.** Also known as female-pattern hair loss, this is a gradual, diffuse thinning of hair at the crown of the head.

As with male-pattern baldness, androgenetic alopecia in women often occurs when there is a family history of hair loss (in a female or male relative). Female-pattern baldness, which affects 20% to 40% of American women, may worsen after menopause due to declining levels of estrogen and a relative increase in testosterone (the condition is linked to male hormones known as androgens).

Diagnosis: In addition to taking a clinical history and asking about your family's hair loss, your doctor may perform a scalp biopsy to look for smaller-than-normal hair follicles—a sign of androgenetic alopecia.

Treatment: Minoxidil, applied topically, twice daily. Because female-pattern baldness is progressive, continued treatment is usually required. Your doctor may also prescribe the diuretic *spironolactone* (Aldactone), which is typically used to treat high blood pressure. The pill, which is not FDA-approved for hair loss, blocks certain male hormones.

Caution: Talk to your doctor if you have a personal or family history of any type of cancer. Spironolactone has been shown in animal studies to significantly increase cancer risk.

•**Alopecia areata.** This condition, which affects at least one million American women, is characterized by patches of hair loss that can affect the entire scalp or body. It is thought to be an autoimmune disorder in which the immune system attacks hair follicles. A certain combination of genes may predispose some people to alopecia areata. Hair usually grows back by itself within six months. However, women who lose their hair at an early age due to this condition are more likely to have extensive hair loss long-term.

Diagnosis: A clinical examination and possibly a scalp biopsy.

Treatment: Monthly cortisone injections or a topical steroid, applied to the skin daily, may halt the inflammation that usually accompanies alopecia areata and help the hair grow back.

For more diffuse hair loss caused by alopecia areata, contact immunotherapy can be used. With this procedure, a compound (squaric acid) is applied topically (initially by your dermatologist, followed up by you at home) to induce an allergic reaction (a mild, itchy, eczema-type rash) that is thought to "distract" your immune system from attacking your hair.

The procedure works in about 40% of cases, with new hair growth usually occurring in six months. Insurance typically covers the cost. Side effects may include an itchy rash and swelling.

Wigs, hair extensions and/or hair pieces are another option. There are also products that, when sprinkled on, stick to the remaining hairs and scalp to camouflage bald spots.

In cases of extensive hair loss, some women find it acceptable—and sometimes liberating—to go bald.

Unusual Hair Growth—Get to the Root Of the Problem

Lubna Pal, MD, reproductive endocrinologist, an associate professor in the department of obstetrics, gynecology and reproductive sciences, and the director of the Polycystic Ovary Program at Yale School of Medicine in New Haven, Connecticut.

I f you notice a rapid or significant increase in body hair (typically on the inner thighs, upper arms, middle of the chest, upper lip and/or chin), alert your doctor—because there may be an underlying medical cause that should be evaluated and treated.

Lubna Pal, MD, a reproductive endocrinologist at Yale School of Medicine, explained the possible causes…

•**Excess androgens.** Women normally produce low levels of androgens (male hormones), such as testosterone. *Excess body and facial hair can be a sign that androgen levels are too high, perhaps due to one of the following conditions…*

•Polycystic ovary syndrome (PCOS) is a common condition in which a woman's eggs, rather than maturing normally and being released from the ovaries monthly, stay in the ovaries. The ovarian follicles (structures in which the immature egg is surrounded by ovarian cells) form multiple tiny cysts. PCOS primarily affects women in their reproductive years, but it can affect older women, too. "The extra androgens are primarily of ovarian origin, although in some PCOS patients, they may be produced by the adrenal gland," Dr. Pal said.

•Ovarian *hyperthecosis*, an uncommon condition, usually is seen in postmenopausal women. Androgen levels in the blood may be much higher than with PCOS. Along with body hair growth, patients occasionally experience deepening of the voice, loss of scalp hair and/or enlargement of the clitoris.

•Steroid cell tumor, an androgen-secreting ovarian tumor, is potentially serious but, fortunately, is quite rare.

•**Cushing's syndrome.** This occurs when the body produces or is exposed to too much of the hormone *cortisol*. Other signs may include a face that grows rounder, upper body obesity, pink or purple stretch marks (unrelated to pregnancy) on the torso and arms, easy bruising and a fatty hump between the shoulder blades. Patients also may develop high blood pressure, diabetes and/or osteoporosis. This condition is relatively uncommon but, if untreated, can be life-threatening.

•**Hypothyroidism.** Producing too little thyroid hormone can cause coarsening of body hair. Other warning signs include fatigue, sensitivity to cold, constipation, unexplained weight gain and muscle aches.

•**Medication side effects.** Drugs that may cause new body hair growth and/or coarsening of existing hair include *diazoxide* (Micromedex) for hypoglycemia…*phenytoin* (Dilantin) for seizures…the immunosuppressant *cyclosporine* and corticosteroids, often used for autoimmune disorders such as psoriasis or rheumatoid arthritis…estrogen/testosterone combinations, such as Estratest, for menopausal symptoms… and over-the-counter "antiaging" supplements containing the hormone *dehydroepiandrosterone* (DHEA). Women also may notice increased body hair after reducing the dosage or halting use of estrogen replacement therapy.

Important: Tell your doctor if your partner uses a topical cream or gel containing testosterone. Your partner's medication can get rubbed onto your skin accidentally and cause you to experience increased body hair growth.

Good news: Getting appropriate treatment for the problems above not only will protect health, but in most cases, will cause excess hair to gradually lessen, lighten and soften. Your doctor also can advise you on methods for minimizing body hair, such as laser treatment, waxing and depilatory creams…and/or use of antiandrogen medication or birth control pills, both of which reduce androgen levels.

Still Suffering from That Long-Ago Episiotomy?

Dana R. Gossett, MD, MSCI (master of science in clinical investigation), is an assistant professor and chief of the division of general obstetrics and gynecology at Northwestern University Feinberg School of Medicine, and chief of gynecology at Northwestern Memorial Hospital, both in Chicago.

According to the Agency for Healthcare Research and Quality, there was a 60% decrease in the use of episiotomy between 1997 and 2008. Why the change? Although in special circumstances the procedure may be appropriate, recent studies show that routine episiotomy usually has no benefits for mother or baby. In fact, making a cut may increase a mother's chances of getting a severe tear in the perineum (the tissue between the vaginal opening and anus) during delivery.

The change in routine protocol is good news for today's new moms. But what about women

who had their children—and their then-routine episiotomies—decades ago? For some, episiotomy-related complications have led to ongoing problems with fecal incontinence (impaired bowel control) and/or painful intercourse. A woman may develop symptoms after giving birth and continue to suffer, constantly or intermittently, for years…or her symptoms may arise or return in midlife or later, triggered by hormonal changes and/or muscle weakening associated with aging.

Dana R. Gossett, MD, MSCI, chief of the division of general obstetrics and gynecology at Northwestern University Feinberg School of Medicine in Chicago, discussed solutions to episiotomy-related health problems…

FECAL INCONTINENCE

Dr. Gossett explained that a very large tear in the perineum can damage the anal sphincter (the muscle surrounding the anus), compromising bowel control. There are three basic levels of fecal incontinence—when the person can hold in stool but not gas…when she can hold solid stool but not diarrhea…or when she cannot hold in stool at all.

Self-help strategies target the muscles of the anus, perineum and pelvic floor. The muscles of the pelvic floor form a sling to hold pelvic organs in place, allowing the organs—including those that control bowel function—to work properly. *Try the following…*

•**Do two types of Kegel exercises daily.** You know that Kegels improve urinary control—but they also improve bowel control, Dr. Gossett noted, if in addition to squeezing your pelvic floor muscles (the ones used to halt your urine stream), you also focus your squeeze on the muscles of the anus and buttocks (as if trying to stop stool from passing).

Exercise #1: Squeeze your anal and pelvic floor muscles and hold for five seconds… relax. Repeat 10 times. During the course of the day, do 10 sets of 10 squeezes.

Exercise #2: Do a chain of 10 quick squeezes, holding for one second and then releasing for one second. Do this 10 times daily. You should start to see improvement after a few weeks, Dr. Gossett said.

•**Sit, don't "hover," in public restrooms.** Squatting puts undue pressure on pelvic floor muscles, compromising them further.

•**Avoid constipation.** You may think that being a bit constipated would aid bowel control, but straining on the toilet puts pressure on pelvic floor muscles.

Helpful: Eat more fiber from fruits, vegetables and whole grains…drink plenty of fluids… limit fats and processed foods…and get regular exercise.

If the above steps do not relieve your symptoms…

•**Consider pelvic floor physical therapy.** The effects of this targeted form of physical therapy (PT) can be "quite miraculous," Dr. Gossett said. *Treatment sessions may include…*

•Additional exercises that strengthen the pelvic floor and anal sphincter.

•Biofeedback, which aims to improve the strength and coordination of anal muscles and increase awareness of rectal sensations. A pressure probe placed in the anus or a sensing electrode on the skin is attached to a visual or sound display that tells you when you are succeeding in engaging the right muscles.

•*Percutaneous tibial nerve stimulation,* in which a fine needle electrode inserted into the leg sends an electrical pulse through the nerves that affect pelvic floor muscles, improving their function.

To find a practitioner: Visit the Web site of the American Physical Therapy Association at *www.apta.org*, click on "Find a PT," then search the "women's health" practice area.

•**Talk to your doctor about surgery.** If fecal incontinence does not respond to other therapies, options may include surgical repair of the anal sphincter or construction of an internal sling to support pelvic organs that have dropped from their normal position.

New: The FDA recently approved an implanted device called InterStim, which uses mild electrical stimulation (like a pacemaker) of the sacral nerves that affect pelvic muscles to improve bowel control.

Referrals: You can find a specialist in urogynecology and female reconstructive surgery through the American Urogynecologic Society (*www.augs.org*).

PAINFUL INTERCOURSE
Another possible long-term consequence of episiotomy is pain during sex. That's because scar tissue can form at the incision site…and scar tissue is inflexible. Symptoms often worsen at menopause, when the effects of scarring combine with reduced lubrication due to declining estrogen. Surgery is not the answer because it generally produces more scar tissue, Dr. Gossett said. *What can help…*

•**Use a long-lasting nonprescription vaginal moisturizer,** such as Replens, several times per week (not just during sex).

•**Do Kegels.** While they do not address the scar tissue problem directly, Kegels may help make sex more pleasurable overall by intensifying orgasms.

•**Try pelvic floor PT.** This therapy can incorporate perineal massage techniques that help soften and release old scar tissue, Dr. Gossett said.

Bottom line: Don't give up. With the right treatment, you can overcome—at long last—the lingering effects of that long-ago episiotomy.

Good News About Pregnancy After a Miscarriage

Sohinee Bhattacharya, MBBS, MSc, is a lecturer in obstetric epidemiology at the University of Aberdeen in Scotland and leader of a study of 30,937 women.

Women who have suffered a miscarriage are sometimes told by their doctors to wait six months before conceiving again to reduce the risk for another miscarriage.

But: New research suggests that this advice, which is based on recommendations from the World Health Organization, is misguided.

The new study included more than 30,000 women who had miscarried in their first pregnancies.

Findings: Compared with women who delayed their second pregnancies for six months or more, those who conceived again within six months were significantly less likely to have another miscarriage…have an ectopic pregnancy (in which the embryo starts to grow in a fallopian tube or elsewhere outside the womb)…need a Cesarean section…give birth prematurely…or have a baby with a low birth weight.

Caveat: It is possible that some of the women who conceived more than six months after their miscarriages did so not by choice or on the advice of their doctors, but rather because they had trouble getting pregnant again—and that this fertility problem also negatively affected their birth outcomes. However, given the large number of women included in this study, it is unlikely that this would be the only explanation for the results.

Bottom line: This study is good news, especially for women over age 35. Given that fertility decreases with age, not having to wait six months after a miscarriage can significantly boost the chances of being able to conceive again.

Editor's note: Some US doctors advise waiting two months to conceive again so that the uterine lining has time to regenerate—talk to your obstetrician.

Princeton University Study Sheds Light On Women's Fertility

American Society for Cell Biology, news release

Different molecular mechanisms may regulate the aging of the human body and the aging of the reproductive system, new research with worms suggests.

The findings may help explain why a woman's fertility begins to decline after age 35 but other cells in her body don't show major signs of aging until decades later, according to study author Coleen Murphy, assistant professor of molecular biology at Princeton University.

Professor Murphy and her colleagues studied the roundworms, called *C. elegans,* to compare the types of genes that affect lifespan and the types that keep immature egg cells (oocytes) healthy.

The findings were presented at the 2012 annual meeting of the American Society for Cell Biology, in Denver.

RESEARCH FINDINGS

The researchers found that both body aging and reproductive aging in *C. elegans* involve the insulin regulation pathway, but there are marked differences in the molecular mechanisms that maintain youthful oocyte function and those that affect body ("somatic") aging.

"It seems that maintaining protein and cell quality is the most important component of somatic longevity in worms, while chromosomal/DNA integrity and cell cycle control are the most critical factors for oocyte health," Professor Murphy said.

IMPLICATIONS

Professor Murphy explained that finding ways to delay oocyte aging could reduce older women's risk of giving birth to a child with birth defects.

Because this study was presented at a medical meeting, the data and conclusions should be viewed as preliminary until published in a peer-reviewed journal.

info The US Department of Health and Human Services has more information about infertility at WomensHealth.gov.

■ ■ ■ ■

Middle-Age STD

A new study found that 13% of women age 50 and older were infected with *Trichomonas vaginalis,* a sexually transmitted parasite. The infection, which often causes no symptoms, is easily treated with antibiotics.

Johns Hopkins Medical Institutions.

Women's Sexual Satisfaction Often Rises With Age

The American Journal of Medicine, news release

Sexual satisfaction increases with age among sexually active older women, according to a new study, while those who don't have sex are satisfied with their sex lives.

The study included 806 older women who live in a planned community in the San Diego area and whose health has been tracked for 40 years. The study participants' average age was 67 years and 63% of them were postmenopausal.

The University of California, San Diego School of Medicine and Veterans Affairs San Diego Healthcare System researchers evaluated the women's sexual activity and satisfaction and found that half of the women with a romantic partner had been sexually active in the previous four weeks.

The investigators also found that the likelihood of sexual activity decreased with age, that 67% of sexually active women always or usually achieved orgasm, and that the youngest and oldest women reported the highest frequency of orgasm satisfaction.

SEX WITHOUT DESIRE

Forty percent of the women in the study said they never or almost never felt sexual desire, and one-third of sexually active women reported low sexual desire, according to the study in *The American Journal of Medicine.*

"Despite a correlation between sexual desire and other sexual function domains, only one in five sexually active women reported high sexual desire," said lead investigator Elizabeth Barrett-Connor, MD, chief of the division of epidemiology at the UCSD School of Medicine.

"Approximately half of the women aged 80 years or more reported arousal, lubrication and orgasm most of the time, but rarely reported sexual desire. In contrast with the traditional linear model in which desire precedes sex, these results suggest that women engage in sexual activity for multiple reasons, which may include affirmation or sustenance of a relationship," Dr. Barrett-Connor said.

Sixty-one percent of the women in the study were satisfied with their overall sex life, regardless of whether they had a partner or were sexually active.

PREVALENT VIEWS CHALLENGED

Older age is considered a predictor of low sexual satisfaction, but the percentage of sexually satisfied women in the study actually increased with age. About half the women older than 80 reported sexual satisfaction almost always or always.

Not only were the oldest women the most sexually satisfied overall, the oldest women who were sexually active had orgasm satisfaction rates similar to those of the youngest women.

"In this study, sexual activity was not always necessary for sexual satisfaction. Those who were not sexually active may have achieved sexual satisfaction through touching, caressing, or other intimacies developed over the course of a long relationship," said study author Susan Trompeter, MD, associate clinical professor in the division of general internal medicine at UCSD School of Medicine, and a staff physician at the VA San Diego Healthcare System.

"Emotional and physical closeness to the partner may be more important than experiencing orgasm. A more positive approach to female sexual health focusing on sexual satisfaction may be more beneficial to women than a focus limited to female sexual activity or dysfunction," Dr. Trompeter concluded.

info To learn more about sexuality later in life, visit the Web site of the US National Institute on Aging at *http://www.nia.nih.gov/health/publication/sexuality-later-life.*

Sex After Years Of Abstinence

Barbara Bartlik, MD, is a sex therapist and assistant clinical professor of psychiatry at Weill Cornell Medical College in New York City. She is the author of numerous scientific publications, medical advisor for the book *Extraordinary Togetherness: A Woman's Guide to Love, Sex and Intimacy. www.barbarabartlikmd.com*

Intercourse is likely to be uncomfortable at first if you've been without a partner for a long time. The vagina can atrophy from lack of activity. Also, if you are postmenopausal, vaginal tissues can become thin and dry due to the natural decline in estrogen and testosterone levels, exacerbating the discomfort of penetration. Fortunately, there is a lot you can do now to prepare yourself so that intercourse will be enjoyable. *Try any or all of the following…*

•**Start using a nonhormonal over-the-counter vaginal moisturizer,** which is a topical suppository, cream or gel with long-lasting effects. Routinely applied two or three times per week, it helps rejuvenate the vaginal tissues, making them more moist and resilient.

Good brand: Replens.

•**Once daily, use a pin to pierce a vitamin E gel-cap supplement (500 IU), squeeze the oil onto your fingertips, then rub it onto the labia and around the vaginal opening.** This plumps up and strengthens the cells.

•**Ask your gynecologist whether a prescription topical estrogen cream or suppository is appropriate for you.** Topical estrogen can improve the integrity of the vaginal lining, reducing the chances of tearing and lessening any discomfort you might experience during sex—and because very little gets into the bloodstream, it does not carry the same level of risk for systemic side effects as oral estrogen does. (Topical estrogen generally is not recommended for women at high risk for breast or ovarian cancer, but there are exceptions.) Also ask about specially compounded testosterone cream to be applied to the vulva. Though not FDA-approved for this purpose, doctors have been prescribing this to women for many years.

•**Keep a water-based or silicone-based personal lubricant on hand** so you'll have it when you need it. Used during foreplay and intercourse, it helps minimize pain and heighten pleasure. Some lubricants contain ingredients that can irritate delicate tissues, particularly in menopausal women, so look for a product that is organic, hypoallergenic and/or paraben-free.

Excellent brands include Hathor Aphrodisia, Pink and Sliquid.

•**Do Kegel exercises, aiming for 20 minutes or 200 repetitions per day.** Repeatedly squeezing and then releasing the muscles you use to start and stop the flow of urine can increase the flow of blood, oxygen and nutrients to the pelvic floor, strengthening not only the muscles but also the tissues in that area.

Bonus: Kegels help prevent incontinence and may intensify orgasms.

•**Masturbate on your own, with a vibrator if desired, to rediscover what makes you feel aroused.** Sometimes getting back in the game takes practice.

•**Consider talking to your gynecologist about a vaginal dilator, which is a set of smooth cylindrical probes in varying sizes.** You use the dilator at home to gradually stretch the vagina—so that by the time you want to have intercourse, you are physically ready.

Don't Have Sex If You Have a Yeast Infection

Cherie A. LeFevre, MD, is an associate professor of gynecology and director of the Vulvar and Vaginal Disorders Specialty Center at Saint Louis University School of Medicine.

It's not a great idea to have sex if you have a vaginal yeast infection. For one thing, a yeast infection usually causes vaginal tissues to become red, swollen, itchy and dry. When you add the friction of intercourse, odds are that you'll experience an uncomfortable burning sensation…and vaginal tissues may develop tiny tears that slightly increase your risk of contracting a blood-borne sexually transmitted disease, such as HIV or hepatitis B or C. There is also a chance that the yeast infection could spread to your partner. And if you are being treated for the infection with antifungal vaginal cream, sex will be messy.

So, overall, it is better to wait to have sex until your treatment is done. Over-the-counter and prescription antifungal vaginal preparations typically require three to seven days of use to clear the infection. If you or your partner cannot wait that long, the oral prescription medication *fluconazole* (Diflucan) is available as a single-dose pill. Two days after you have taken it, the yeast should be gone and you can have sex again—comfortably.

Caution: Oral antifungals carry a small risk of causing liver problems, so if you develop jaundice (yellow skin or eyes), dark urine, flulike symptoms and/or abdominal pain, alert your doctor.

How to Look 10 Years Younger in 1.3 Seconds

Laurie Steelsmith, ND, is the author of *Natural Choices for Women's Health* (Three Rivers) and a medical reviewer for *HealthyWoman* from Bottom Line. Her private practice in naturopathic and Chinese medicine is in Honolulu. *www.naturalchoicesforwomen.com*

You can look younger without much effort, expense or scary plastic surgery. Honolulu-based naturopathic physician Laurie Steelsmith, ND, author of *Natural Choices for Women's Health,* offers an abundance of creative suggestions. Some take just minutes, others take almost no time at all…yet they can take as much as 10 years off a woman's appearance.

Youth-restoring options for when you have only 1.3 seconds to spare…

•**Project your "love glow."** A new study from Syracuse University shows that falling in love takes only one-fifth of a second! Remember how new love could light you up from the inside, projecting youth and vitality? OK, maybe it's not possible to fall in love just now. But you can think a loving thought and give a big smile, Dr. Steelsmith said, which will bring a youthful sparkle to your face.

•**Check your posture.** Nothing reads old like slumping. For an instantly improved figure, stand up straight, raise your chin, throw those shoulders back and pull in your tummy.

•**Do a facial exercise.** Open your mouth and eyes wide…then scrunch up your face… then release. This gets the blood flowing, putting roses in your cheeks.

•**Brighten your eyes.** Use two drops of homeopathic Similasan eyedrops in each eye every three hours, as needed. This remedy, which is generally safe for everyone, reduces redness and soothes dryness and irritation, Dr. Steelsmith noted.

•**Dash on the right lipstick**—a light-colored one. Dark lipstick seems old-ladyish and actually emphasizes tiny lip lines.

•**Take a pass on heavy makeup.** Pancake foundation and too-bright blush look unnatural and make wrinkles more noticeable.

What to try when you have three minutes…

•**Exfoliate your face.** Getting rid of dead cells with a facial scrub makes your complexion glow.

Natural option: Combine a spoonful of ground oatmeal with enough honey to make a paste, then gently rub it onto your clean face. Rinse.

•**Use contrast hydrotherapy.** To rinse your face, use two splashes of medium-hot water followed by two splashes of cold water. The hot/cold contrast increases circulation and tones skin, Dr. Steelsmith explained.

Next: Moisten a cotton ball with a natural astringent, such as rose water, aloe vera juice or green tea, and stroke it across your face to remove lingering residue and restore the skin's proper pH.

•**Combat sun damage.** Smooth a dab of vitamin C serum over your face—its antioxidants protect against ultraviolet rays and environmental toxins. Dr. Steelsmith recommended the brands Obagi (*www.obagi.com*) and SkinCeuticals (*www.skinceuticals.com*).

•**Counteract saggy eyelids.** Curling your eyelashes is a simple beauty technique that makes eyes appear larger.

If you can indulge yourself for 10 minutes…

•**Make your hair shine.** Rosemary essential oil gives tresses an extra sheen and a scent that's light and clean. It is particularly helpful for dry, brittle or frizzy hair.

After shampooing: Add a few drops of rosemary oil to your conditioner, work through your hair for a few minutes, then rinse…or towel-dry your hair, rub a dab of rosemary oil between your palms and stroke it onto your damp hair. Then style as usual. Repeat after each shampoo (as Dr. Steelsmith does to keep her long hair frizz-free despite the Hawaiian humidity) or as often as desired.

• **Clear up blemishes.** Even if pimples remind you of being a teen, they don't make you look any younger.

The fix: Use your fingertips to spread honey over your face, avoiding the eye area. Leave on for five minutes…rinse off with water…then cleanse your face as usual. "For people prone to acne, this works like a charm if used every day," Dr. Steelsmith said.

• **Ease eye puffiness.** Dampen cotton balls with diluted witch hazel, then lie down with eyes closed and place the cotton balls over your eyes for five minutes (be careful not to let the witch hazel get into your eyes). Witch hazel contains *catechol tannin*, which reduces puffiness by constricting tiny capillaries just below the skin's surface.

■ ■ ■ ■

Got Insomnia? Go to Bed Later

Researchers gave 79 women with insomnia (average age 72) printed material on good sleep habits or four weeks of behavioral therapy that included in-person counseling.

Result: Those who received therapy significantly improved sleep by going to bed later, waking up at the same time each morning and limiting time in bed.

Theory: Turning in later increases one's natural sleep drive.

If you have insomnia: Go to bed later, when sleepy, and get up at your usual time each day. Your total time in bed should equal your average amount of actual sleep plus no more than 30 minutes.

Daniel Buysse, MD, professor of psychiatry, Sleep Medicine Institute, University of Pittsburgh School of Medicine.

■ ■ ■ ■

Sleep Right to Fight Breast Sag

Do you usually sleep on your side? If you want to keep your breasts as perky as possible, you might want to rethink that habitual position. "Side-sleeping leaves the breasts hanging, so over time, it encourages them to sag," says Christopher Rose, MD, medical director of the sleep center at Covenant Medical Center in Lubbock, Texas.

Sleeping on your stomach isn't smart, either. It squashes the breasts and promotes wrinkling—not to mention distorting the alignment of your neck and spine.

Best for breasts (and the rest of your body): Sleep on your back, Dr. Rose advises.

Exception: Pregnant women should avoid back-sleeping in the later months to keep the weight of the growing fetus off the intestines and major blood vessels (the aorta and vena cava), so that blood flows more freely to the fetus.

Christopher Rose, MD, is medical director of the sleep center at Covenant Medical Center in Lubbock, Texas.

Breast Implants: Safety Still Under Fire

William Maisel, MD, deputy director for science and chief scientist, Center for Devices and Radiological Health, US Food and Drug Administration, Silver Spring, Maryland.

The ongoing debate about the long-term safety of silicone breast implants—which were removed from the US market from 1992 to 2006 (except for breast reconstruction or to replace existing ones)—has reared up again. It was revealed this year that two long-term studies currently addressing the issue have, so far, analyzed only a fraction of the women that they were supposed to be following. The FDA, which regulates the silicone breast implants as medical devices, has recently concluded that they are safe when used as intended. But maybe the more accurate characterization would be: safe enough—as far as we know.

WHY THE SUDDEN WORRY?

There are two brands of silicone gel-filled breast implants on the market in the US—one is made by a company called Allergan and the other is made by Mentor Corporation. Data on how well women with these implants fare over the long term (for 10 years or longer) is scarce. So when the FDA approved the devices for use in 2006, there was a condition: Each company was required to begin a 10-year study of safety data on 40,000 women who got their silicone gel-filled implants between 2006 and 2016. In 2011 the FDA held a two-day meeting in Washington, DC, to get an update on their progress... and it's not so impressive.

Over the past five-plus years, Allergan has collected survey data on only 60% of the women that it was supposed to be following, and Mentor Corporation's patient response rate is even worse—a mere 21%. Therefore many fewer women are being studied than expected. One main problem is that women participating in these studies are being asked to complete a massive, 27-page questionnaire each year following surgery.

MAKING SENSE OF THE DATA (OR LACK THEREOF)

Silicone implants are quite popular. In fact, in 2010, about 150,000 women got them in the US for cosmetic reasons. Many women obviously feel that the benefits outweigh the risks (or lack of scientific data). And risks and problems still occur. William Maisel, MD, deputy director for science and chief scientist with the FDA's Center for Devices and Radiological Health in Silver Spring, Maryland, offered his views on the safety of implants.

RISKS VS. BENEFITS

Many medical devices and drugs that are FDA-approved, as we all know, carry serious risks. In the case of breast implants, Dr. Maisel readily acknowledged that they can cause problems that include scarring, pain, infection, a hardening of the tissue around them, and even rupturing—which can cause silicone to leak into a woman's body (that's one of the reasons that they were removed from the market in 1992).

Past research shows that the longer a woman has implants, the more likely she is to experience complications. In fact, one in five women who chooses to get implants for cosmetic reasons will likely need to have them removed within 10 years! But all of those risks are old news and not enough to make the FDA keep silicone implants off the market.

"Not every patient is the same, which is why we always encourage patients to talk to their doctors," said Dr. Maisel. After all, there is evidence supporting patient happiness, too. In the FDA's recent review of research, studies showed that more than 90% of women with silicone implants are satisfied. Plus, body image improves in the majority of women who receive silicone implants, and this feeling lasts for at least two years post-implant. "Based on the total scientific data available right now, we believe that implants are safe and effective," said Dr. Maisel.

Although there is a little bit of long-term data, the thorough research that we thought we were going to have in five years from Allergan and Mentor Corporation doesn't seem likely to provide the big-picture information that doctors were hoping it would. So what's a woman who is considering getting silicone implants supposed to do, since aspects of the implants' long-term safety are still largely unknown (and may be for a while)?

Simply put: It depends on how much of a risk-taker you are. Are there other implant options to consider getting? Besides silicone, the only other type of implant on the market is saline, but "saline implants have a similar risk profile," said Dr. Maisel.

If you already have silicone implants, said Dr. Maisel, keep a close eye on them and schedule follow-up appointments with your doctor. The FDA recommends that you have periodic MRI scans (three years after your surgery and then every two years after that) to help detect "silent ruptures" that you may not be able to feel. So talk to your doctor about scheduling those tests—especially since Dr. Maisel said that many doctors don't tell patients about this MRI recommendation. Maybe it's because MRIs aren't cheap: An MRI could set you back $2,000 or more—and insurance may or may not cover any of the cost.

Also: Notify your doctor if you develop any unusual symptoms, like pain, asymmetry, lumps, hardness or swelling, because it could mean that your implants have become defective—and you may need to have them removed or replaced.

Natural Relief for Fibrocystic Breasts

Cindee Gardner, PhD, DHom (doctor of homeopathy), is a registered and certified homeopathic practitioner, molecular biologist, herbalist and nutritional counselor in private practice in Pittsburgh. *www.cindeegardner. com* and *www.homeohelpline.com*

Among the challenges that come with being a woman, having fibrocystic breasts may seem like a minor one. Unless, that is, your breasts often feel achy and tender…you experience significant pain and swelling before your period…and/or your mammogram is too murky to read, requiring you to have further tests to screen for cancer.

Fibrocycstic breasts have ropy, dense tissue and lumpy, fluid-filled cysts. Frustratingly, Western medicine doesn't have much to offer other than over-the-counter pain medication and, in cases where a large cyst causes extreme pain, drainage with needle aspiration or surgery—but these won't help prevent further cysts from forming. So, it's a relief to hear that alternative therapies can ease symptoms and even help resolve the root causes that lead to fibrocystic breasts, according to Cindee Gardner, PhD, DHom, a homeopathic practitioner, molecular biologist and herbalist in Pittsburgh.

The following natural therapies have long traditions of use and (unlike drugs and surgical procedures) have no adverse side effects or risks when used as directed, so there's no harm in trying them to see if they relieve your symptoms and/or help prevent future flare-ups. The products mentioned below are available without a prescription at health-food stores and/or online…the treatments can be used alone or together in any combination. *Options…*

•**Homeopathy.** Homeopathic remedies are tailored to address a particular combination of symptoms, so choose whichever one of the following most closely matches your situation. *If…*

•**Your breasts often feel heavy, hard, stony and swollen**—try the homeopathic remedy called *Phytolacca decandra.*

•**Aching and lumpiness worsen before your period and tend to be accompanied by tearful moods**—opt for *Pulsatilla.*

•**Cysts and soreness occur mainly in the left breast**—consider *Calcarea phosphorica.*

•**Symptom flare-ups are accompanied by itching**—use *Silica.*

For moderate pain, Dr. Gardner recommended using a 30x or 30c remedy three times per day as needed, following the directions on the label…for severe pain, use the remedy every 30 minutes as needed, lessening the frequency as symptoms improve.

Important: When using any of the remedies above, avoid drinking strong coffee or inhaling strong scents of mint or camphor (for instance, from mothballs)—these can counteract a remedy's effects.

If a nonprescription remedy doesn't help or you need to use it more than a few days per month, it is best to consult a professional homeopath. As Dr. Gardner noted, there are about 45 different remedies for fibrocystic breasts listed in the Homeopathic Materia Medica (the homeopath's version of the Physician's Desk Reference)—so identifying the most effective one for you may require expert guidance. To find a practitioner, visit the Web site of the National Center for Homeopathy (*www.homeopathic. org/practitioners*) or The National United Professional Association of Trained Homeopaths (*www.nupath.org*).

•**Breast massage.** This practice relieves fibrocystic breast symptoms and helps prevent flare-ups because it stimulates the endocrine system to balance female hormones, keeps breast tissue from getting overly congested and reduces stagnation in the breast glands and ducts, Dr. Gardner said. She recommended massaging the breasts with a topical product called Vita-Cal with Poke, available from *www. archeusonline.com,* which contains vitamins A,

D3 and E and organic cold-pressed oils (sesame, avocado, mango, nut, etc.). This rich cream, which is easily absorbed through the skin, is designed to help break up cysts and relieve lymph stagnation.

At least once a week: Lie down, breathe deeply and relax. With a dab of the cream, massage each breast for five minutes or more, moving outward from the nipple and using circular motions, first in one direction and then the other.

•**Dietary changes.** Many women report that fibrocystic symptoms ease significantly when they avoid caffeine and limit high-fat foods, particularly meat and dairy products, Dr. Gardner noted. It also is helpful to drink plenty of water between meals and to increase intake of high-fiber, high-water-content foods such as fruits and vegetables.

•**Herbal tonic.** Dr. Gardner also recommended an oral product called Cystic Breast Tonic (from *www.archeusonline.com*), which combines extracts from various herbs including burdock, echinacea and poke root. It works by thinning the lymphatic fluid so that it can more effectively remove toxins and by aiding the breakdown of fibrous tissue, she explained. For acute symptom flare-ups, take 30 to 60 drops four times per day as needed, continuing for up to one week...for chronic discomfort, take 40 drops twice daily. If symptoms persist for more than three months, consult a trained herbalist.

Referrals: American Herbalists Guild, *www.americanherbalistsguild.com*.

New Concern for Women With Endometriosis

Maurice Cerulli, MD, program director of gastroenterology, hepatology and nutrition at the North Shore-Long Island Jewish Health System, New Hyde Park, New York.

The 5.5 million women in North America who have endometriosis—an inflammatory disorder of the female reproductive system that often leads to abdominal pain and infertility—already endure a lot. Now, a new study is telling us that women with endometriosis also have a higher-than-normal risk of developing *inflammatory bowel disease* (IBD), an umbrella term for two horrid conditions, Crohn's disease and ulcerative colitis.

FINDING THE CONNECTION

Previous studies had suggested an association between endometriosis and autoimmune diseases such as multiple sclerosis. With that in mind, researchers at the Statens Serum Institut in Copenhagen decided to investigate the possibility of an association between endometriosis and IBD, another autoimmune disease. They gathered the medical records of 37,661 women who had been diagnosed with endometriosis between 1977 and 2007 and looked through these records to answer this question—during that 30-year span, how many of these women went on to develop IBD?

The results: 228 of the women had developed Crohn's disease and 92 had developed ulcerative colitis. Those numbers might seem small, but that's only because IBD in the general population is rare. Compared with the general population, these women were, on average, 50% more likely to develop IBD.

Another interesting finding: Endometriosis occurs when the uterine lining abnormally grows outside the uterus. Having a hysterectomy or going through menopause can make endometriosis symptoms either disappear completely or lessen. So the researchers were curious to know whether women who had undergone menopause would still be at greater risk for IBD. It turns out that, unfortunately, they were. The mean age of endometriosis diagnosis in the study was 39, and the findings showed that even 20 years after diagnosis (when women were 59, on average, and likely past menopause), they still had a 50% higher risk for IBD.

SYMPTOMS TO LOOK OUT FOR

Although no one knows for sure why endometriosis raises the risk for IBD, Maurice Cerulli, MD, program director of gastroenterology, hepatology and nutrition at the North Shore-Long Island Jewish Health System in New Hyde Park, New York, described one intriguing possibility. Having endometriosis (or having had it in the past) can cause scarring that makes bowel movement more difficult. This, in turn, can lead to bacterial overgrowth that could contribute to the development of IBD, he said. Drinking lots of fluids, said Dr. Cerulli, may make your bowel movements softer and easier and, therefore, potentially limit bacterial overgrowth. So if you have endometriosis, try to sip on water throughout the day. And ask your doctor if taking probiotics is a good idea.

Dr. Cerulli also said that it's extremely important for women with endometriosis to be aware of the connection between endometriosis and IBD because many IBD symptoms are strikingly similar to those of endometriosis—so it would be all too easy for both a doctor and a patient to not realize that a woman has both health problems. Two symptoms in particular are common among endometriosis, Crohn's disease and ulcerative colitis—chronic abdominal pain and diarrhea. But some distinguishing features of both Crohn's disease and ulcerative colitis include rectal pain, bleeding, bloody diarrhea, an urgent need to have a bowel movement and an inability to move the bowels.

So if you have or have had endometriosis, note your symptoms carefully—and tell your doctor if you start experiencing any IBD-like symptoms. If testing reveals IBD, then your physician may help you find relief with treatment.

Do You Have a Hidden Hernia?

Shirin Towfigh, MD, is an associate professor of surgery and a faculty surgeon in the division of general surgery and the Center for Minimally Invasive Surgery at Cedars-Sinai Medical Center in Los Angeles.

Imagine living for years with debilitating pelvic pain that often worsens when you exercise, stand for a while or bend over…or get your period…or even just sneeze or cough. Imagine undergoing numerous tests and treatments for suspected gynecological problems, from ovarian cysts to pelvic inflammatory disease to endometriosis, only to have your gynecologist and other specialists shrug in confusion when all test results turn up negative and no treatment seems to help.

This is a scenario that female patients frequently describe to Shirin Towfigh, MD, an associate professor of surgery at Cedars-Sinai Medical Center in Los Angeles. Patients come to her, desperate to learn what is causing their mysterious symptoms—yet the answer turns out to be rather straightforward. These women are suffering from hernias.

The condition is vastly underdiagnosed in women. Dr. Towfigh explained that many doctors simply do not think of hernias when they examine women, considering hernias to be a "man's problem"—even though certain types of hernias actually are more common among women. Also, since hernia symptoms can mimic pelvic pain and may worsen during menstrual periods, the signs often are mistakenly attributed to gynecological disorders. Misdiagnosis leads to unnecessary suffering and increased risk for complications, including tissue death. *Here's what women need to know to protect themselves…*

•**Types of hernias.** A hernia occurs when part of an internal organ or fat tissue bulges through a hole, tear or weak area of muscle, most commonly in the abdomen. *A hernia is classified by location…*

•Inguinal hernia occurs in the groin area where the torso meets the thigh (called the inguinal crease).

•Femoral hernia develops just below the inguinal crease toward the inner thigh. It is more common in women due to the wider bone structure of the female pelvis.

•Umbilical hernia, in the belly button area, also is more common among women, especially after pregnancy.

•Epigastric hernia occurs between the navel and breastbone.

•Hiatal hernia develops when part of the stomach protrudes through the diaphragm.

•Incisional hernia forms at the site of a previous abdominal surgery.

•**Who's at risk?** Often doctors cannot pinpoint why a particular patient has a hernia, but there are known risk factors, Dr. Towfigh said. Anything that increases pressure on the abdominal area can contribute to risk—for instance, pregnancy and vaginal childbirth... chronic cough from smoking, asthma, bronchitis, postnasal drip or gastroesophageal reflux disease...frequent constipation with straining... heavy lifting...or being overweight. Additional risk factors include genetics (hernias tend to run in families)...aging, because tissues weaken over time...smoking...and a history of abdominal surgery, such as a C-section or abdominal hysterectomy.

•**Warning signs.** In men, a hernia usually creates a visible bulge that doctors can easily detect—but in women, hernias tend to be tiny and internal. The lack of a distinguishable bulge is another reason why hernias are underdiagnosed in women, Dr. Towfigh noted.

What to watch for: A hernia typically causes burning or sharp pain in the affected area. Pain worsens when there is an increase in abdominal pressure, such as when you bend over, and can be reproduced by pressing directly on the spot...pain improves when you lie flat on your back. The pain can be constant if a piece of fat or tissue is caught in the hernia hole, or intermittent if tissue gets pinched only occasionally (for instance, during certain activities).

If you have any such symptoms, see your primary care physician first and ask whether the problem could be a hernia. You may then be referred to a general surgeon for further evaluation. "Among general surgeons, a small number have a special interest in hernias—they are referred to as herniologists. This type of doctor is most likely to correctly suspect hernias in women and to order radiologic testing if needed to confirm the diagnosis," Dr. Towfigh said.

Referrals: American Hernia Society (*www.americanherniasociety.org*).

•**Help for hernias.** Once a hernia develops, it will not go away on its own. Hernia surgery usually consists of an open or laparoscopic procedure in which mesh is used to patch the hole.

Good news: After a hernia is surgically corrected, Dr. Towfigh said, the pain typically disappears quickly and completely.

■ ■ ■ ■

Alcohol More Dangerous for Women Than Men

Women who drink to excess are at much greater risk for liver, brain and heart damage than men who drink to excess. Women have more body fat than men, less water in their systems and lower levels of an enzyme that breaks down alcohol, so the effects of alcohol are more acutely concentrated in women. Excessive drinking is an average of four or more drinks within two hours for women and five or more drinks within two hours for men.

Deidra Roach, MD, program director, division of treatment and recovery research, National Institute on Alcohol Abuse and Alcoholism, Bethesda, Maryland. *www.niaaa.nih.gov*

Alcohol: How Much Can A Woman Safely Drink?

Wendy Chen, MD, assistant professor of medicine at Harvard Medical School and associate physician at Brigham and Women's Hospital, and Dana-Farber Cancer Institute, all in Boston.
Robert Stark, MD, cardiologist, Greenwich, Connecticut, and medical director, cardiovascular prevention program, Greenwich Hospital/Yale New Haven Health.

You've probably already heard that about one drink of alcohol a day may reduce a woman's chances of developing heart disease. And you've probably also heard that drinking alcohol can raise the risk for breast cancer—in fact, a new study shows that as few as three drinks a week can have that life-threatening effect. How are women supposed to live with such conflicting health advice?

HOW BOOZE AFFECTS BREAST HEALTH

Wendy Chen, an oncologist and epidemiologist at Brigham and Women's Hospital and Dana-Farber Cancer Institute, conducted the recent study on breast cancer and alcohol. She analyzed data from almost 106,000 women, ages 34 to 59, who participated in the US Nurses' Health

Study. Participants were followed from 1980 through 2008, and one thing that was tracked was their alcohol consumption. Dr. Chen found that those who reported having just three to six drinks per week were 15% more likely to develop breast cancer, compared with teetotalers—and the type of alcohol didn't matter. Slightly heavier drinkers did worse—with those averaging about 11 or 12 drinks a week having a 51% higher risk for breast cancer. (That's just under two drinks a day on average!) Alcohol is associated with higher estrogen levels and may make breast tissue more sensitive to the effects of estrogen, which can fuel cancer growth, said Dr. Chen. The findings were published in the *Journal of the American Medical Association*.

"We already knew that alcohol upped breast cancer risk, but this study gives us a better idea of the threshold," Dr. Chen said. The study found that having two or fewer drinks a week was not "statistically significant" in terms of leading to an increased risk for breast cancer. It also provides a more long-term view of the effects of alcohol consumption, compared with prior research, since this study followed women for almost three decades. It's important, she said, to focus on the common thread among those most at risk for breast cancer—drinking alcohol regularly over the course of many years. In other words, in terms of breast cancer risk, don't worry about occasional drinking or even occasionally overdoing it—like at a holiday party—because that type of consumption wasn't linked to increased risk.

HOW IT AFFECTS HEART HEALTH

But how do we balance this news about breast cancer with the fact that one drink per day—especially red wine, which contains the antioxidant resveratrol—might keep the cardiologist away? Robert Stark, MD, medical director of the cardiovascular prevention program at Greenwich Hospital/Yale New Haven Health, noted that a glass of alcohol a day has been shown in prior studies to help fend off cardiovascular problems by raising levels of HDL "good" cholesterol. But make no mistake, he said, aerobic exercise, such as walking or running, does a better job at raising our levels of HDL cholesterol than drinking red wine. And there is no downside to a sensible program of regular exercise.

SO WHAT'S THE SOLUTION?

As you might have guessed, there's no single answer to whether or not you should hesitate to fill your wine glass, and a lot has to do with the individual risk factors that you have for either condition. For example, Dr. Stark said, women with one or more cardiovascular risk factors should do several things to reduce their risk for heart disease—and having a nightly glass of red wine could be one of them.

But for women at high risk for breast cancer, drinking should probably be a rare indulgence, said Dr. Chen. Who else may want to cut back? Women under age 38, because their estrogen levels are at their peak, said Dr. Stark.

What if you carry risk factors for both cardiovascular disease and breast cancer? Now that's a tougher question to answer.

But keep this one uplifting thought in mind: There are so many risk factors that you can't control, like age and genetics—focus on the fact that drinking alcohol is at least a modifiable risk factor, one that you can control. Talk to your doctor—maybe even bring along a copy of this article—and together, figure out your best sipping strategy.

■ ■ ■ ■

IUDs Reduce Cervical Cancer Risk

Women who used an intrauterine device (IUD) for birth control had only about half the risk for cervical cancer, compared with women who had not used one. Research suggests that IUDs—possibly because they cause chronic low-grade inflammation—may boost a woman's immune system, helping to fight off human papillomavirus (HPV) infections that can progress to cancer.

Xavier Castellsagué, MD, PhD, unit chief, Institut Català d'Oncologia, Barcelona, Spain, and leader of an analysis of 26 studies of a total of more than 20,000 women, published in *The Lancet Oncology*.

■ ■ ■ ■

New HPV Test Catches Cancer Earlier

The FDA-approved Cobas test is the only HPV test able to determine whether a woman has HPV types 16 and 18—the forms that are most likely to lead to cervical cancer. Women age 30 and older should have an HPV test along with a Pap test—usually every three years. Ask your doctor for details.

Health, 2100 Lake Shore Dr., Birmingham, Alabama 35209. *www.health.com*

■ ■ ■ ■

How to Prevent Recurrence Once You've Had Cervical Cancer

It's a huge relief for any woman to put cervical cancer behind her and get on with life, of course.

But: Even more than four decades after being successfully treated, women who have undergone radiation therapy for cervical cancer have a 30% increased risk of developing a second cancer. The most vulnerable areas are those near the cervix—including the colon, rectum, anus, bladder, ovaries and genitals.

Cancer defense: Researchers urge cervical cancer survivors to scrupulously adhere to their oncologists' recommendations for getting periodic follow-up cancer screenings of organs near the cervix.

Anil K. Chaturvedi, PhD, MPII, is a researcher in the infections and immunoepidemiology branch of the National Cancer Institute in Bethesda, Maryland, and lead author of a study of 104,760 cervical cancer survivors.

Should You Be Screened For Uterine Cancer?

Debbie Saslow, PhD, director, Breast and Gynecologic Cancer, American Cancer Society, Atlanta.

A test for an insidious, lethal cancer isn't used very much even though it has been around for years and has a very high success rate of detecting risk. Why is that?

The cancer is uterine cancer, which sometimes can progress quickly and dangerously. So why is this test not being recommended as a screening for all postmenopausal women, who are the most likely to get uterine cancer?

For answers to these questions, we turned to Debbie Saslow, PhD, director of breast and gynecologic cancer at the American Cancer Society in Atlanta.

THICK AND THIN

Also known as endometrial cancer, since it begins in the endometrium (the lining of the uterus), uterine cancer is the most common gynecological cancer, affecting more than 43,000 women and causing nearly 8,000 deaths in this country each year.

You may not realize that one physiological characteristic that a gynecologist is attuned to is the thickness of your uterine lining. It's normal for the lining of a woman's uterus to atrophy and grow thin with menopause, Dr. Saslow explained. There are several reasons why a woman might have a thickened uterine lining, but cancer is one of them, so the condition should be monitored. A test called transvaginal ultrasound (TVS) is one way this can be done.

How it works: A technician inserts a specially designed ultrasound probe into a woman's vagina and captures an image, which is sent to a display, enabling the technician to measure the thickness of the uterine lining. Though it can be somewhat uncomfortable, this test is not painful.

Researchers in the UK administered TVS to nearly 37,000 postmenopausal women, measuring the thickness of their uterine linings and then following them for a year to see how many developed cancer. The study, which was published in *The Lancet,* found that women with a uterine lining that was 5mm or thicker were indeed at about 80% higher risk for uterine cancer within a year.

Even so, the study authors oppose using TVS for mass screening and, said Dr. Saslow, so does the American Cancer Society. One reason, she said, is that the risk of a false-positive result is high. Nearly 15% of women who undergo TVS and are found to have abnormally thick uterine linings will then end up having to endure an uncomfortable (and expensive) biopsy, with all the accompanying mental turmoil that it brings—but they will not have cancer. Meanwhile, she said, the vast majority (90%) of women who do have endometrial cancer also will have abnormal bleeding as an early warning sign. These factors have led the researchers and other experts to conclude that it is unlikely there will be much benefit to screening asymptomatic women. "We found that there is no proof that detection through screening improves outcome over detection from symptoms (vaginal bleeding)," Dr. Saslow explained.

ARE YOU A CANDIDATE?

While TVS is not a routine test, it is widely available. Risk factors for uterine cancer include obesity…never having been pregnant…and exposure to synthetic estrogens, such as hormone replacement therapy, or *tamoxifen* (for breast cancer). Dr. Saslow said that at present the American Cancer Society is focused on limiting the number of false-positives and therefore recommends screening only for women with a rare hereditary disease called Lynch syndrome that increases the risk for both uterine and colorectal cancers.

Cancer screening tests remain a controversial topic, and this story sheds light on the complexities that make it so difficult—the risk-versus-benefits equation does not always present a clear case for making a recommendation. The one thing that every woman absolutely should know is that the most important warning sign of uterine cancer is vaginal bleeding after menopause—if you experience this symptom, call your doctor immediately.

■ ■ ■ ■

Better Ovarian Cancer Detection

Among 37,000 healthy women (average age 57) who took part in studies to investigate the effectiveness of transvaginal ultrasound screening, 72 ovarian cancers were detected. Of these, 70% were early stage, and 88% of these women had a five-year survival rate, compared with about 50% of unscreened women who were diagnosed with ovarian cancer.

Theory: Ultrasound detects changes in size and structure of the ovary. Women at risk for ovarian cancer (due to family history, for example) should discuss transvaginal screening with their doctors.

Edward J. Pavlik, PhD, director, Ovarian Screening Research Program, University of Kentucky, Lexington.

■ ■ ■ ■

Hysterectomy May Raise Kidney Cancer Risk

Researchers compared rates of a common kidney cancer in about 185,000 women who had undergone hysterectomies with about 657,000 who had not.

Result: Those who had undergone hysterectomies were up to 50% more likely to develop kidney cancer—with women age 44 or younger when they had the hysterectomy at highest risk.

Theory: Hysterectomy may alter urine flow, setting the stage for kidney cells to become cancerous.

If a doctor recommends hysterectomy for a noncancerous condition: Discuss kidney cancer risk and other nonsurgical options for treating your problem.

Daniel Altman, PhD, associate professor of medical epidemiology, Karolinska Institute, Stockholm, Sweden.

Ways to Fight Lingering Shingles Pain

Salim M. Hayek, MD, PhD, is chief of the division of pain medicine at University Hospitals Case Medical Center and an associate professor at Case Western Reserve University School of Medicine, both in Cleveland. He is board-certified in pain medicine and anesthesiology.

Women have the unfortunate distinction of being more susceptible than men to the painful skin disease *herpes zoster,* otherwise known as shingles.

Surprising: Though shingles has long been considered a once-in-a-lifetime affliction, a recent Mayo Clinic study revealed that more than

5% of sufferers experienced a second bout within the follow-up period, which averaged eight years...and that recurrences were 60% more likely in women.

Shingles develops when the *varicella-zoster virus*—the same virus that causes chicken pox and then goes into hiding in nerve cells—becomes reactivated at a time when a person's immune function is reduced. Shingles risk rises with age as immunity gradually declines. The virus follows a nerve path that leads out from the spine, traveling around one side of the body and surfacing at nerve endings in the skin. The inflamed nerve becomes extremely painful and the affected skin (which reflects the location of that nerve path) erupts in clusters of fluid-filled blisters that take two to four weeks to crust over and heal.

Bad as shingles can be, an even scarier threat is a complication called *postherpetic neuralgia* (PHN) that develops in about 20% of shingles patients. PHN is characterized by intense nerve pain that lingers for months or years after the blisters themselves have healed. According to Salim M. Hayek, MD, PhD, chief of the division of pain medicine at University Hospitals Case Medical Center in Cleveland, the burning, stabbing sensations of PHN can be so severe that even the feeling of clothing or a breeze against the skin can be unbearable—and PHN sufferers often experience depression, isolation and concentration problems. *Self-defense...*

For prevention: Get vaccinated. The FDA recently lowered the approved age for receiving the shingles vaccine, Zostavax, from 60 to 50. The vaccine reduces shingles risk by an estimated 55% to 70%...and it reduces PHN risk by 67%. Vaccinated people who do develop shingles typically experience milder outbreaks and may be less vulnerable to recurrences than unvaccinated ones.

For a shingles outbreak: The first sign of shingles usually is a tingling, burning or itching sensation on the skin, most often on one side of the torso (though it can develop anywhere). This usually is followed within a few days by a red, blotchy rash that later blisters...some patients also have a headache and fever.

Important: If you have possible symptoms of shingles, see your physician immediately, Dr. Hayek advised—if taken within 72 hours of the onset of the rash, a prescription antiviral drug such as *acyclovir* (Zovirax), *famciclovir* (Famvir) or *valacyclovir* (Valtrex) can lessen the severity of shingles and significantly reduce PHN risk.

For pain relief: If over-the-counter painkillers don't do the job, ask your doctor about taking prescription-strength *ibuprofen, acetaminophen with codeine, tramadol* (Ultram) or other pain medication.

For PHN: There is no cure (except, in some cases, time), but there are ways to manage the persistent pain of PHN, Dr. Hayek said. *These include...*

•**Mindfulness-based stress reduction.** A program developed at the University of Massachusetts Medical School combines yoga, meditation, support groups and individually tailored instruction to improve quality of life for PHN patients and other pain sufferers. Visit *www.umassmed.edu/cfm/stress* for information, then check your local hospitals for similar programs.

•**Topical medications.** These inhibit damaged nerve cells in the skin from sending pain messages to the brain. The prescription skin patch Lidoderm, which contains lidocaine, is applied at home and worn for up to 12 hours per day. The prescription skin patch Qutenza, which contains *capsaicin* (the "hot" substance in chili peppers), is applied at the doctor's office in a one-hour procedure and replaced after three months. Nonprescription topical capsaicin products, such as the ointment Zostrix, may help—but patients should follow instructions carefully and some still may not be able to tolerate the burning sensation when capsaicin is first applied, Dr. Hayek said.

•**Oral medications.** Options include the neuropathic pain drug *pregabalin* (Lyrica)...the anticonvulsant *gabapentin* (Neurontin)...the SNRI antidepressant *duloxetine* (Cymbalta)...a tricyclic antidepressant, such as *amitriptyline* (Elavil)... and opioids, such as *oxycodone* (Oxycontin).

Topical and oral PHN medications can have potentially serious side effects, Dr. Hayek cautioned—so it is important to work closely with your physician when using such drugs to manage PHN pain.

∎ ∎ ∎ ∎

Supplements That Reduce Your Risk of Melanoma

Women with a history of nonmelanoma skin cancer who took 400 international units (IU) of vitamin D and 1,000 milligrams (mg) of calcium daily had about half the risk for melanoma as women given a placebo.

Best: Consume the recommended daily dose of vitamin D (600 IU up to age 70…800 IU if older) and calcium (1,000 mg for women up to age 50 and men up to age 70…1,200 mg if older).

Study of 36,282 postmenopausal women by researchers at Stanford University School of Medicine, Redwood City, California, published in *Journal of Clinical Oncology*.

Women's Surgeons Aren't as Careful as They Should Be

Jason D. Wright, MD, Levine Family Assistant Professor of Women's Health and the Florence Irving Assistant Professor of Obstetrics and Gynecology in the division of gynecologic oncology at Columbia University College of Physicians and Surgeons in New York City and lead author of a study on VTE risk published in *Obstetrics & Gynecology*.

If you have to have surgery, you naturally want to feel confident that your surgeon is doing everything possible to prevent complications that could put you in harm's way…or at death's door. Yet for an alarmingly high number of women having gynecologic surgery, such confidence would be sadly misplaced, a recent study showed.

Background: About 16% of women who undergo major gynecologic surgery develop *venous thromboembolism* (VTE), a postsurgical hazard in which a blood clot blocks a blood vessel. VTE can lead to pain, swelling, blood vessel damage—and to the potentially fatal *pulmonary embolism* (blood clot in the lungs). To reduce this risk, doctors can prescribe prophylactic VTE care in the form of anticlotting medication and/or mechanical devices (such as compression stockings or pneumatic compression equipment that promotes circulation by massaging the legs) before and after surgery. VTE is a risk with many types of surgery—however, evidence suggests that gynecological surgeons are less likely to comply with VTE prevention guidelines than surgeons in other high-risk specialties.

New 10-year study: Investigators examined hospital records of 738,150 women who had major gynecologic surgery, such as removal of the uterus, fallopian tubes and/or ovaries. Among these patients, 40% received *no* prophylactic VTE care at all—a shocking finding, given how often this potentially deadly complication develops. The only encouraging news is that the situation seems to be improving. In 2000, 47% of the patients received no prophylactic VTE care…by 2010, that number had fallen to 33%, which is better but still disturbingly high.

If you need gynecologic surgery: Choose a surgeon who operates frequently, and have your surgery in a hospital that does a high volume of gynecologic procedures—the research showed that those factors upped the odds that a woman would receive prophylactic VTE care. Also, ask your doctor specifically what he or she will do—and whether there is anything you can do yourself—to lower your risk for a postsurgical clot.

info The Agency for Healthcare Research and Quality publishes blood-clot prevention guidelines at *www.guideline.gov/content. aspx?id=11429*.

Index